SONOGRAPHY

Edited by **Kerry Thoirs**

Sonography
Edited by Kerry Thoirs

Published by InTech
Janeza Trdine 9, 51000 Rijeka, Croatia

Notice
Statements and opinions expressed in the chapters are these of the individual contributors and not necessarily those of the editors or publisher. No responsibility is accepted for the accuracy of information contained in the published chapters. The publisher assumes no responsibility for any damage or injury to persons or property arising out of the use of any materials, instructions, methods or ideas contained in the book.

Publishing Process Manager Romana Vukelic

Technical Editor Teodora Smiljanic

Cover Designer InTech Design Team

Additional hard copies can be obtained from orders@intechopen.com

Sonography, Edited by Kerry Thoirs
p. cm.
ISBN 978-953-307-947-9

Meet the editor

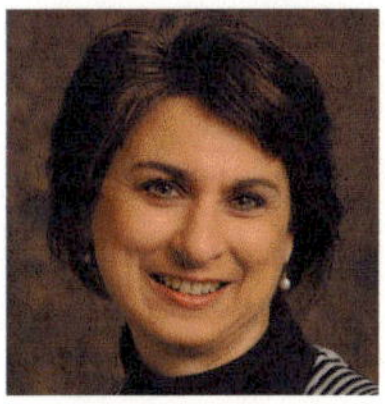

Dr Kerry Thoirs is a Senior Lecturer in Medical Sonography at the School of Health Sciences, University of South Australia. She has extensive clinical experience as a Medical Sonographer, having worked in a large private radiologic practice for over twenty years. More recently, academia has become a greater focus for her, with interests in teaching, research and academic leadership. She is eager to encourage independent research amongst sonographers, and also has an interest in innovative teaching practices in sonography. Kerry Thoirs has published widely, is a regular presenter at Sonography conferences within Australia and is an active member of the Australian Sonographers Association.

Contents

Preface

Medical sonography is a medical imaging modality used across many medical disciplines because of its relative low cost and easy accessibility, with its use constantly growing. Currently, there are many high quality ultrasound imaging systems available that are easily transportable, making it a diagnostic tool amenable to bedside and office scanning. This book includes sonography applications usable across a number of medical disciplines including radiology, thoracic medicine, urology, rheumatology, obstetrics and fetal medicine and neurology.

The book is divided into two sections. The first section is comprised of author contributions that revisit established applications in medical sonography such as biliary, testicular and breast sonography, and sonography in early pregnancy. The second section outlines some interesting applications of sonography that are still in their early stages, such as fetal yawning as an indicator of safe neurological development, and transcranial sonography used to assess the intracranial arteries and also to investigate mental effort and cognitive competence. A number of chapters look at applications and techniques used to assess tissue perfusion, and three- and four-dimensional sonography are also featured.

Considering the rapid advances in technology and sonography applications, it is important that the users regularly update their professional knowledge. The final chapter looks at preferred ways for achieving this for health professionals using sonography.

Dr. Kerry Thoirs
School of Health Sciences
University of South Australia
Australia

Part 1

Current Applications of Sonography

1

Sonography of the Scrotum

Chee-Wai Mak and Wen-Sheng Tzeng
Department of Medical Imaging, Chi Mei Medical Center, Tainan, Taiwan
Central Taiwan University of Science and Technology, Taichung, Taiwan
Chung Hwa University of Medical Technology, Tainan, Taiwan
Republic of China

1. Introduction

Although the development of new imaging modality such as computerized tomography and magnetic resonance imaging have open a new era for medical imaging, high resolution sonography remains as the initial imaging modality of choice for evaluation of scrotal disease. Many of the disease processes, such as testicular torsion, epididymo-orchitis, and intratesticular tumor, produce the common symptom of pain at presentation, and differentiation of these conditions and disorders is important for determining the appropriate treatment. High resolution ultrasound helps in better characterize some of the intrascrotal lesions, and suggest a more specific diagnosis, resulting in more appropriate treatments and avoiding unnecessary operation for some of the diseases.

2. Imaging technique

For any scrotal examination, thorough palpation of the scrotal contents and history taking should precede the sonographic examination. Patients are usually examined in the supine position with a towel draped over his thighs to support the scrotum. Warm gel should always be used because cold gel can elicit a cremasteric response resulting in thickening of the scrotal wall; hence a thorough examination is difficult to be performed. A high resolution, near-focused, linear array transducer with a frequency of 7.5 MHz or greater is often used because it provides increased resolutions of the scrotal contents. Images of both scrotum and bilateral inguinal regions are obtained in both transverse and longitudinal planes. Color Doppler and pulsed Doppler examination is subsequently performed, optimized to display low-flow velocities, to demonstrate blood flow in the testes and surrounding scrotal structures. In evaluation of acute scrotum, the asymptomatic side should be scanned first to ensure that the flow parameters are set appropriately. A transverse image including all or a portion of both testicles in the field of view is obtained to allow side-to-side comparison of their sizes, echogenicity, and vascularity. Additional views may also be obtained with the patient performing Valsalva maneuver.

3. Anatomy

The normal adult testis is an ovoid structure measuring 3 cm in anterior-posterior dimension, 2–4 cm in width, and 3–5 cm in length. The weight of each testis normally ranges from 12.5 to 19 g. Both the sizes and weights of the testes normally decrease with age. At ultrasound, the normal testis has a homogeneous, medium-level, granular echotexture. The testicle is surrounded by a dense white fibrous capsule, the tunica albuginea, which is often not visualized in the absence of intrascrotal fluid. However, the tunica is often seen as an echogenic structure where it invaginates into the testis to form the mediastinum testis [Fig. 1]. In the testis, the seminiferous tubules converge to form the rete testes, which is located in the mediastinum testis. The rete testis connects to the epididymal head via the efferent ductules. The epididymis is located posterolateral to the testis and measures 6–7 cm in length. At sonography, the epididymis is normally iso- or slightly hyperechoic to the normal testis and its echo texture may be coarser. The head is the largest and most easily identified portion of the epididymis. It is located superior-lateral to the upper pole of the testicle and is often seen on paramedian views of the testis [Fig. 2]. The normal epididymal body and tail are smaller and more variable in position.

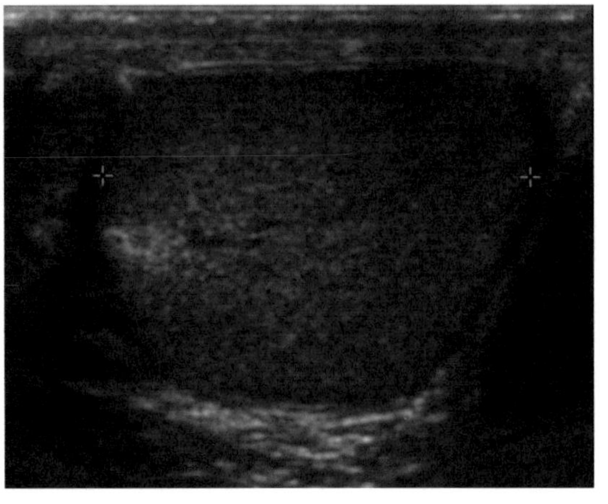

Fig. 1. Sonography of a normal testis. The normal testis presents as a structure having homogeneous, medium level, granular echotexture. The mediastinum testis appears as the hyperechoic region located at the periphery of the testis as seen in this figure

The testis obtains its blood supply from the deferential, cremasteric and testicular arteries. The right and left testicular arteries, branches of the abdominal aorta, arise just distal to the renal arteries, provide the primary vascular supply to the testes. They course through the inguinal canal with the spermatic cord to the posterior superior aspect of the testis. Upon reaching the testis, the testicular artery divides into branches, which penetrate the tunica albuginea and arborize over the surface of the testis in a layer known as tunica vasculosa. Centripetal branches arising from the capsular arteries carry blood toward the mediastinum, where they divide to form the recurrent rami that carry blood away from the mediastinum into the testis. The deferential artery, a branch of the superior vesicle artery and the cremasteric artery, a branch of the inferior epigastric artery, supply the epididymis, vas deferens, and peritesticular tissue.

Four testicular appendages have been described: the appendix testis, the appendix epididymis, the vas aberrans, and the paradidymis. They are all remnants of embryonic ducts (Dogra et al 2003, as cited in Cook and Dewbury, 2000). Among them, the appendix testis and the appendix epididymis are usually seen at scrotal US. The appendix testis is a mullerian duct remnant and consists of fibrous tissue and blood vessels within an envelope of columnar epithelium. The appendix testis is attached to the upper pole of the testis and found in the groove between the testis and the epididymis. The appendix epididymis is attached to the head of the epididymis. The spermatic cord, which begins at the deep inguinal ring and descends vertically into the scrotum is consists of vas deferens, testicular artery, cremasteric artery, deferential artery, pampiniform plexuses, genitofemoral nerve, and lymphatic vessel.

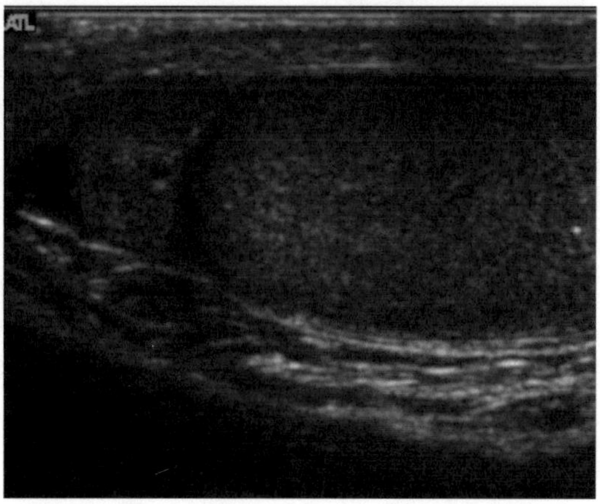

Fig. 2. Normal epididymal head. The epididymal head, usually iso- or slightly hyperechoic than the testis is seen located cephalad to the testis

4. Intratesticular tumors

One of the primary indications for scrotal sonography is to evaluate for the presence of intratesticular tumor in the setting of scrotal enlargement or a palpable abnormality at physical examination. It is well known that the presence of a solitary intratesticular solid mass is highly suspicious for malignancy. Conversely, the vast majority of extratesticular lesions are benign.

4.1 Germ cell tumors

Primary intratesticular malignancy can be divided into germ cell tumors and non-germ cell tumors. Germ cell tumors are further categorized as either seminomas or nonseminomatous tumors. Other malignant testicular tumors include those of gonadal stromal origin, lymphoma, leukemia, and metastases.

4.1.1 Seminoma

Approximately 95% of malignant testicular tumors are germ cell tumors, of which seminoma is the most common. It accounts for 35%-50% of all germ cell tumors (Woodward et al, 2002). Seminomas occur in a slightly older age group when compared with other nonseminomatous tumor, with a peak incidence in the forth and fifth decades. They are less aggressive than other testicular tumors and usually confined within the tunica albuginea at presentation. Seminomas are associated with the best prognosis of the germ cell tumors because of their high sensitivity to radiation and chemotherapy (Kim et al, 2007).

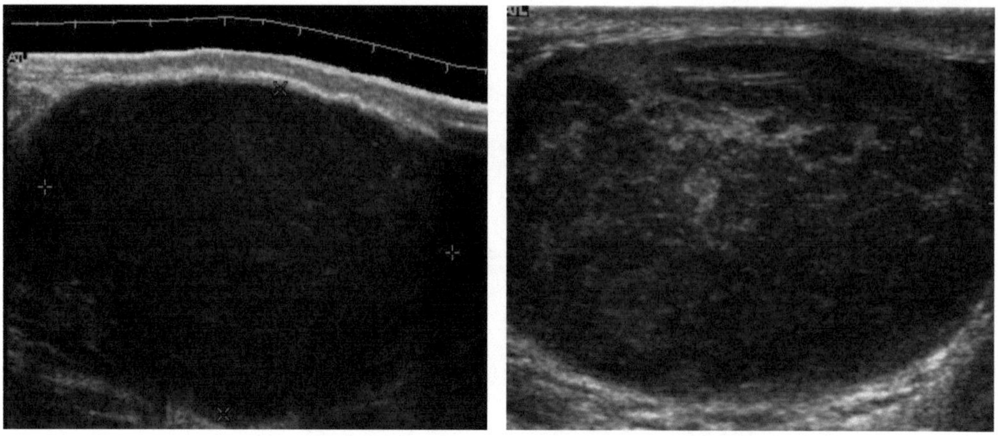

(a) (b)

Fig. 3. Seminoma. (a) Seminoma usually presents as a homogeneous hypoechoic nodule confined within the tunica albuginea. (b) Sonography shows a large heterogeneous mass is seen occupying nearly the whole testis but still confined within the tunica albuginea, it is rare for seminoma to invade to peritesticular structures

Seminoma is the most common tumor type in cryptorchid testes. The risk of developing a seminoma is increased in patients with cryptorchidism, even after orchiopexy. There is an increased incidence of malignancy developing in the contralateral testis too, hence sonography is sometimes used to screen for an occult tumor in the remaining testis.

On US images, seminomas are generally uniformly hypoechoic, larger tumors may be more heterogeneous [Fig. 3]. Seminomas are usually confined by the tunica albuginea and rarely extend to peritesticular structures. Lymphatic spread to retroperitoneal lymph nodes and hematogenous metastases to lung, brain, or both are evident in about 25% of patients at the time of presentation (Dogra et al 2003, as cited in Guthrie & Fowler, 1992)

4.1.2 Nonseminomatous germ cell tumors

Nonseminomatous germ cell tumors most often affect men in their third decades of life. Histologically, the presence of any nonseminomatous cell types in a testicular germ cell tumor classifies it as a nonseminomatous tumor, even if most of the tumor cells belong to seminona. These subtypes include yolk sac tumor, embryonal cell carcinoma, teratocarcinoma, teratoma, and choriocarcinoma. Clinically nonsemionatous tumors usually present as mixed germ cell tumors with variety cell types and in different proportions.

Embryonal cell carcinoma --- Embryonal cell carcinomas, a more aggressive tumor than seminoma usually occurs in men in their 30s. Although it is the second most common testicular tumor after seminoma, pure embryonal cell carcinoma is rare and constitutes only about 3 percent of the nonseminomatous germ cell tumors. Most of the cases occur in combination with other cell types.

At ultrasound, embryonal cell carcinomas are predominantly hypoechoic lesions with ill defined margins and an inhomogeneous echotexture. Echogenic foci due to hemorrhage, calcification, or fibrosis are commonly seen. Twenty percent of embryonal cell carcinomas have cystic components (Dogra et al, 2003). The tumor may invade into the tunica albuginea resulting in contour distortion of the testis [Fig. 4].

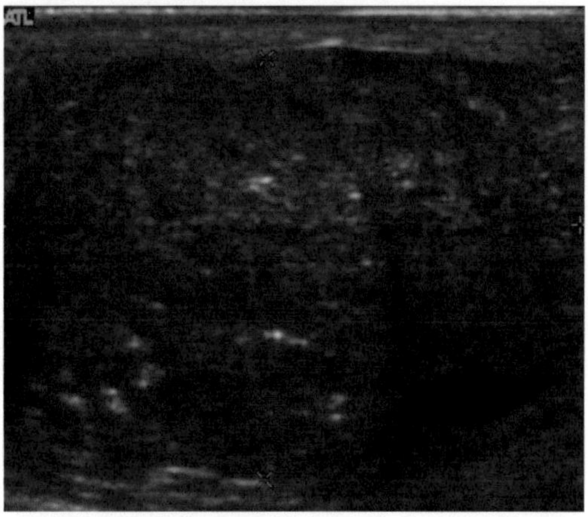

Fig. 4. Embryonal cell carcinoma. Longitudinal ultrasound image of the testis shows an irregular heterogeneous mass that forms an irregular margin with the tunica albuginea

Yolk sac tumor --- Yolk sac tumors also known as endodermal sinus tumors account for 80% of childhood testicular tumors, with most cases occuring before the age of 2 years (Woodward et al, 2002, as cited in Frush & Sheldon 1998). Alpha-fetoprotein is normally elevated in greater than 90% of patients with yolk sac tumor (Woodward et al, 2002, as cited in Ulbright et al, 1999). In its pure form, yolk sac tumor is rare in adults; however yolk sac elements are frequently seen in tumors with mixed histologic features in adults and thus indicate poor prognosis. The US appearance of yolk sac tumor is usually nonspecific and consists of inhomogeneous mass that may contain echogenic foci secondary to hemorrhage.

Choriocarcinoma --- Choriocarcinoma is a highly malignant testicular tumor that usually develops in the 2nd and 3rd decades of life. Pure choriocarcinomas are rare and represent only less than 1 percent of all testicular tumors (Woodward et al, 2002). Choriocarcinomas are composed of both cytotrophoblasts and syncytiotrophoblasts, with the latter responsible for the clinical elevation of human chorionic gonadotrophic hormone level. As microscopic vascular invasion is common in choriocarcinoma, hematogeneous metastasis, especially to the lungs is common (Dogra et al, 2003, as cited in Geraghty et al, 1998). Many choriocarcinomas show extensive hemorrhagic necrosis in the central portion of the tumor; this appears as mixed cystic and solid components (Dogra et al 2003, as cited in Hamm, 1997) at ultrasound.

Teratoma --- Although teratoma is the second most common testicular tumor in children, it affects all age groups. Mature teratoma in children is often benign, but teratoma in adults, regardless of age, should be considered as malignant. Teratomas are composed of all three germ cell layers, i.e. endoderm, mesoderm and ectoderm. At ultrasound, teratomas generally form well-circumscribed complex masses. Echogenic foci representing calcification, cartilage, immature bone and fibrosis are commonly seen [Fig. 5]. Cysts are also a common feature and depending on the contents of the cysts i.e. serous, mucoid or keratinous fluid, it may present as anechoic or complex structure [Fig. 6].

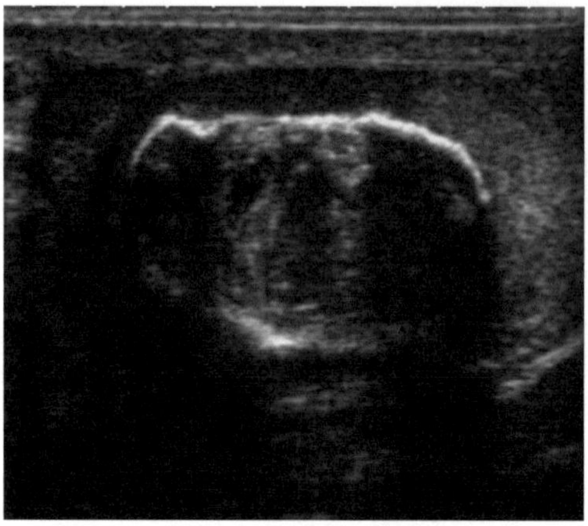

Fig. 5. Teratoma. A plaque like calcification with acoustic shadow is seen in the testis

4.2 Non-germ cell tumours

4.2.1 Sex cord-stromal tumours

Sex cord-stromal (gonadal stromal) tumors of the testis, account for 4 per cent of all testicular tumors (Dogra et al, 2003). The most common are Leydig and Sertoli cell tumors. Although the majority of these tumors are benign, these tumors can produce hormonal changes, for example, Leydig cell tumor in a child may produce isosexual virilization. In adult, it may have no endocrine manifestation or gynecomastia, and decrease in libido may result from production of estrogens. These tumors are typically small and are usually discovered incidentally. They do not have any specific ultrasound appearance but appear as well-defined hypoechoic lesions. These tumors are usually removed because they cannot be distinguished from malignant germ cell tumors.

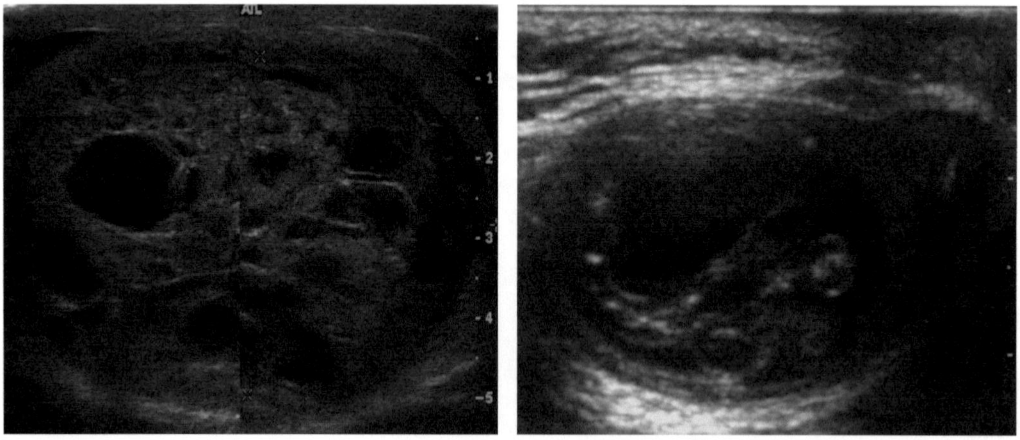

(a) (b)

Fig. 6. Mature cystic teratoma. (a) Composite Image. Mature cystic teratoma in a 29 year-old man. Longitudinal sonography image of the right testis shows a multilocular cystic mass. (b) Mature cystic teratoma in a 6 year-old boy. Longitudinal sonography of the right testis shows a cystic mass contains calcification with no obvious acoustic shadow

Leydig cell tumors are the most common type of sex cord–stromal tumor of the testis, accounting for 1%–3% of all testicular tumors. They can be seen in any age group, they are generally small solid masses, but they may show cystic areas, hemorrhage, or necrosis (Woodward et al 2002, as cited in Ulbright et al, 1999). Their sonographic appearance is variable and is indistinguishable from that of germ cell tumors (Woodward et al 2002, as cited in Avery et al, 1991)

Sertoli cell tumors are less common, constituting less than 1% of testicular tumors. They are less likely than Leydig cell tumors to be hormonally active, but gynecomastia can occur (Woodward et al 2002, as cited in Ulbright et al, 1999). Sertoli cell tumors are typically well circumscribed, unilateral, round to lobulated masses.

4.2.2 Lymphoma

Clinically lymphoma can manifest in one of three ways: as the primary site of involvement, or as a secondary tumor such as the initial manifestation of clinically occult disease or recurrent disease. Although lymphomas constitute 5% of testicular tumors and are almost exclusively diffuse non-Hodgkin B-cell tumors, only less than 1 % of non-Hodgkin lymphomas involve the testis (Doll and Weiss 1986).

Patients with testicular lymphoma are usually old aged around 60 years of age, present with painless testicular enlargement and less commonly with other systemic symptoms such as weight loss, anorexia, fever and weakness. Bilateral testicle involvements are common and occur in 8.5% to18% of cases (Dogra et al, 2003, as cited in Horstman et al, 1992). At sonography, most lymphomas are homogeneous and diffusely replace the testis [Fig. 7]. However focal hypoechoic lesions can occur, hemorrhage and necrosis are rare. At times, the sonographic appearance of lymphoma is indistinguishable from that of the germ cell tumors [Fig. 8], then the patient's age at presentation, symptoms, and medical history, as well as multiplicity and bilaterality of the lesions, are all important factors in making the appropriate diagnosis.

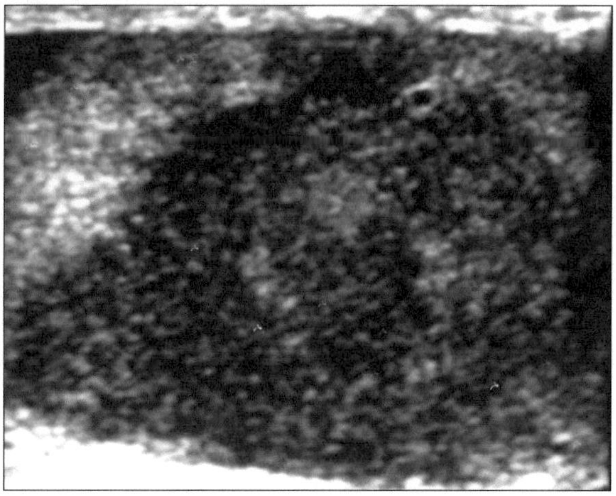

Fig. 7. Lymphoma. Lymphoma in a 61 year-old man. Longitudinal sonography shows an irregular hypoechoic lesion occupied nearly the whole testis

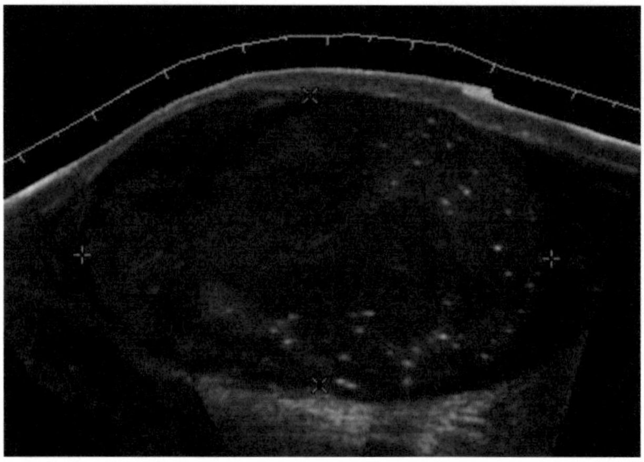

Fig. 8. Primary Lymphoma. Longitudinal sonography of a 64 year-old man shows a lymphoma mimicking a germ cell tumor

4.2.3 Leukemia

Primary leukemia of the testis is rare. However due to the presence of blood-testis barrier, chemotherapeutic agents are unable to reach the testis, hence in boys with acute lymphoblastic leukemia, testicular involvement is reported in 5% to 10% of patients, with the majority found during clinical remission (Dogra et al, 2003). The sonographic appearance of leukemia of the testis can be quite varied, as the tumors may be unilateral or bilateral, diffuse or focal, hypoechoic or hyperechoic (Woodward et al, 2002). These findings are usually indistinguishable from that of the lymphoma [Fig. 9].

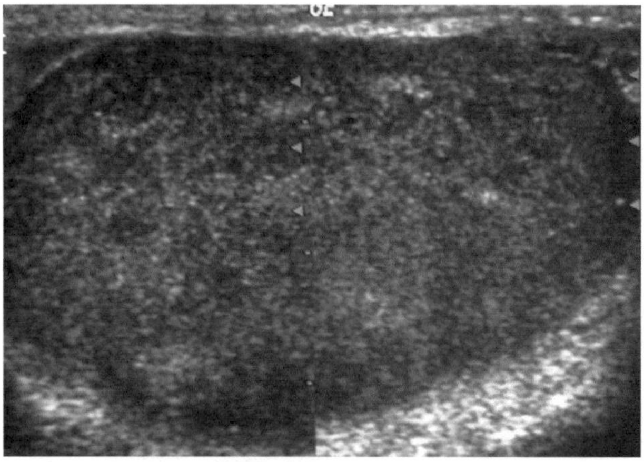

Fig. 9. Leukemia. Diffuse hypoechoic infiltrative lesions are seen involving the whole testis, indistinguishable from that of the lymphoma

4.3 Epidermoid cyst

Epidermoid cysts, also known as keratocysts, are benign epithelial tumors which usually occur in the second to fourth decades and accounts for only 1-2% of all intratesticular tumors. As these tumors have a benign biological behavior and with no malignant potential, preoperative recognition of this tumor is important as this will lead to testicle preserving surgery (enucleation) rather than unnecessary orchiectomy.

Clinically, epidermoid cyst cannot be differentiated from other testicular tumors, typically presenting as a non-tender, palpable, solitary intratesticular mass. Tumor markers such as serum beta-human chorionic gonadotropin and alpha-feto protein are negative.

The ultrasound patterns of epidermoid cysts are variable and include:

i. A mass with a target appearance, i.e. a central hypoechoic area surrounded by an echolucent rim (Mak et al, 2007a, as cited in Maxwell & Mamtora, 1990);
ii. An echogenic mass with dense acoustic shadowing due to calcification; (Mak et al, 2007a, as cited in Meiches & Nurenberg 1991);
iii. A well-circumscribed mass with a hyperechoic rim (Mak et al, 2007a, as cited in Cohen 1984);
iv. Mixed pattern having heterogeneous echotexture and poor-defined contour (Mak et al, 2007a, as cited in Atchley & Dewbury, 2000) and
v. An onion peel appearance consisting of alternating rings of hyperechogenicities and hypoechogenicities (Mak et al, 2007a, as cited in Malvica, 1993).

However, these patterns, except the latter one, may be considered as non-specific as heterogeneous echotexture and shadowing calcification can also be detected in malignant testicular tumors (Mak et al, 2007a). The onion peel pattern of epidermoid cyst [Fig. 10] correlates well with the pathologic finding of multiple layers of keratin debris produced by the lining of the epidermoid cyst. This sonographic appearance should be considered characteristic of an epidermoid cyst and corresponds to the natural evolution of the cyst. Absence of vascular flow is another important feature that is helpful in differentiation of epidermoid cyst from other solid intratesticular lesions.

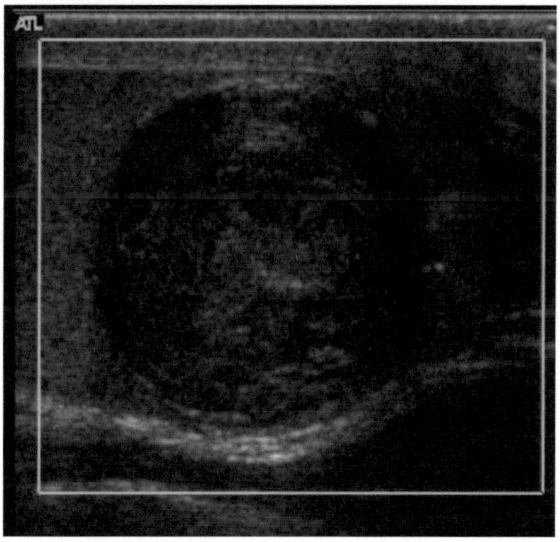

Fig. 10. Epidermoid cyst. Onion peel appearances of the tumor together with absence of vascular flow are typical findings of epidermoid cyst

5. Extratesticular tumors

Although most of the extratesticular lesions are benign, malignancy does occur; the most common malignant tumors in infants and children are rhabdomyosarcomas (Mak et al 2004, as cited in Green, 1986). Other malignant tumors include liposarcoma, leiomyosarcoma, malignant fibrous histiocytoma and mesothelioma.

5.1 Rhabdomyosarcoma

Rhabdomyosarcoma is the most common tumor of the lower genitourinary tract in children in the first two decades, it may develop anywhere in the body, and 4% occur in the paratesticular region (Mak et al 2004a, as cited in Hamilton et al, 1989) which carries a better outcome than lesions elsewhere in the genitourinary tract. Clinically, the patient usually presents with non-specific complaints of a unilateral, painless intrascrotal swelling not associated with fever. Transillumination test is positive when a hydrocele is present, often resulting in a misdiagnosis of epididymitis, which is more commonly associated with hydrocele.

The ultrasound findings of paratesticular rhabdomyosarcoma are variable. It usually presents as an echo-poor mass [Fig. 11a] with or without hydrocele (Mak et al 2004a, as cited in Solvietti et al, 1989). With color Doppler sonography [Fig. 11b] these tumors are generally hypervascular (Mak et al, 2004a).

5.2 Mesothelioma

Malignant mesothelioma is an uncommon tumor arising in body cavities lined by mesothelium. The majority of these tumors are found in the pleura, peritoneum and less frequently pericardium. As the tunica vaginalis is a layer of reflected peritoneum, mesothelioma can occur in the scrotal sac. Although trauma, herniorrhaphy and long term

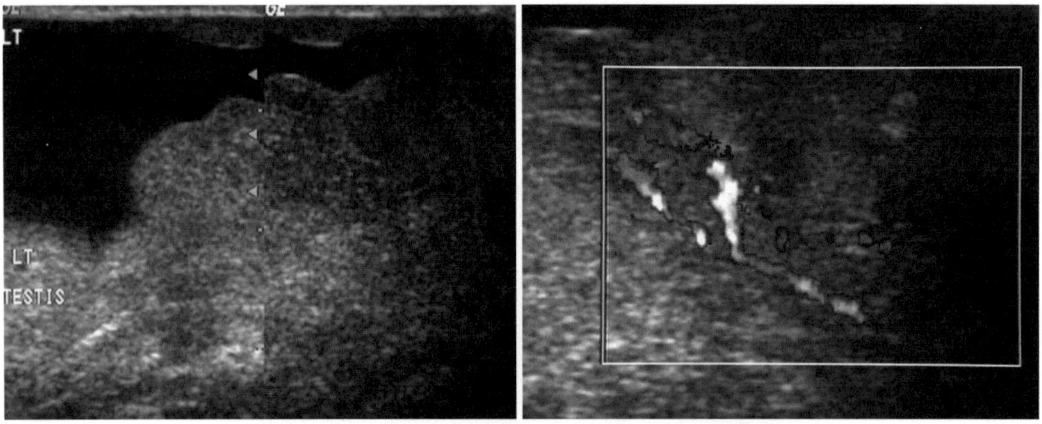

(a) (b)

Fig. 11. Rhabdomyosarcoma (Reproduced with permission from British Institute of Radiology, British Journal of Radiology 2004; 77: 250–252). (a) Longituidinal section (composite image) of high resolution ultrasound of a 14 year-old boy shows a well defined hypoechoic extratesticular mass is found in the left scrotum, hydrocele is also present. (b) Color Doppler ultrasound shows that the mass is hypervascular hydrocele (Mak et al, 2004b, as cited in Gurdal & Erol, 2001) have been considered as the predisposing factors for development of malignant mesothelioma, the only well established risk factor is asbestos exposure (Boyum & Wasserman, 2008). Patients with malignant mesothelioma of the tunica vaginalis frequently have a progressively enlarging hydrocele and less frequently a scrotal mass, rapid re-accumulation of fluid after aspiration raises the suggestion of malignancy (Mak et al, 2004b, as cited in Wolanske & Nino-Murcia, 2001).

The reported ultrasound features of mesothelioma of the tunica vaginalis testis are variable. Hydrocele, either simple or complex is present and may be associated with: (1) multiple extratesticular papillary projections of mixed echogenicity (Boyum & Wasserman 2008, as cited in Fields et al, 1992); (2) multiple extratesticular nodular masses of increased echogenicity (Boyum & Wasserman, 2008, as cited in Bruno et al, 2002 and Tyagi et al, 1989); (3) focal irregular thickening of the tunica vaginalis testis (Bruno et al, 2002); (4) a simple hydrocele as the only finding (Boyum & Wasserman, 2008, as cited in Jalon et al, 2003) and (5) A single hypoechoic mass located in the epididymal head (Boyum & Wasserman, 2008; Mak et al, 2004b). With color Doppler sonography, mesothelioma is hypovascular [Fig. 12] (Bruno et al, 2002; Mak et al, 2004b; Wang et al, 2005).

5.3 Leiomyoma

Leiomyomas are benign neoplasms that may arise from any structure or organ containing smooth muscle. The majority of genitourinary leiomyomas are found in the renal capsule, but this tumor has also been reported in the epididymis, spermatic cord, and tunica albuginea. Scrotal leiomyomas have been reported in patients from the fourth to ninth decades of life with most presenting during the fifth decade. These tumors are generally slow growth and asymptomatic. The sonographic features of leiomyomas have been reported as solid hypoechoic or heterogeneous masses that may or may not contain

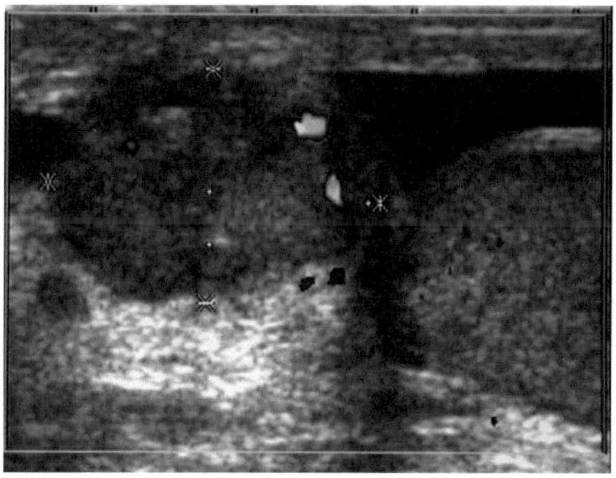

Fig. 12. Mesothelioma arising from the tunica vaginalis (Reproduced with permission from British Institute of Radiology, British Journal of Radiology 2004:77:780–781). Color Doppler ultrasound demonstrates a well-defined hypoechoic nodule occupying the left epididymal head, with a few areas of color flow demonstrated. The left testis is intact with no focal nodule detected. Hydrocele is also present

shadowing calcification (Mak et al, 2004c, as cited in Hricak & Filly, 1983 & Leonhardt, 1993). Other findings include whorl shaped configuration [Fig. 13a] of the nodule (Mak et al, 2004c) and multiple, narrow areas of shadowing not cast by calcifications [Fig. 13b], but corresponding to transition zones between the various tissue components of the mass (Mak et al, 2004c, as cited in Hertzberg et al, 1996) are characteristic of leiomyoma and may help differentiate it from other scrotal tumors.

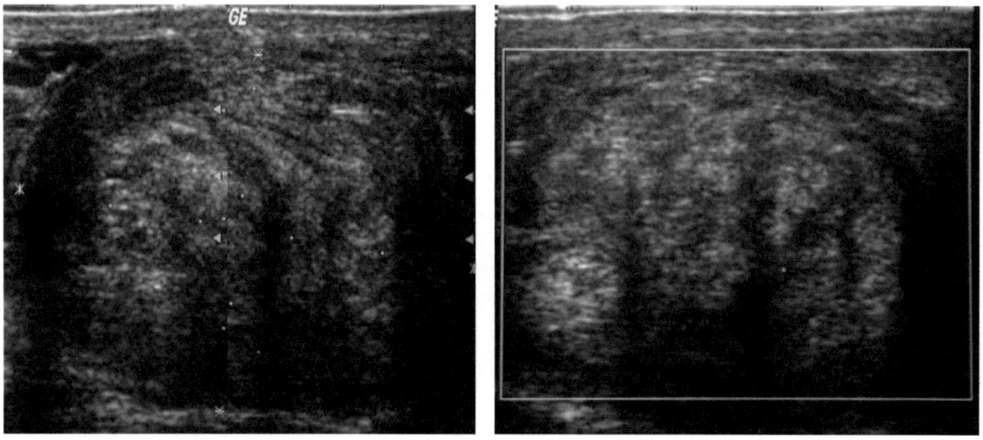

(a) (b)

Fig. 13. Leiomyoma arising from tunica albuginea (Reproduced with permission from John Wiley and Sons publishing company License number 2643411100095, Journal of Clinical Ultrasound 2004; 32:309–311). (a) Montage of 2 contiguous sonograms of a 67 year-old man shows a well-defined extratesticular mass with a whorl-shaped echotexture. (b) Color Doppler sonogram shows no internal vascularity. Note the presence of multiple shadows not associated with echogenic foci in the mass

5.4 Fat containing tumors

5.4.1 Lipoma

Lipoma is the most common nontesticular intrascrotal tumor. It can be divided into 3 types depending upon the site of origination and spread:

1. Originate in the spermatic cord with spread to the scrotum;
2. Originate and develop within the cord (most common type) and
3. Originate and develop within the scrotum (Rosenberg & Williamson, 1989).

At ultrasound, lipoma is a well–defined, homogeneous, hyperechoic paratesticular lesion of varying size [Fig. 14]. The simple finding of an echogenic fatty mass within the inguinal canal, while suggestive of a lipoma, should also raise a question of fat from the omentum secondary to an inguinal hernia. However lipomas are well-defined masses, whereas herniated omentum appears to be more elongated and can be traced to the inguinal area, hence scanning along the inguinal canal as well as the scrotum is necessary to make the differential diagnosis. Magnetic resonance imaging and computerized tomography are helpful in doubtful cases.

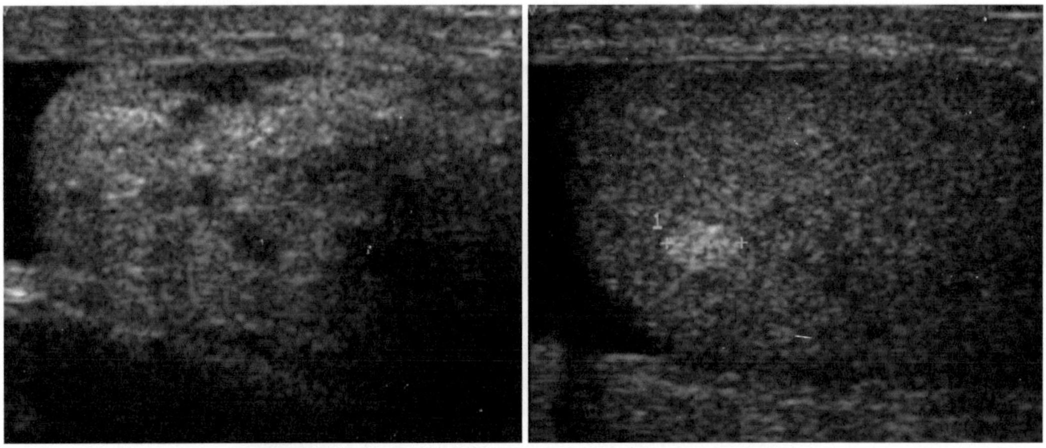

(a) (b)

Fig. 14. Lipoma at spermatic cord and testiscle. (a) Longitudinal scrotal sonography of a 61 year-old patient shows a well defined hyperechoic nodule is seen in the scrotum. (b) Scrotal sonography of the same patient shows a hyper echoic nodule in the left testis, pathology proved that this is a lipoma too

5.4.2 Liposarcoma

Malignant extratesticular tumors are rare. Most of the malignant tumors are solid and have nonspecific features on ultrasonography. The majority of the malignant extratesticular tumors arise from spermatic cord with liposarcoma being the most common in adults (Woodward et al, 2003). On gross speciemen, liposarcoma is a solid, bulky lipomatous tumor with heterogeneous architecture, often containing areas of calcification (Bostwick & Eble, 1997). Although the sonographic appearances of liposarcoma are variable and nonspecific, it still provides a clue about the presence of lipomatous matrix. Echogenic areas corresponding to fat often associated with poor sound transmission and areas of heterogeneous

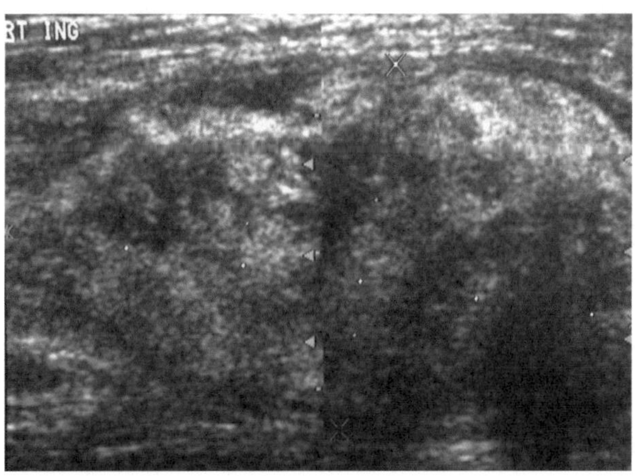

Fig. 15. Liposarcoma. A heterogeneous mass consists of an upper hyperechoic portion corresponds to lipomatous matrix and areas of hypoechogenicity corresponds to nonlipomatous component is seen

echogenicity corresponding to nonlipomatous component are present [Fig. 15]. Some liposarcomas may also mimic the sonographic appearance of lipomas [Fig. 16] and hernias that contain omentum, but lipomas are generally smaller and more homogeneous and hernias are elongated masses that can often be traced back to the inguinal canal. CT and MR imaging are more specific, as they can easily recognize fatty component along with other soft tissue component more clearly than ultrasound.

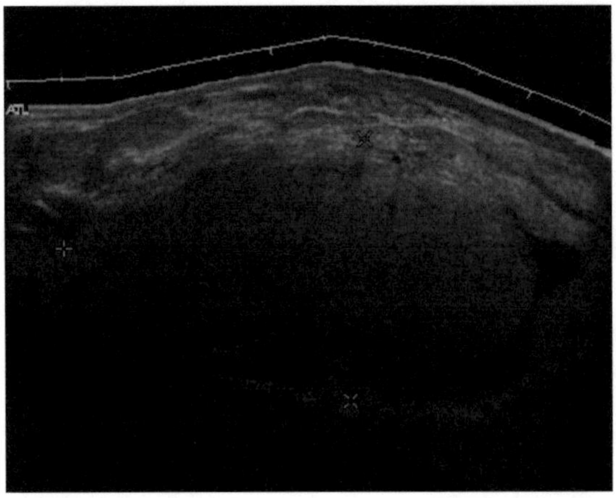

Fig. 16. Liposarcoma mimicking lipoma. A homogeneous hypoechoic mass presents with the same appearance of lipoma, rapid growth of this tumors grants surgical intervention with pathology proved to be well differentiated liposarcoma

5.5 Adenomatoid tumor

Adenomatoid tumors are the most common tumors of the epididymis and account for approximately 30% of all paratesticular neoplasms, second only to lipoma (Bostwick & Eble, 1997). They are usually unilateral, more common on the left side, and usually involve the epididymal tail. Adenomatoid tumor typically occurs in men during the third and fourth decades of life. Patients usually present with a painless scrotal mass that is smooth, round and well circumscribed on palpation. They are believed to be of mesothelial origin and are universally benign. Their sonographic appearance is that of a round shaped, well-defined, homogeneous mass with echogenicity ranging from hypo- to iso- to hyperechoic [Fig. 17] (Mak et al, 2001).

5.6 Fibrous pseudotumor

Fibrous pseudotumors, also known as fibromas are thought to be reactive, nonneoplastic lesions. They can occur at any age, about 50% of fibromas are associated with hydrocele, and 30% are associated with a history of trauma or inflammation (Akbar et al, 2003). Although the exact cause of this tumor is not completely understood, it is generally believed that these lesions represent a benign reactive proliferation of inflammatory and fibrous tissue, in response to chronic irritation (Garriga et al, 2009).

Sonographic evaluation generally shows one or more solid nodules arising from the tunica vaginalis, epididymis, spermatic cord and tunica albuginea [Fig. 18]. A hydrocele is frequently present too. The nodules may appear hypoechoic or hyperechoic, depending on the amount

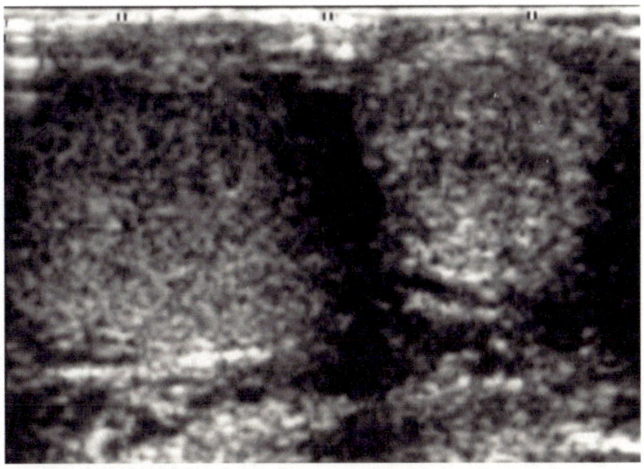

Fig. 17. Adenomatoid tumor at epididymis. A nodule that is isoechoic to the testis is seen occupying nearly the entire epididymal tail

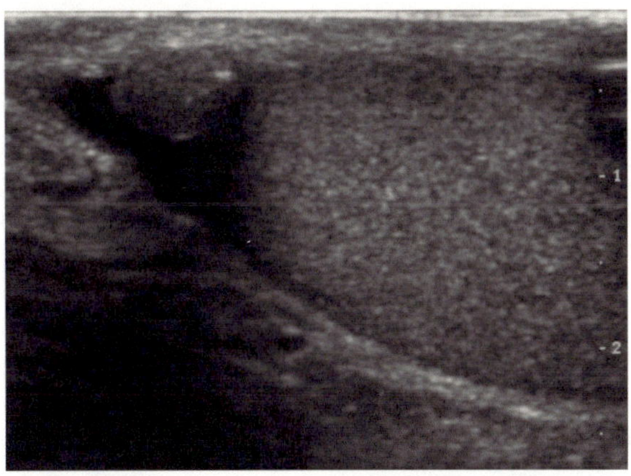

Fig. 18. Fibrous pseudotumor. A homogeneous hypoechoic nodular lesion is seen attached to the tunica associated with minimal amount of hydrocele

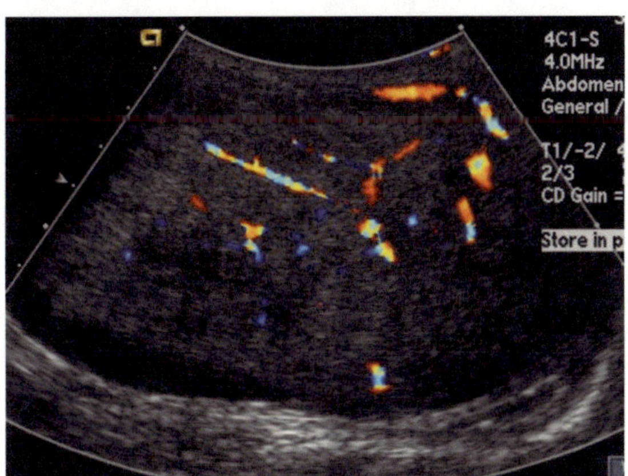

Fig. 19. Fibrous pseudotumor. With color Doppler, a little vascular flow is seen in this fibrous pseudotumor

of collagen or fibroblast present (Garriga et al, 2009, as cited in Tobias-Machado et al, 2000). Acoustic shadowing may occur in the absence of calcification due to the dense collagen component of this tumor. With color Doppler sonography, a small to moderate amount of vascularity may be seen (Garriga et al 2009, as cited in Germaine and Simerman, 2007) [Fig. 19].

6. Inflammation

6.1 Epididymitis and epididymo-orchitis

Epididymitis and epididymo-orchitis are common causes of acute scrotal pain in adolescent boys and adults. At physical examination, they usually are palpable as tender and enlarged structures. Clinically, this disease can be differentiated from torsion of the spermatic cord by elevation of the testes above the pubic symphysis. If scrotal pain decreases, it is more likely to be due to epidiymitis rather than torsion (Prehn's sign). Most cases of epididymitis are secondary to sexually transmitted disease or retrograde bacteria infection from the urinary bladder. The infection usually begins in the epididymal tail and spreads to the epididymal body and head. Approximately 20% to 40 % of cases are associated with orchitis due to direct spread of infection into the testis (Kim et al, 2007, as cited in Horstman et al, 1991).

At ultrasound, the findings of acute epididymitis include an enlarged hypoechoic or hyperechoic (presumably secondary to hemorrhage) epididymis [Fig. 20a]. Other signs of inflammation such as increased vascularity, reactive hydrocele, pyocele and scrotal wall thickening may also be present. Testicular involvement is confirmed by the presence of testicular enlargement and an inhomogeneous echotexture. Hypervascularity on color Doppler images [Fig. 20b] is a well-established diagnostic criterion and may be the only imaging finding of epididymo-orchitis in some men (Kim et al, 2007, as cited in Horstman et al, 1991).

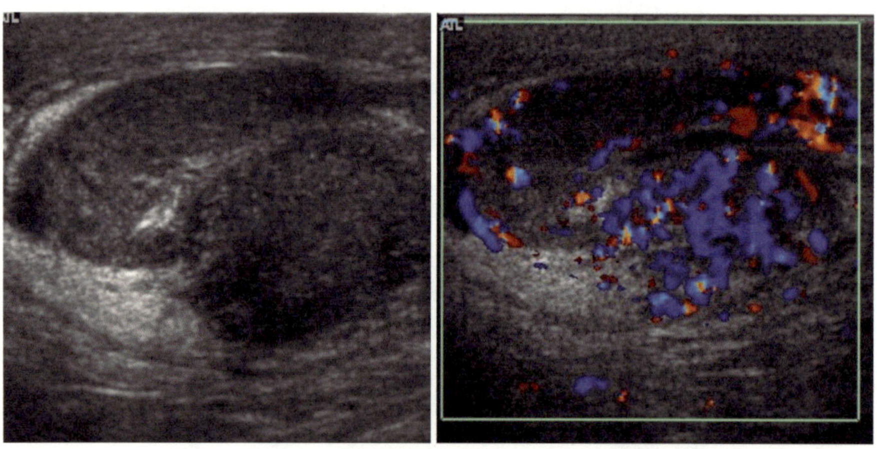

(a) (b)

Fig. 20. Epididymo-orchitis in a 77 year-old man. (a) Transverse sonography shows enlargement of the epididymis with hypoechogenicity noted over the testis and epididymis associated with scrotal wall thickening. (b) Color Doppler sonography showed hyperemic change of the testis and epididymis, presenting as an "inferno" vascular flow pattern

6.2 Tuberculous epididymo-orchitis

Although the genitourinary tract is the most common site of extra-pulmonary involvement by tuberculosis, tuberculous infection of the scrotum is rare and occurs in approximately 7% of patients with tuberculosis (Muttarak and Peh, 2006, as cited in Drudi et al, 1997). At the initial stage of infection, the epididymis alone is involved. However if appropriate antituberculous treatment is not administered promptly, the infection will spreads to the ipsilateral testis. The occurrence of isolated testicular tuberculosis is rare (Muttarak and Peh, 2006, as cited in Riehle & Jayaraman, 1982). Clinically patients with tuberculous epididymo-orchitis may present with painful or painless enlargement of the scrotum, hence they cannot be distinguished from lesions such as testicular tumor, testicular infarction and may mimic testicular torsion.

At ultrasound, tuberculous epididymitis is characterized by an enlarged epididymis with variable echogenicity. The presence of calcification, caseation necrosis, granulomas and fibrosis can result in heterogeneous echogenicity [Fig. 21a]. The ultrasound findings of tuberculous orchitis are as follow: (a) diffusely enlarged heterogeneously hypoechoic testis (b) diffusely enlarged homogeneously hypoechoic testis (c) nodular enlarged heterogeneously hypoechoic testis and (d) presence of multiple small hypoechoic nodules in an enlarged testis [Fig. 21b] (Muttarak and Peh, 2006).

Although both bacterial and tuberculous infections may involve both the epididymis and the testes, an enlarged epididymis with heterogeneously hypoechoic pattern favors a diagnosis of tuberculosis (Muttarak and Peh, 2006, as cited in Kim et al, 1993 and Chung et al, 1997). With color Doppler ultrasound, a diffuse increased blood flow pattern is seen in bacterial epididymitis, whereas focal linear or spotty blood flow signals are seen in the peripheral zone of the affected epididymis in patients with tuberculosis (Muttarak and Peh, 2006, as cited in Yang et al, 2000).

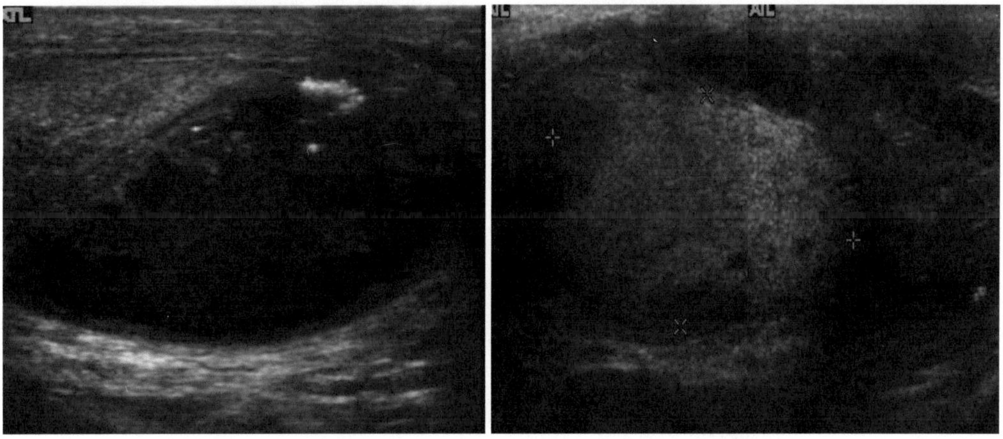

(a) (b)

Fig. 21. Tuberculous epididymo-orchitis. (a) Transverse sonography of a surgically proved tuberculous epididymitis shows an enlarged epididymis containing calcification and necrosis. (b) Composite image: Transverse sonography of the same patient shows multiple hypoechoic nodules in the left testis associated with surrounding reactive hydrocele

6.3 Fournier gangrene

Fournier gangrene is a polymicrobial necrotizing fascitis involving the perineal, perianal, or genital regions and constitutes a true surgical emergency with a potentially high mortality rate. It usually develops from a perineal or genitourinary infection, but can arise following local trauma with secondary infection of the wound. 40–60% of patients are being diabetic. Although the diagnosis of Fournier gangrene is often made clinically, diagnostic imaging is useful in ambiguous cases.

The sonographic hallmark of Fournier gangrene is presence of subcutaneous gas within the thickened scrotal wall. At ultrasound, the gas appears as numerous, discrete, hyperechoic foci with reverberation artifacts [Fig. 22]. Evidence of gas within the scrotal wall may be seen prior to clinical crepitus. The only other condition manifesting with gas at sonographic examination is an inguinoscrotal hernia. This can be differentiated from Fournier gangrene by the presence of gas within the protruding bowel lumen and away from the scrotal wall. (Levenson et al, 2008).

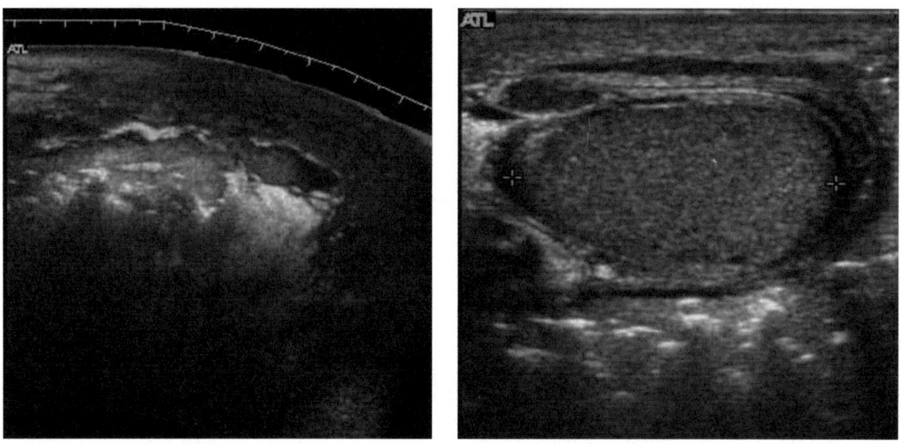

(a) (b)

Fig. 22. Fournier gangrene. (a) Transverse sonography image shows echogenic areas with dirty shadowing representing air in the perineum. (b) Gas presented as numerous, discrete, hyperechoic foci with reverberation artifacts are seen at scrotal wall

7. Other benign lesions of the scrotum

7.1 Tubular ectasia

The normal testis consists of several hundred lobules, with each lobule containing several seminiferous tubules. The seminiferous tubules of each lobule merge to form the straight tubes, which in turn converge to form the rete testis. The rete testis tubules, which lie within the mediastinum testis, are an anastomosing network of irregular channels with a broad lumen, which then empties into the efferent ductules to give rise to the head of the epididymis. Obstruction in the epididymis or efferent ductules may lead to cystic dilatation of the efferent ductules, which usually presents as an epididymal cyst on ultrasound. However, in the more proximal portion this could lead to the formation of an intratesticular cyst or dilatation of the tubules, so called tubular ectasia. Factors contributing to the development of tubular ectasia include epididymitis, testicular biopsy, vasectomy or an aging process (Mak et al 2007b). Clinically this lesion is usually asymptomatic. The ultrasound appearance of a microcystic or multiple tubular-like lesions located at the mediastinal testis [Fig. 23] and associated with an epididymal cyst in a middle-aged or elderly patient should alert the sonographer to the possibility of tubular ectasia.

The differential diagnosis of a multicystic lesion in testis should include a cystic tumor, especially a cystic teratoma. A cystic teratoma is usually a palpable lesion containing both solid and cystic components; and the cysts are normally larger than that of tubular ectasia, which appear microcystic [Fig. 24]. Furthermore, the location of tubular ectasia in the mediastinum testis is also helpful in making the differential diagnosis.

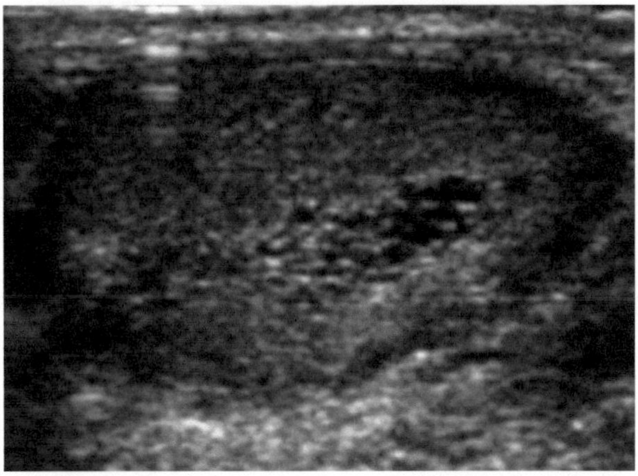

Fig. 23. Tubular ectasia of the testis. Honey-comb shaped cystic lesion at mediastinum testis

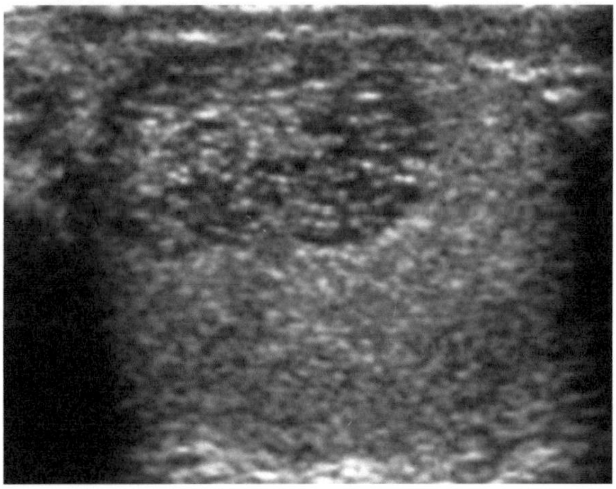

Fig. 24. Tubular ectasia of the testis (Reproduced with permission from British Institute of Radiology, British Journal of Radiology 2007; 80: 67-68). Lesion in the testis mimicking testicular tumor, but the microcystic appearance of this lesion is suggestive of tubular ectasia

7.2 Testicular microlithiasis

Histologically, testicular microlithiasis refers to the scattered laminated calcium deposits in the lumina of the seminiferous tubules. These calcifications arise from degeneration of the cells lining the seminiferous tubules. At ultrasonography, microliths appear as tiny punctate echogenic foci, which typically do not shadow. Although minor microcalcification within a testis is considered normal, the typical US appearance of testicular microlithiasis is of multiple nonshadowing echogenic foci measuring 2-3 mm and randomly scattered throughout the testicular parenchyma [Fig. 25] (Dogra et al, 2003, as cited in Janzen et al, 1992). The clinical significance of testicular microlithiasis is that it is associated with increased risk of testicular malignancy, thus follow up of affected individuals with scrotal sonography is necessary to ensure that a testicular tumor does not develop.

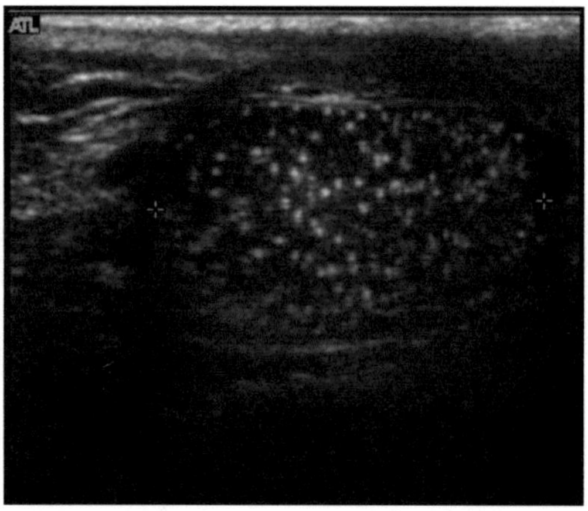

Fig. 25. Testicular microlithiasis. Multiple hyperechoic foci without acoustic shadow presenting as a starry sky appearance is seen in the testis

7.3 Testicular torsion

The normal testis and epididymis are anchored to the scrotal wall. If there is a lack of development of these attachments, the testis is free to twist on its vascular pedicle. This will result in torsion of the spermatic cord and interruption of testicular blood flow. Testicular torsion occurs most commonly at 12 to 18 years but can occur at any age. Torsion results in swelling and edema of the testis, and as the edema increases, testicular perfusion is further altered. The extent of testicular ischemia depends on the degree of torsion, which ranges from 180° to 720° or greater. The testicular salvage rate depends on the degree of torsion and the duration of ischemia. A nearly 100% salvage rate exists within the first 6 hours after the onset of symptoms; a 70% rate, within 6–12 hours; and a 20% rate, within 12–24 hours (Dogra et al, 2003, as cited in Patriquin et al, 1993). Therefore testicular torsion is a surgical emergency and the role of ultrasound is to differentiate it from epididymitis as both disease presents with acute testicular pain clinically.

There are two types of testicular torsion: extravaginal and intravaginal. Extravaginal torsion occurs exclusively in newborns. Ultrasound findings include an enlarged heterogeneous testis, ipsilateral hydrocele, thickened scrotal wall and absence of vascular flow in the testis and spermatic cord (Dogra et al 2003, as cited in Brown et al, 1990). The ultrasound findings of intravaginal torsion vary with the duration and the degree of rotation of the spermatic cord. Gray scale ultrasound may appear normal if the torsion is just occurred. At 4-6 hours after onset of torsion, enlarged testis with decreased echogenicity is seen. At 24 hours after onset, the testis appears heterogeneous due to vascular congestion, hemorrhage and infarction (Dogra et al, 2003). As gray scale ultrasound is often normal during early onset of torsion, Doppler sonography is considered as essential in early diagnosis of testicular torsion. The absence of testicular flow at color and power Doppler ultrasound is considered diagnostic of ischemia [Fig. 26], provided that the scanner is set for detection of slow flow, the sampling box is small and the scanner is adjusted for the lowest repetition frequency and the lowest possible threshold setting.

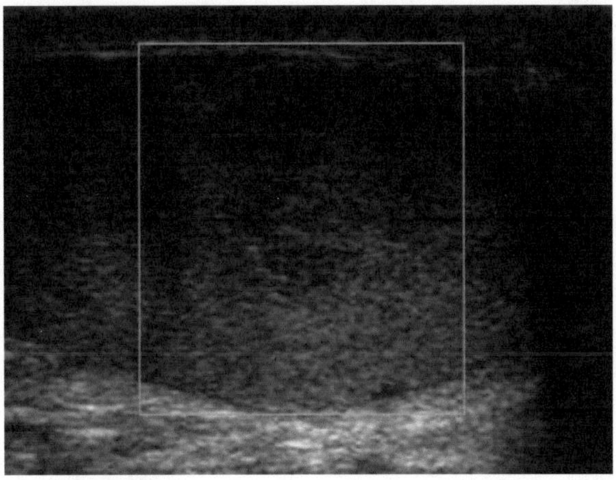

Fig. 26. Testicular torsion of the right testis. Absence of vascular flow and ill-defined hypoechoic lesions are seen in the testis

7.4 Varicocele

Varicocele refers to an abnormal dilatation of the veins of the spermatic cord due to incompetence of valve in the spermatic vein. This results in impaired blood drainage into the spermatic vein when the patient assumes a standing position or during Valsalva's maneuver. Varicoceles are more common on the left side due to the following reasons (a) The left testicular vein is longer, (b) the left testicular vein enters the left renal vein at a right angle; (c) the left testicular artery in some men arches over the left renal vein, thereby compressing it; and (d) the descending colon distended with feces may compress the left testicular vein (Mehta and, Dogra, 1998).

The US appearance of varicocele consists of multiple, hypoechoic, serpiginous, tubular like structures of varying sizes larger than 2 mm in diameter that are usually best visualized superior or lateral to the testis [Fig. 27a]. Color flow and duplex Doppler US optimized for low-flow velocities help confirm the venous flow pattern, with phasic variation and retrograde filling during a Valsalva's maneuver [Fig. 27b]. Intratesticular varicocele may appear as a vague hypoechoic area in the testis or mimics tubular ectasia. With color Doppler, this intratesticular hypoechoic area also showed reflux of vascular flow during Valsalva's maneuver [Fig. 28]

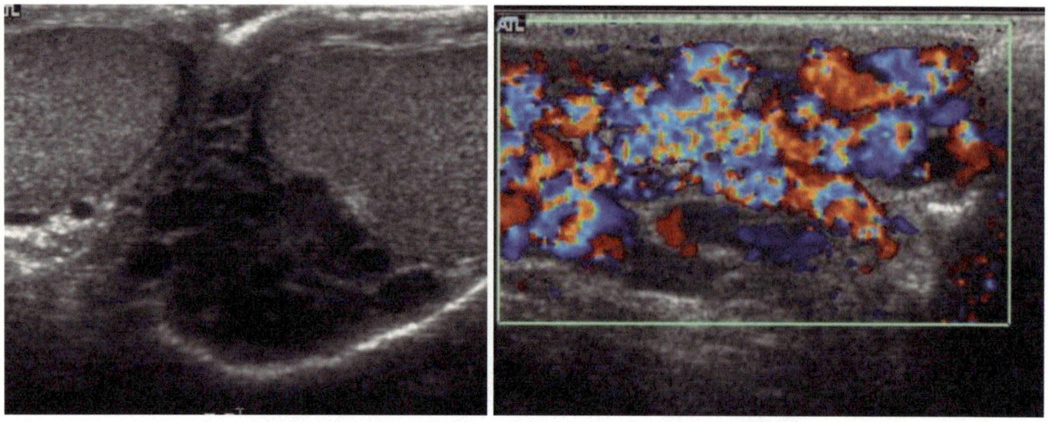

(a) (b)

Fig. 27. Varicocele. (a) Multiple tortuous tubular like structure are seen in the left scrotum. (b) Color Doppler sonography shows vascular reflux during Valsalva's maneuver

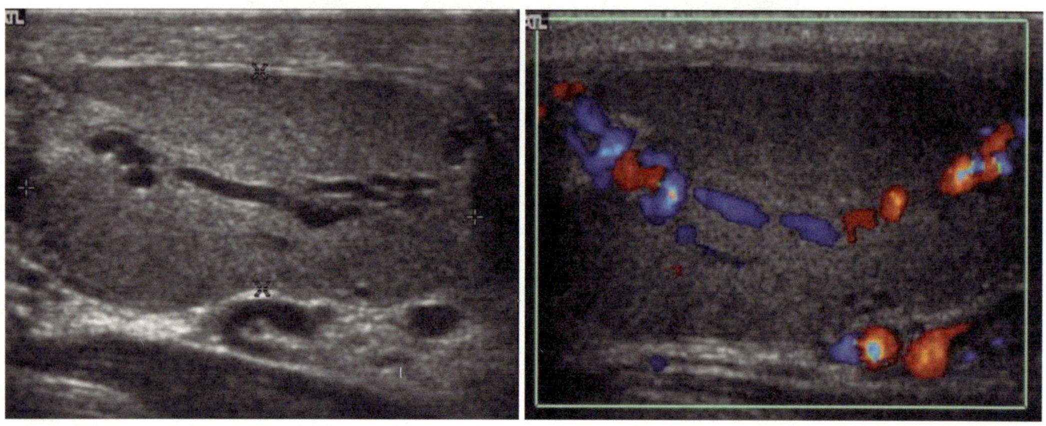

(a) (b)

Fig. 28. Intratesticular varicocele. (a) Dilated tubular structures are seen within the testis. (b) Presence of vascular reflux is noted during Valsalva's maneuver

7.5 Undescended testis (Cryptorchidism)

Normally the testes begin its descent through the inguinal canal to the scrotum at 36 weeks' of gestation and completed at birth. Failure in the course of testes descent will result in undescended testes. Undescended testis is found in 4% of full-term infants and only 0.8% of males at the age of 1 year have true cryptorchidism. Although an undescended testis can be found anywhere along the pathway of descent from the retroperitoneum to the scrotum, the inguinal canal is the most common site for an undescended testis. Deviation of testis from the normal pathway of descent will result in ectopic testis that is commonly seen in pubopenile, femoral triangle and perineal regions.

Besides infertility, undescended testes carry an increased risk of malignancy even for the normally located contralateral testis. The risk of malignancy is estimated to be as high as 10 times the normal individual with seminoma being the most common malignancy. The incidence of infertility is decreased if surgical orchiopexy is carried out before the 1-3 years but the risk of malignancy does not change.

Because of the superficial location of the inguinal canal in children, sonography of undescended testes should be performed with a high frequency transducer. At ultrasound, the undescended testis usually appears small, less echogenic than the contralateral normal testis and usually located in the inguinal region [Fig. 29]. With color Doppler, the vascularity of the undescended testis is poor.

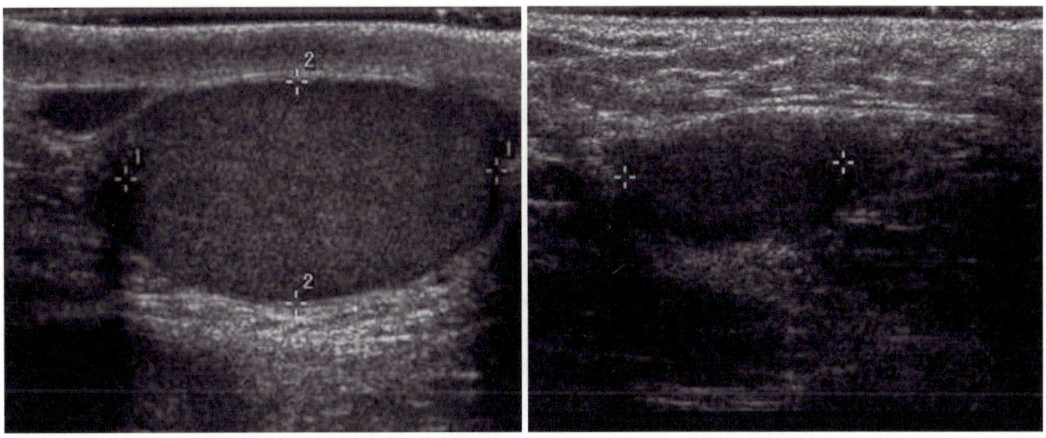

(a) (b)

Fig. 29. Undescended testis. (a) Normal testis in the scrotum. (b) Atrophic and decreased echogenicity of the contralateral testis of the same patient seen in the inguinal region

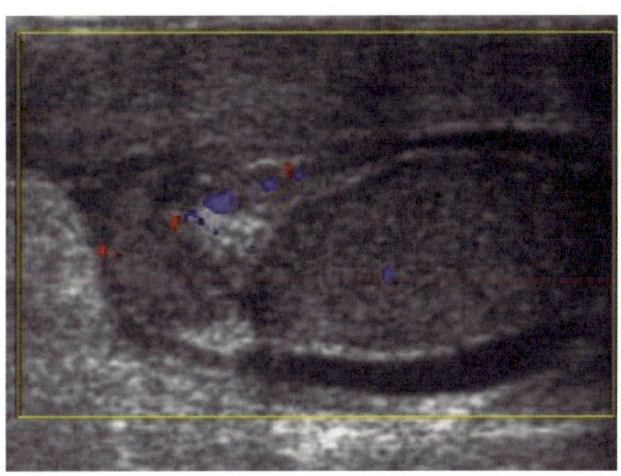

Fig. 30. Testicular appendiceal torsion. A hyperechoic lesion with surrounding vascularity is seen in the groove between the testis and epididymis

7.6 Testicular appendiceal torsion

At sonography, the appendix testis usually appears as a 5 mm ovoid structure located in the groove between the testis and the epididymis. Normally it is isoechoic to the testis but at times it may be cystic. The appendix epididymis is of the same size as the appendix testis but is more often pedunculated. Clinically pain may occur with torsion of either appendage. Physical examination showed a small, firm nodule is palpable on the superior aspect of the testis and a bluish discoloration known as "blue dot" sign may be seen on the overlying skin (Dogra and Bhatt 2004, as cited in Skoglund et al 1970). Torsion of the appendiceal testis most frequently involved in boys aged 7-14 years (Dogra and Bhatt 2004).

The sonographic features of testicular appendiceal torsion includes a circular mass with variable echogenicity located adjacent to the testis or epididymis [Fig. 30], reactive hydrocele and skin thickening of the scrotum is common, increased peripheral vascular flow may be found around the testicular appendage on color Doppler ultrasound. Surgical intervention is unnecessary and pain usually resolves in 2 to 3 days with an atrophied or calcified appendages remaining.

8. Conclusion

Ultrasound remains as the mainstay in scrotal imaging not only because of its high accuracy, excellent depiction of scrotal anatomy, low cost and wide availability, it is also useful in determining whether a mass is intra- or extra-testicular, thus providing us useful and valuable information to decide whether a mass is benign or malignant even though malignancy do occur in extratesticular tumors and vice versa. Furthermore, ultrasound also provides information essential to reach a specific diagnosis in patients with testicular torsion, testicular appendiceal torsion and inflammation such as epididymo-orchitis, Fournier gangrene etc, thus enabling us to avoid unnecessary operation.

9. Acknowledgments

The authors acknowledge Miss Lee Ying-Fang for her expert technical support in preparation of this manuscript. We are also thankful to British Institute of Radiology and John Wiley and Sons publishing company in granting us permission to reuse some of the figures previously published in British Journal of Radiology and Journal of Clinical Ultrasound.

10. References

Akbar SA (2003), Sayyed TA, Jafri SZ, Hasteh F & Neill JS. Multimodality Imaging of Paratesticular Neoplasms and Their Rare Mimics. *Radiographics*, Vol. 23, No. 6, (November-December 2003), pp. 1461-1476, ISSN 0271-5333

Bostwick DG (1997). Spermatic Cord and Testicular Adnexa, In: *Urologic Surgical Pathology* , Bostwick DG, Eble JN, pp. 647-674 Mosby, ISBN 978080167 St Louis, Missouri.

Boyum J (2008) & Wasserman NF. Malignant Mesothelioma of the Tunica Vaginalis Testis. *Journal of ultrasound in Medicine*, Vol. 27, No. 8, (August 2008), pp.1249-1255. ISSN 0278-4297

Bruno C (2002), Minniti S & Procacci C. Diagnosis of Malignant Mesothelioma of the Tunica Vaginalis Testis by Ultrasound Guided Fine Needle Aspiration. *Journal of Clinical Ultrasound*, Vol. 30, No.3, (March-April 2002), pp.181-183. ISSN 0091-2751

Dogra VS (2003), Gottlieb RH, Oka M & Rubens DJ. Sonography of the Scrotum. *Radiology*, Vol.227, No.1, (April 2003), pp.18–36. ISSN 0033-8419

Dogra V (2004) & Bhatt S. Acute Painful Scrotum. *Radiologic Clinics of North America*, Vol.42, (2004), pp. 349– 363, ISSN 0033-8389

Doll DC (1986) & Weiss RB Malignant Lymphoma of the Testis. *American Journal of Medicine*, Vol.81, No. 3, (September 1986), pp.515-524, ISSN 0002-9343

Garriga V (2009), Serrano A, Marin A, Medrano S, Roson N & Pruna X. US of the Tunica Vaginalis Testis: anatomic relationships and pathologic conditions. *Radiographics*, Vol.29, No.7, pp.2017-2032, (November, 2009), ISSN0271-5333

Kim W (2007), Rosen MA, Langer JE, Banner MP, Siegelman ES & Ramchandani P. US–MR Imaging Correlation in Pathologic Conditions of the Scrotum. *Radiographics,* Vol.27, No.5, (September 2007), pp.1239–1253, ISSN 0271-5333.

Levenson RB (2008), Singh AK & Novelline RA. Fournier Gangrene: Role of Imaging. *Radiographics*, Vol.28, No.2, (March-April 2008), pp.519-528, ISSN0271-5333

Mak CW (2001), Wu TC, Chou CK, Tzeng WS, Sia YL, Chang JM & Lin CN. Ultrasonographic Appearance of an Adenomatoid Tumor in the Epididymis: Report of a Case. *Journal of Medical Ultrasound*, Vol.9, No.4, (December 2001), pp. 202-205, ISSN 0929-6441

Mak CW (2004a), Chou CK, Su CC, Huan SK & Chang JM. Ultrasound Diagnosis of Paratesticular Rhabdomyosarcoma. *British Journal of Radiology*, Vol.77, No. 915, (March 2004), pp.250–252, ISSN 0007-1285

Mak CW (2004b), Cheng TC, Chuang SS, Wu RH, Chou CK & Chang JM. Malignant Mesothelioma of the Tunica Vaginalis Testis. *British Journal of Radiology*, Vol.77, No.921, (September2004), pp.780–781, ISSN 0007-1285

Mak CW (2004c), Tzeng WS, Chou CK, Chen CY, Chang JM & Tzeng CC. Leiomyoma Arising from the Tunica Albuginea of the Testis: Sonographic Findings. *Journal of Clinical Ultrasound*, Vol.32, No.6, (July-August 2004), pp.309–311, ISSN 0091-2751

Mak CW (2007a), Chen CY, Tzeng WS & Li CF. Epidermoid Cyst of the Testis. *Australasian Radiology*, Vol.51, No.Supplement S1, (October 2007), pp.B74–B76, ISSN 0004-8461

Mak CW (2007b), Tzeng WS & Chou CK. Microcystic Lesion of the Testis. *British. Journal. Radiology*, Vol.80, No. 949, (January 2007) pp.67-68, ISSN 0007-1285.

Mehta AL (1998) & Dogra VS. Intratesticular Varicocele. *Journal of Clinical Ultrasound*, Vol.26, No.1, pp.49-51, (January 1998), ISSN 0091-2751

Muttarak M(2006) & Peh WC. Case 91: Tuberculous Epididymo-orchitis. *Radiology*, Vol.238, No.2, (February 2006), pp.748-751, ISSN 0033-8419

Rosenberg R (1989) & Williamson MR. Lipomas of the Spermatic cord and Testis: Report of Two Cases. *Journal of Clinical Ultrasound*, Vol.17, No.9, (November-December 1989), pp.670-674, ISSN 0091-2751

Wang MT (2005), Mak CW, Tzeng WS, Chen JC, Chang JM & Lin CN. Malignant Mesothelioma of the Tunica Vaginalis Testis: Unusual Sonographic Appearance. *Journal of Clinical Ultrasound*, Vol.33, No.8, (October, 2005), pp.418–420, ISSN 0091-2751

Woodward PJ (2002), Sohaey, R, O'Donoghue MJ & Green DE. Tumors and Tumorlike Lesions of the Testis: Radiologic-Pathologic Correlation. *RadioGraphics*, Vol.22, No.1, (January-February 2002), pp.189–216, ISSN 0271-5333.

Woodward PJ (2003), Schwab CM & Sesterhenn IA. Extratesticular scrotal masses: Radiologic-pathologic correlation. *Radiographics*, Vol.23, No.1, (January-February 2003), pp. 215-40, ISSN 0271-5333.

2

Clinical Perspectives of Scrotal Ultrasound in Urology

Shou-Hung Tang, Tai-Lung Cha and Guang-Huan Sun
Tri-Service General Hospital, National Defense Medical Center, Taiwan, R.O.C.

1. Introduction

Scrotal ultrasound is widely used in modern hospitals as the first-line evaluation of almost all scrotal abnormalities. It provides useful and timely information for physicians to make management decisions without delay. This chapter is written in accordance with the clinical perspectives of urologists, as opposed to the technical interpretation of radiologists, in order to provide practical assistance to practicing physicians. An assessment of the commonest scrotal disorders will be discussed in this chapter.

Quick guide to ultrasound equipment and common imaging techniques
Normal ultrasound anatomy of the testis and epididymus
Identify scrotal and testicular emergencies that require surgical attention
Testicular torsion
Acute epididymitis, orchitis, and epididymo-orchitis
Testicular trauma
Fournier's gangrene
Neoplasm of the testis
Malignant neoplasms of the testis
Benign neoplasms of the testis
Non-neoplastic disease of the scrotum and testis
Varicocele
Hydrocele
Spermatocele
Testicular microlithiasis
Scrotal wall abscess

Table 1. Chapter highlights

2. Quick guide to ultrasound equipment and common imaging techniques

It is generally recommended that a high frequency (7 to 12 MHz) ultrasound transducer should be used whenever possible, set to the "small parts" setting, in order to examine scrotal contents (Bluth et al., 2001). Transducers with higher frequencies (e.g., >17 MHz) may help to obtain greater resolutions of fine anatomical details and are therefore particularly useful in pediatric patients. A machine that has the ability to perform color Doppler scans is always included as a standard setting. Color Doppler scans are required to diagnose vascular abnormalities, such as varicoceles, or more importantly, testicular torsion. Combined high-frequency scans and color Doppler images are sufficient for the diagnosis of most cases (Sandor et al., 2011). Advanced ultrasound techniques include contrast-enhanced studies, power Doppler scanning, and down-shifted Doppler frequencies in specific clinical situations. However, we do not recommend their use in routine daily practice.

Prior to the ultrasound examination, it is crucial that the patient should be calmed and that the procedure has been fully explained to them. The examiner should obtain a clear clinical history of the patient and any major past medical history should be known about before the study begins. It is recommended that the patient should be placed in the supine position with their thighs slightly abducted, described as the "frog-legs" posture. We have found that putting a rolled towel underneath the scrotum is helpful, but this maneuver should be individualized and only performed when the findings will not be affected by any compressive force.

Routine scanning procedures include the following scans as a minimum: long-axis (longitudinal), short-axis (transverse), and color-Doppler scans of both testicles, the epididymis and the spermatic cords. Care must be taken not to overlook lesions underneath or within the scrotal wall. In most cases, the content of the contralateral scrotum is a good reference guide to assessing the side with the lesion, and it is convenient to use the split-screen function for a contemporaneous comparison of both sides.

3. Normal ultrasound anatomy of the testis and epididymis

Normal testes are responsible for both reproductive and endocrine functions. In the adult human, the testes are ovoid in shape, with a size of approximately 4 x 3 x 2.5 cm (30 ml volume). Each testis is composed of approximately 250-300 lobules that contain seminiferous tubules. The lobules are separated by septa that cannot be visualized under sonography. These septa attach to the inner side of the tunica albuginea and connect to the mediastinum of the testis. At the mediastinum, the convoluted seminiferous tubules become straightened (the so-called "rete testis") and form 10-15 ductules that drain into the epididymis (Campbell et al., 2007).

The epididymis tightly attaches to the posterior lateral aspect of each testis. Grossly, this organ resembles an earthworm with an overall length of 4 to 5 cm. The epididymis contains a head (upper pole), body (mid-part), and a tail which connects to the vas deferens.

4. Identify scrotal and testicular emergencies that require surgical attention

4.1 Testicular torsion

Testicular torsion, or more precisely, torsion of the spermatic cord, is a true urological emergency. It affects approximately 1 in 4,000 young males before the age of 25 years (Datta et al., 2011). Almost all patients with testicular torsion present with excruciating pain, which usually wakes them up during sleep. The pain occurs as a result of testicular ischemia, and in some cases, the pain might have resolved as a result of spontaneous detorsion.

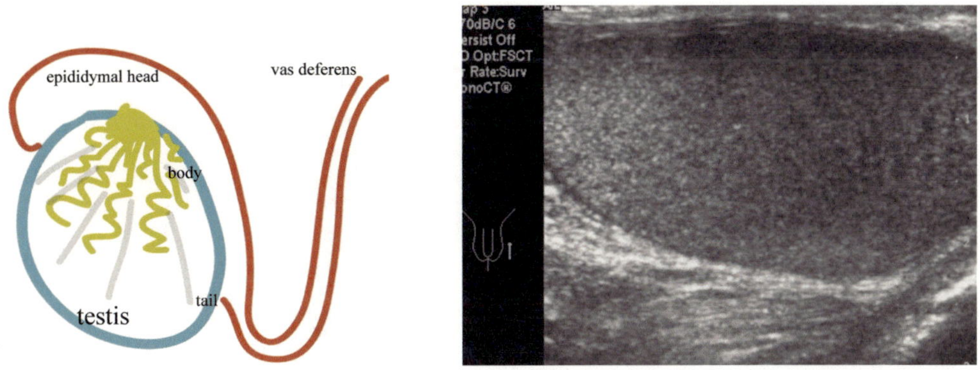

(a) (b)

Fig. 1. (a) Simplified anatomy of the testis and epididymis; (b) normal appearance of the left-sided testis on a longitudinal scan

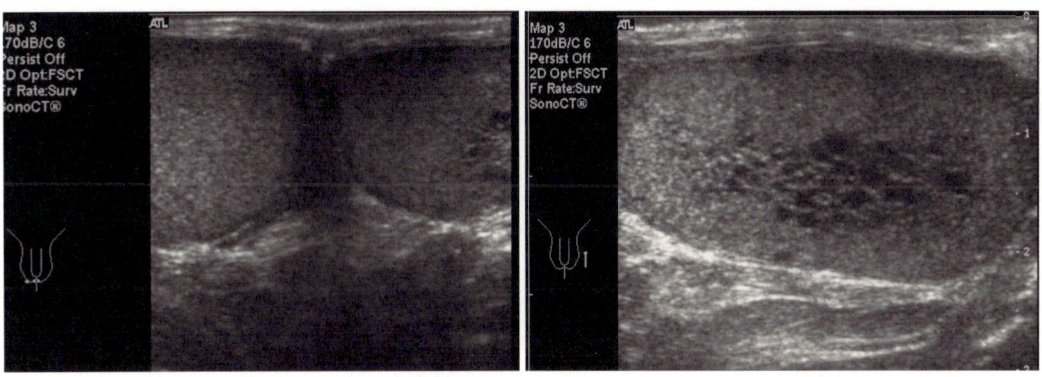

(a) (b)

Fig. 2. The rete testis: (a) hypoechoic foci in the left testis were found on a transverse midline scan; (b) multiple tubule-like hypoechoic areas in the area of testicular mediastinum

The etiology of this condition is attributed to an abnormally high or thin attachment of the tunica vaginalis to the spermatic cord, which makes twisting of the cord more likely. This is known as a bell-clapper deformity. Testicular torsion can be intravaginal, which is seen in all age groups, or extravaginal, which is seen exclusively in neonates.

Torsion of the epididymal appendix should also be included in the differential diagnosis of testicular pain, but is seldom treated as a surgical emergency. Physical examination of the affected testis may reveal that its long axis is altered, and it lies more horizontally. Mildly swelling of the scrotum can be expected, and the testis moves in a cephalad direction towards the external inguinal ring. In up to 99% of patients, there is no cremasteric reflex on the affected side (Schmitz, 2009).

Although manual detorsion has been suggested by some authors, this is not considered to be the definite treatment. All patients in which testicular torsion is suspected should undergo surgical detorsion within 6 hours of the symptoms developing, and a concurrent prophylactic orchiopexy should be performed on the contralateral testis.

Ultrasound with color Doppler flow imaging provides the most useful information to urologists within a very short time. Typically, lower or no vascular flow to the affected testis is compatible with the diagnosis, and a detectable blood flow to the peripheral tunica albuginea may be seen. The echogenicity of the testis may vary from normal to hypoechoic, or even heterogeneous, which reflects the severity of injury.

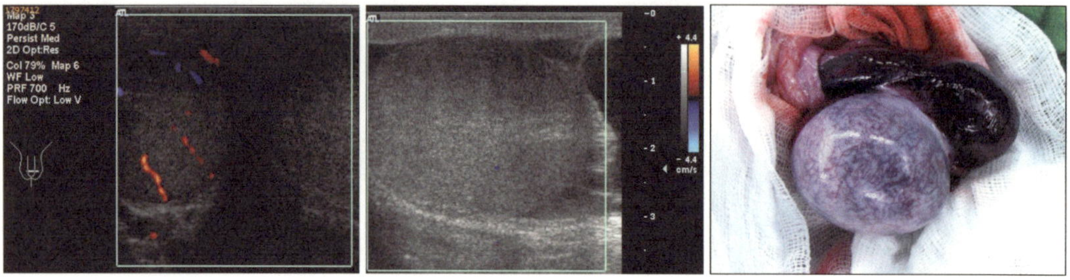

(a) (b) (c)

Fig. 3. Testicular torsion. A 50-year-old male presented to the ER and complained of a sudden painful enlargement of his left testis over 1 day: (a, b) ultrasonography showed absent vascularity with a cystic lesion in the left testis. Testicular echogenicity had not changes; (c) emergent exploration confirmed a 360° torsion and necrotic change of the affected organ. A left-sided orchiectomy was performed

4.2 Acute epididymitis, orchitis, and epididymo-orchitis

Acute epididymitis or epididymo-orchitis is one of the most common urological disorders in males. It primarily occurs in men aged between 18 and 60 years old, but can affect males of any age. This type of inflammatory change is often caused by bacteria (e.g., *E. coli* and *Pseudomonas* species), sexually-transmitted pathogens (e.g., *Neisseria gonorrhea*), or *Mycobacterium tuberculosis*. Ascending infections of pathogens from the urethra is the most common etiology; however, the hematogenous spread of pathogens to the epididymus can occur.

Patients tend to present with unilateral scrotal swelling and pain. Fever and leukocytosis may accompany the pain. If the inflammatory process cannot be controlled during its early phase, the affected epididymis/testis may undergo infarction and necrotic change, which eventually lead to abscess formation. It is not uncommon to see those abscesses ruptured through the scrotal skin.

Scrotal ultrasound with color Doppler imaging offers a clue to making this diagnosis, if present in conjunction with relevant clinical symptoms. During the early phase of inflammation, focal swelling (most commonly, the epididymal tail is the first to become enlarged) and increased focal blood flow can be detected. Later, the testis becomes tense and enlarged, and its blood flow is therefore compromised in certain areas, which results in a heterogeneous sonographic appearance (de Cassio Saito et al., 2004). The formation of a large abscess is usually an indication for surgery.

Chronic inflammatory changes of the epididymis and testes are not uncommon. Diagnosing chronic epididymitis requires the combination of a relevant clinical history for over 3 months, positive urine cultures, and an inflammatory process that observed with sonography.

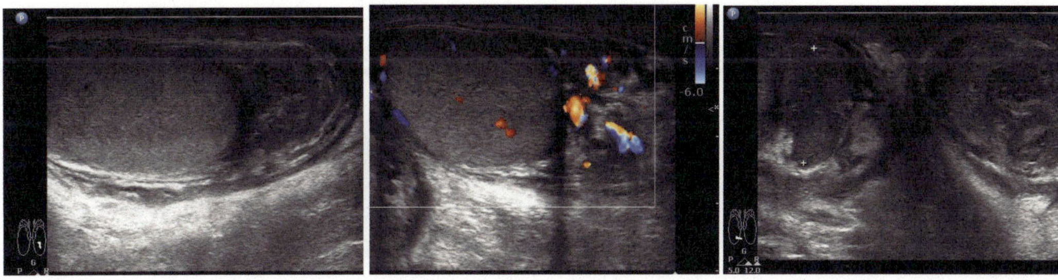

(a) (b) (c)

Fig. 4. Bilateral epididymitis. A 21-year-old with a gonococcal urethritis later developed fever and bilateral painful swelling of testicles. The sonography showed (a, b) swelling and hypervascularity of the left epididymal tail. (c) A short-axis scan at the level of the lower scrotum demonstrated bilateral involvement of the inflammatory process

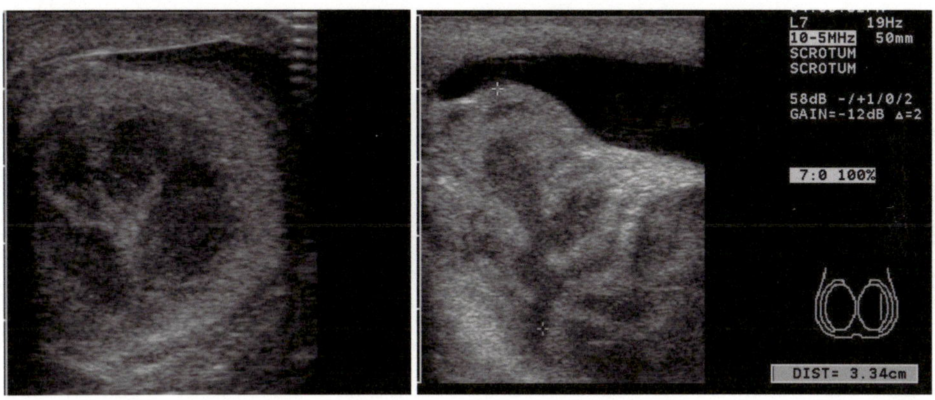

(a) (b)

Fig. 5. A case of chronic epididymo-orchitis with an abscess. An 86-year-old male presented with a low grade fever and painful swelling of his left testicle. (a) A short-axis scan and (b) long-axis scan both revealed a heterogeneous irregularly enlarged epididymis and testis. A hydrocele was also noted. The patient underwent a left-sided orchiectomy and the histopathological findings confirmed a chronic inflammation. It was not sonographically evident to differentiate a neoplasm from the inflammatory changes in this case

4.3 Testicular trauma

4.3.1 Testicular rupture

Testicular trauma is a common presentation to the emergency department. Blunt trauma to the genitalia accounts for more than 80% of these patients, and testicular injury should be considered in any patient with a pelvic fracture.

Patients universally present with a definite mechanism and with pain. At physical examination, the affected testicle is usually enlarged and tender. As only a ruptured tunica albuginea should be surgically corrected, this should be diagnosed as quickly as possible.

Diagnosing testicular rupture with ultrasound has a specificity of over 80% (Cokkinos et al., 2011). The sonography should be focused on the presence of hematocele (fluid between the layers of the tunica vaginalis), a discontinued line of the tunica albuginea, and unequal testicular sizes. It is important to consider that testicular torsion can occur after a minor trauma, and this should not be overlooked.

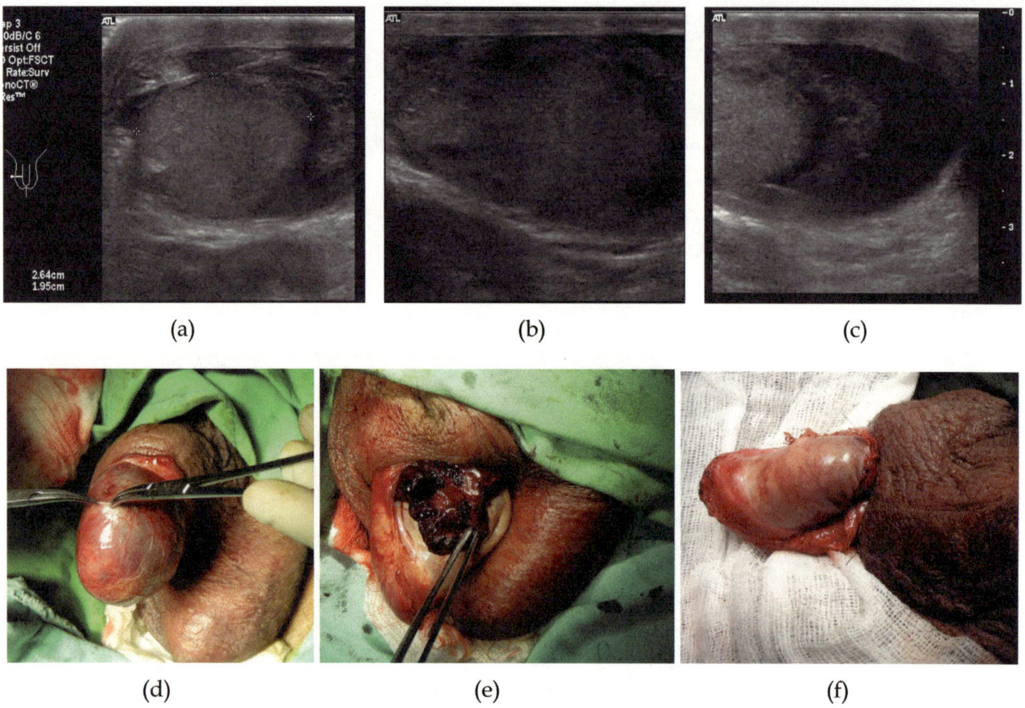

Fig. 6. Testicular rupture. A 46-year-old male sustained a blunt force to the genitalia and scrotal painful swelling developed. (a-c) Ultrasonography showed an ill-defined testicular margin, deformity, heterogeneous echogenicity and swelling of the right testis. A hydrocele or hematocele was also noted. (d) On surgical exploration, the tunica vaginalis was intact and a hematocele was found inside. (e) Testicular rupture through the disrupted tunica albuginea. (f) The tunica albuginea was repaired, and swollen testicular tissues were trimmed away

4.3.2 Intratesticular hematoma

After blunt contusion of the testis, testicular hematoma may occur, rather than a true rupture. The patient may complain of a gradually enlarging testis if he is seen few weeks after the injury. The typical sonographic findings reveal various degrees of heterogeneous echogenicity with a focally decreased pattern of blood flow. It is difficult to diagnose an intratesticular hematoma purely based on image findings.

4.3.3 Testicular contusion

Testicular contusion occurs frequently in active males. Contusion can be accidental, related to sports or as a result of violence. It is therefore important to obtain a clear history in order to estimate the force of injury accurately. Scrotal ultrasound is helpful in diagnosing testicular rupture, but making the diagnosis of a contusion by ultrasound is sometimes difficult.

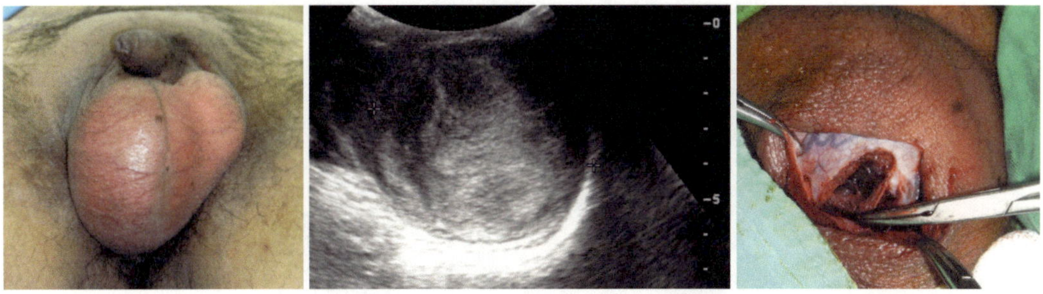

(a) (b) (c)

Fig. 7. Intratesticular hematoma. A 25-year-old male suffered a contused right hemiscrotum while lifting a box 2 weeks before. (a) Gross appearances showed an enlarged right testicle but no scrotal ecchymosis. (b) The right testis was enlarged with a heterogeneous echopattern, diminished blood flow, and an irregular contour that was suspicious of a testicular rupture. (c) Surgical exploration found a tense intratesticular hematoma; decompression was performed

The sonographic pictures may change over the first 72 hours from injury.After a blunt force to the testis, the testis may undergo inflammatory changes and become swollen. Since the tunica albuginea itself is strong and maintains the shape and volume of the testis, blood flow to a tense testis decreases as a result of swelling. Such a mechanism therefore makes the pattern seen on sonography very similar to that of a testicular torsion.

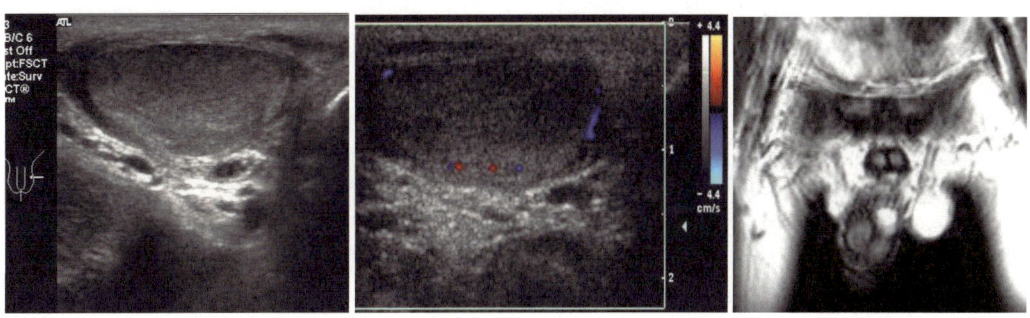

(a) (b) (c)

Fig. 8. A 26-year-old male sustained blunt scrotal injury and presented with left scrotal pain. (a) A transverse sonographic scan showed mild heterogeneous change of the left-sided testis. (b) There was a marked decrease in blood flow to the affected testis. (c) Magnetic resonance imaging: normal testicular perfusion and shape 1 day after the initial sonographic study

4.4 Fournier's gangrene

Fournier's gangrene is the most lethal necrotizing fasciitis that involves the genital and the perianal region. Most of the cases occur in patients between the ages of 20 and 50 years, with a male predominance. The mortality rate remains high at approximately 50% of cases even after aggressive debridement and other modern interventions.

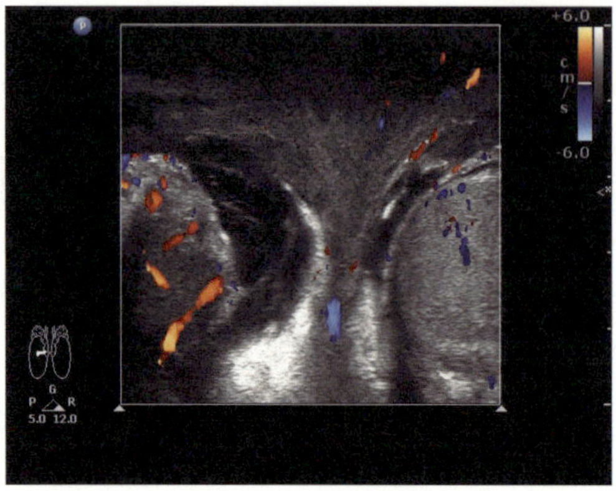

(a)

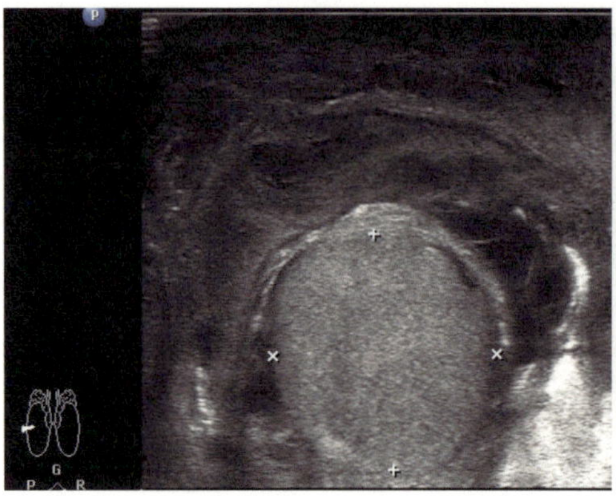

(b)

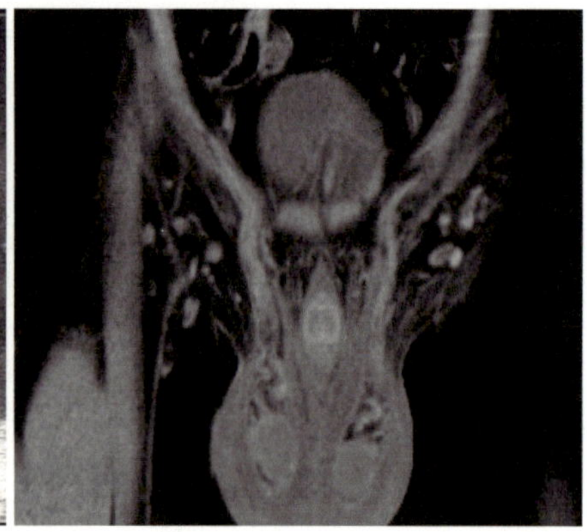

(c)

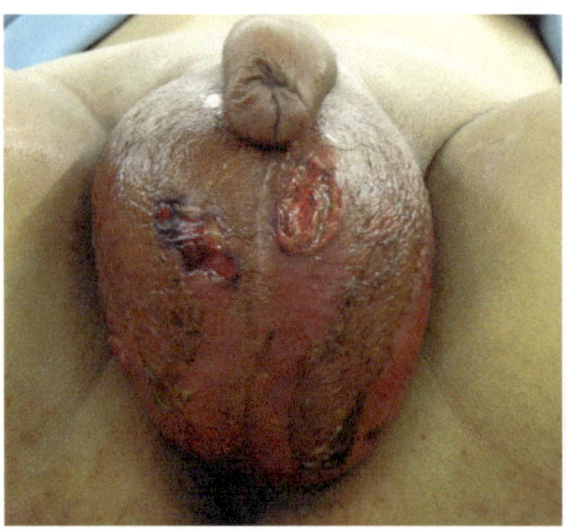

(d)

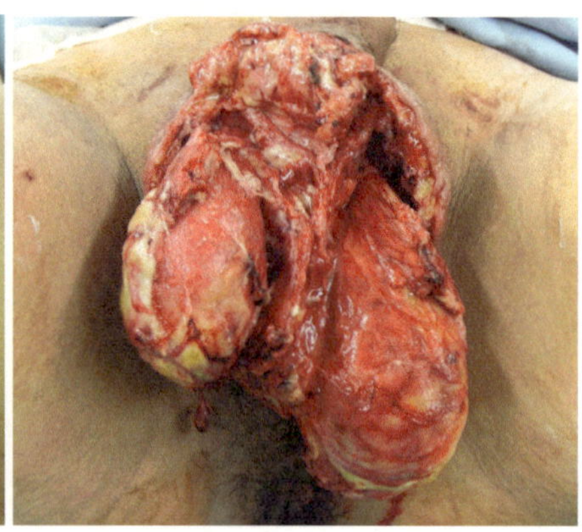

(e)

Fig. 9. A 27-year-old male presented with scrotal pain. (a,b) Enlargement, heterogeneous echogenicity, and increased vascularity of the bilateral epididymis with bilateral scrotal wall thickening on sonography. (c) Edematous scrotal wall on CT scanning. (d) Gross appearance of the scrotum. (e) Intraoperative view, showing that large amount of necrotic tissue should be removed

Urinary tract infection is recognized as the most common etiology, and it is commonly seen in cases that have undergone urethral catheterization; colorectal disease may also progress to Fournier's gangrene. Cases of Fournier's gangrene are associated with mixed flora on bacterial culture and some gas-forming organisms. The diagnosis depends on careful physical examinations, and with the aid of imaging studies to access the extent of the infection. During physical examination, any abnormally red or black skin coloration of the affected area should be observed to indicate ischemia; all examinations should include a test for skin crepitus to assess the presence of subcutaneous air.

Additional imaging study should never delay the timing of surgical intervention, since the infection is characterized by its rapid progression. Scrotal ultrasonography and CT scans of the lower abdomen to pelvic area are usually indicated.

Ultrasound imaging reveals heterogeneous echogenicity and increased vascularity in the affected testis. Thickening of the scrotal wall and areas of fluid-gas accumulation may be observed (Bartolotta et al., 2000). Without additional clear clinical information, a Fournier's gangrene can be mistaken ultrasonographically for acute epididymitis.

5. Neoplasm of the testis

5.1 Malignant neoplasms of the testis

The incidence of malignant neoplasms of the testis is rare compared with the aforementioned disorders. Overall, 90-95% of primary testicular cancers are germ cell tumors. Germ cell tumors can be divided into two major groups: seminomas (35%) and non-seminomatous germ cell tumors (65%). Subgroups that include embryonal cell carcinoma, teratoma, choriocarcinoma, and mixed type tumors are termed as non-seminomatous germ cell tumors (NSGCTs). A small portion of testicular cancers are metastatic lesions of leukemias and lymphomas (Tanagho et al., 2008).

Testicular cancers are more common on the right side, but this is not always the rule. Thirty to fifty percent of primary testicular cancers are seen in patients with a history of cryptorchidism. Approximately 90% of patients have painless enlargement of the testis, while others may present with pain or without symptoms at all. The combination of a sonographic diagnosis and serum tumor markers play an important role in the diagnosis of testicular cancers.

The major role of ultrasonography is to differentiate between malignant and benign testicular enlargement. In difficult cases, testicular cancers may mimic the signs of an infection; both of these share a pattern of increased blood flow of the affected region. However, characteristic sonographic features of malignancy are associated with specific cancer types.

Seminomas are intratesticular lesions, where the size of the lesion ranges from small nodules to the replacement of a whole testis. Seminomas typically appear as homogeneously hypoechoic on ultrasonography. NSGCTs are more aggressive tumors that can distort the contour of the ovoid tunica albuginea. They appear as heterogeneous lesions with irregular margins on ultrasonography. Teratomas consist of all three layers of embryonic tissues; they appear as mixed cysts, heterogeneous masses, and foci of calcification.

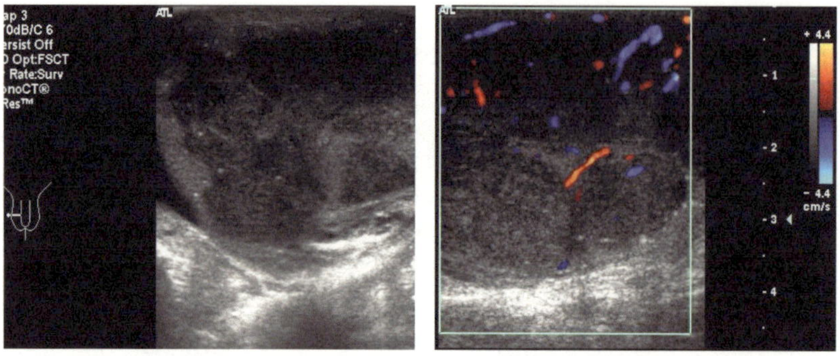

(a) (b)

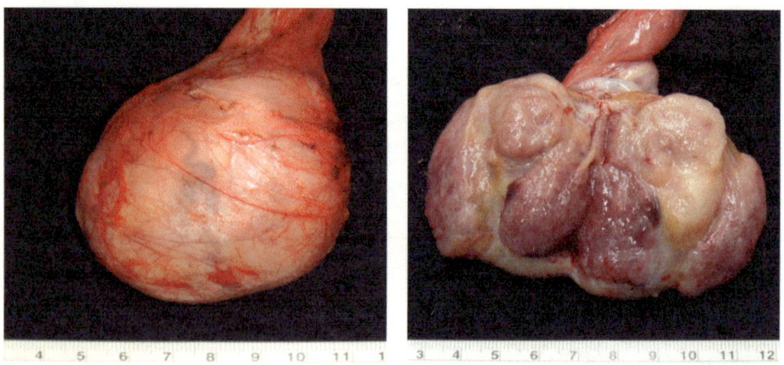

(c) (d)

Fig. 10. Seminoma of the testis. A 31-year-old male presented with a gradual enlargement of the right testicle over several months. Vague pain was also mentioned. (a,b) Transverse ultrasound images showed multiple well-defined homogeneously hypoechoic lesions (the largest one was approximately 2.1 cm in size) in the right testis with increased vascularity in the peripheral region. (c) Radical orchiectomy was performed: the tumor was grossly confined within the tunica vaginalis. (d) The bivalve specimen showed the typical histological pattern of a seminoma

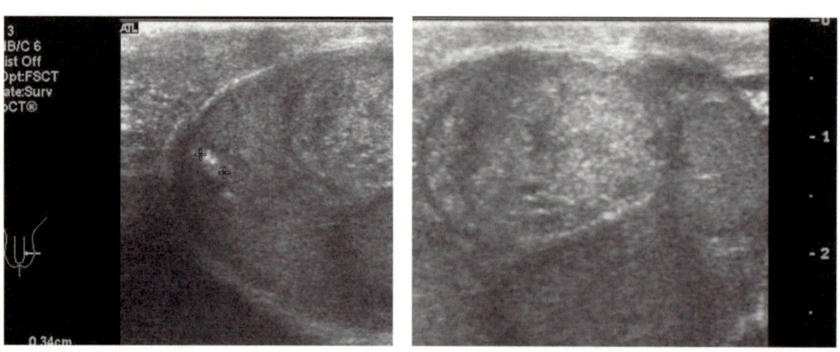

(a) (b)

Fig. 11. A non-seminomatous germ cell tumor of the testis. A 25-year-old male presented with pain over his lower abdomen. (a,b) A heterogenous mass (size: 3.2 x 2.9 cm) was shown to be located in the left testis with a few peripheral calcified spots. Pathology later confirmed that the lesion was a mixed germ cell tumor with embryonal carcinoma and yolk sac tumor components

If a primary testicular cancer is suspected, a biopsy should not be performed before definitive surgery (radical orchiectomy), in order to avoid iatrogenic seeding.

Testicular involvements from leukemia/lymphoma are usually seen in elderly patients. They appear as homogeneous, hypoechoic lesions within the testes, and are usually bilateral. A biopsy is required to make a definite diagnosis. Lung cancer and prostatic cancer can rarely metastasize to the testes, and sonographic findings may vary according to the nature of the cell of origin.

5.2 Benign neoplasms of the testis

Benign tumors of the testis are rare. Among these, epidermoid cysts are the most common disorder. Epidermoid cysts can be diagnosed with ultrasonography, which avoids an orchiectomy. They occur in men aged between 20 and 40 years and are often found during a routine physical check-up or self-examination. Epidermoid cysts usually grow slowly and seldom cause pain. The characteristics of ultrasonography of an epidermoid cyst are a well-circumscribed lesion with a solid central core surrounded by an echogenic rim(s), which sometimes resemble a hollow target or layers of an onion (Meng et al., 2004). Recently magnetic resonance imaging has also played a role in this diagnosis of epidermoid cysts.

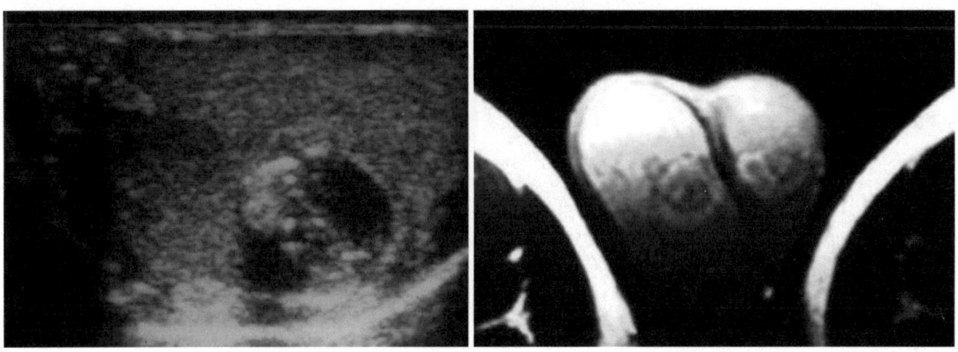

(a) (b)

Fig. 12. Testicular epidermoid cysts. (a) Typical sonographic pattern showing cystic lesion with an echogenic ring and some internal echogenic spots. (b) Magnetic resonance imaging was compatible with the diagnosis. This patient then underwent conservative surgery

6. Non-neoplastic disease of the scrotum and testis

6.1 Varicocele (scrotal varices)

Varicocele is a common cause of scrotal mass, and is estimated to affect 15% of males. It frequently causes symptoms in young males. Symptoms of varicoceles may include dull ache of the affected testis especially after prolonged standing or exercise. Varicoceles have also frequently been diagnosed during studies for male infertility (Tsao et al., 2009).

Varicoceles are more common in left-sided testicles (90%), and can occur bilaterally. By definition, a varicocele is the dilatation of the pampiniform plexus, which are the veins that drain the testis. The testicular vein (internal spermatic vein) drains to the renal vein on the left side and to the inferior vena cava on the right side. The anatomical characteristics of these drainage routes means that there is a steeper insertion of the internal spermatic vein on the left side, which makes it prone to vascular reflux as a result of gravity. It is also believed that incompetent venous valves will cause reflux within the spermatic veins, which can be responsible for venous reflux back into the testis.

Diagnosing varicoceles is straightforward with physical examination. Varicoceles can be classified as mild, moderate or severe. With severe varicocele, one can easily observe "a bag-of-worms" appearance while the patient is standing. When in doubt, or there is a need to evaluate the underlying testes, ultrasonography with color flow imaging can offer clear information. Most authors agree that dilated veins greater than 2-3 mm in diameter with a change in the direction of flow during the Valsalva maneuver are compatible with the diagnosis of a varicocele.

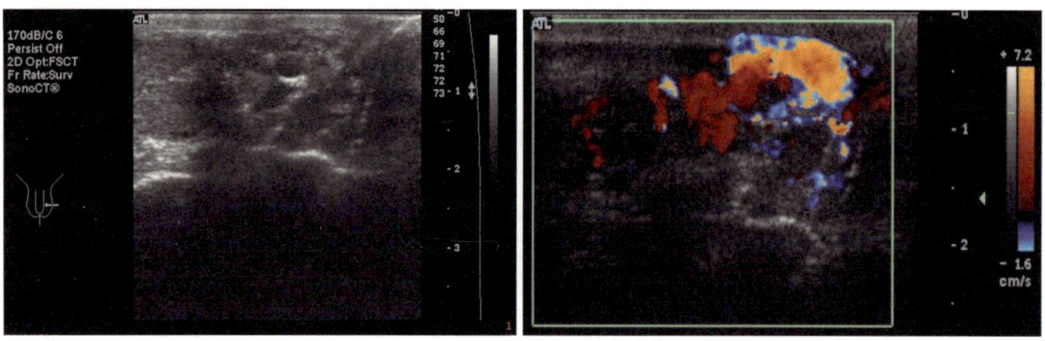

(a) (b)

Fig. 13. Scrotal varices. A 15-year-old male presented with dull ache and a left upper scrotal mass. (a) Upper scrotal transverse scan showed multiple hypoechoic vascular channels. (b) The Valsalva maneuver confirmed the reversed venous flow within the varicocele

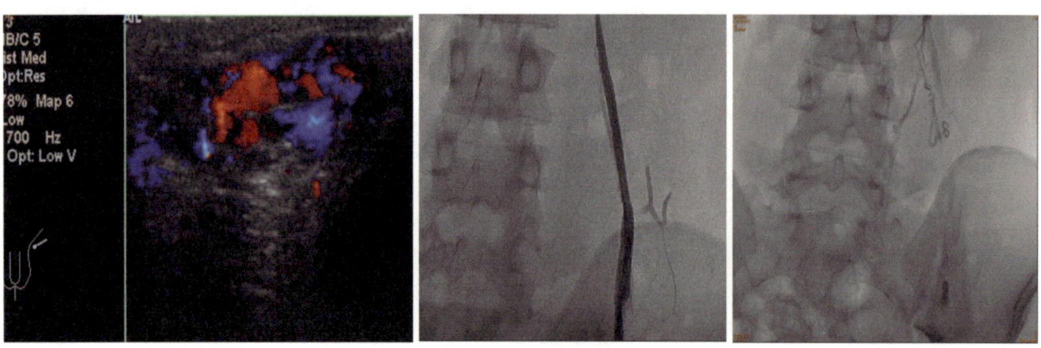

(a) (b) (c)

Fig. 14. Recurrent varicoceles. A 21-year-old male presented with a recurrent scrotal mass after a high ligation of internal spermatic vein (ISV) 2 years previously. (a) Sonographic diagnosis of reflux flow in the dilated left pampiniform plexus; (b) trans-jugular venography demonstrated patency of the left ISV; (c) embolization with coils successfully treated the recurrence

6.2 Hydrocele (hydrocele of the tunica vaginalis)

A hydrocele of the testis indicated fluid accumulation between the two layers of the tunica vaginalis. The tunica vaginalis is a remnant of peritoneum, which should close before birth. In children, a hydrocele is usually congenital and can present with an inguinal hernia. In the adult population, the hydrocele is usually secondary to infections (e.g., epididymitis), renal transplantation, peritoneal dialysis, testicular cancers, or torsion. Hydrocele affects 1% of adult men and is bilateral in 10% of all cases. Bilateral hydroceles should raise the suspicion of other underlying systemic diseases.

A hydrocele typically presents as a gradually enlarged testicle with no obvious pain. Severe and abrupt pain can indicate that the underlying condition should be investigated. During physical examination, good transillumination indicates a fluid content within the scrotum. Definite diagnosis can be made by ultrasonography. Scrotal ultrasound plays an important role not only for the diagnosis of hydrocele, but also to seek other possible etiologies, such as torsion, inflammation or malignancy.

Ultrasonographic findings of hydrocele are of typically pure anechoic fluid collection outside the tunica albuginea (Akin et al., 2004), but the fluid can be mixed with internal echoes in chronic cases. Some complex cases may demonstrate septations and loculations.

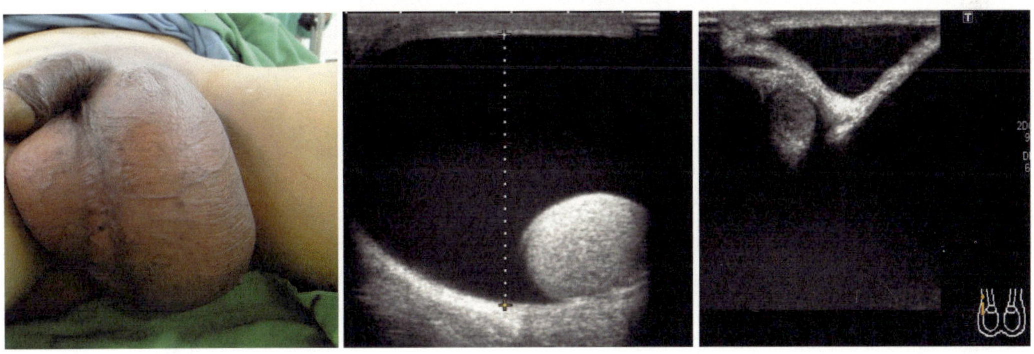

(a) (b) (c)

Fig. 15. A 58-year-old male presented with a feeling of heaviness and a gradually enlarged left scrotum. (a) A grossly enlarged left scrotum that was not tender; (b) transverse scan showed a marked accumulation of anechoic fluid and the testis was pushed aside; and (c) the hydrocele extends to the level of the external inguinal ring

6.3 Spermatocele

A spermatocele is a benign cystic lesion that contains sperm. It is commonly found in the epididymal head. Many spermatoceles are incidental, and are found during ultrasound screening in middle- to old-aged patients. The size of a spermatocele may vary from a few millimeters to several centimeters. Most spermatoceles do not cause symptoms, and the patient may present with a soft palpable mass inside the scrotum. In some cases, discomfort secondary to the mass effect may be present.

The etiology of spermatocele remains unclear. Most authors suggest that an obstruction in the efferent ductules is the origin of the disease. It is expected to grow slowly. Therefore, aspiration of the cystic lesion will not solve the problem, and surgical excision offers the only curative approach for this disorder.

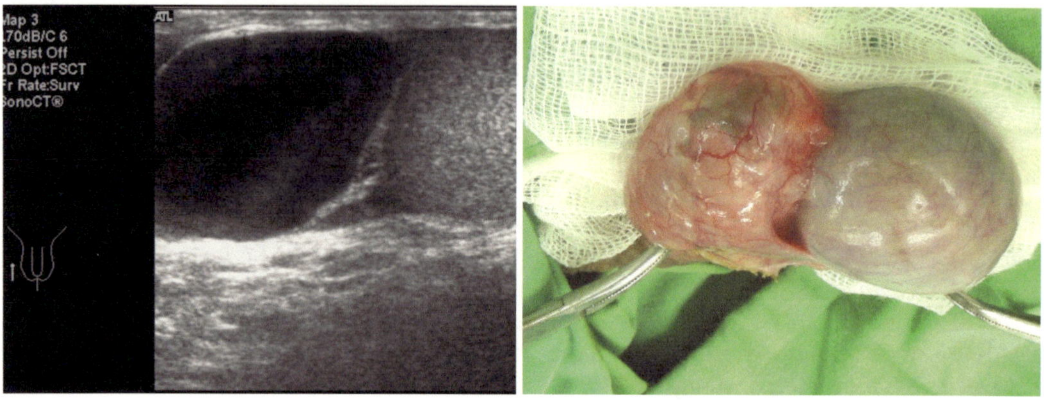

(a) (b)

Fig. 16. Epididymal spermatocele. A 56-year-old male presented with a slow-growing right scrotal mass that developed over several years. (a) Longitudinal scan showed a well-defined, 3-cm cystic lesion at right epididymal head with faint internal echogenicity; (b) scrotal exploration revealed findings that were compatible with the diagnosis of spermatocele

6.4 Testicular microlithiasis

Testicular microlithiasis (TM) is usually incidentally diagnosed by ultrasonography. TM may be correlated with testicular cancer and carcinoma in situ, although this issue remains controversial. In addition, TM is reported to be associated with various conditions, including male infertility, testicular atrophy, cryptorchidism, gonadal dysgenesis, Klinefelter syndrome, male pseudohermaphroditism, testicular torsion and varicocele. By definition, TM consists of small hyperechoic spots that less than 3 mm in size in the testis; the spots are usually multiple. A classic TM was defined as five or more microliths found on an

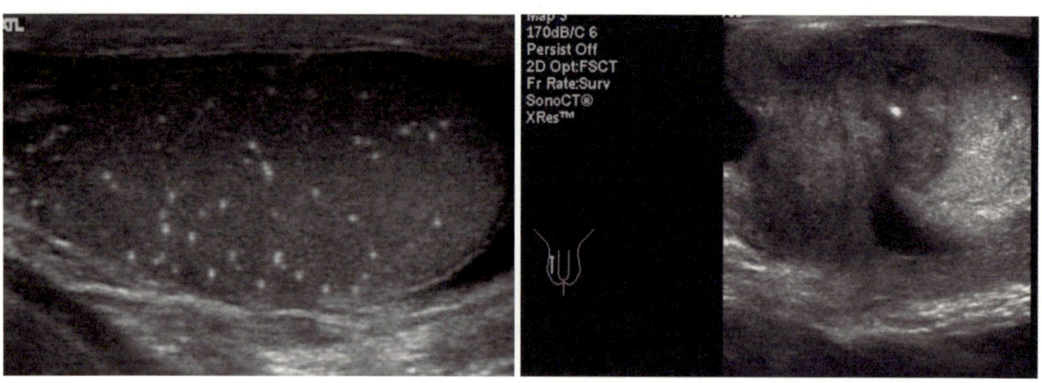

(a) (b)

Fig. 17. Two cases of TM associated with germ cell neoplasms. (a) Classic TM associated with a testicular cancer in the contralateral testis; (b) limited TM associated with an ipsilateral testicular germ cell tumor ultrasound scan, and fewer the five microliths would be recognized as a form of limited TM. Hyperechoic spots on sonography are usually found without acoustic shadows. The incidence of TM ranges from 0.6%-9% in various retrospective studies (Chen et al., 2010). We also noted that patients with a malignant testicular neoplasm have a higher prevalence of TM (Ou et al., 2007).

6.5 Scrotal wall abscess

Abnormal scrotal conditions can be missed on routine ultrasonography if the clinical information is ignored. Detecting common scrotal disorders, such as an abscess, sebaceous cysts, lipomas, and edematous skin, should be the final step of the sonographic evaluation. The examiner is suggested to ask relevant questions to the patient in order to locate scrotal abnormalities accurately.

The sonographic patterns of scrotal abscesses range from anechoic to irregularly hyperechoic, with areas of internal echoes, septae, or even gas. Manually compressing with the ultrasound probe upon the abscess may induce motion within the abscess material.

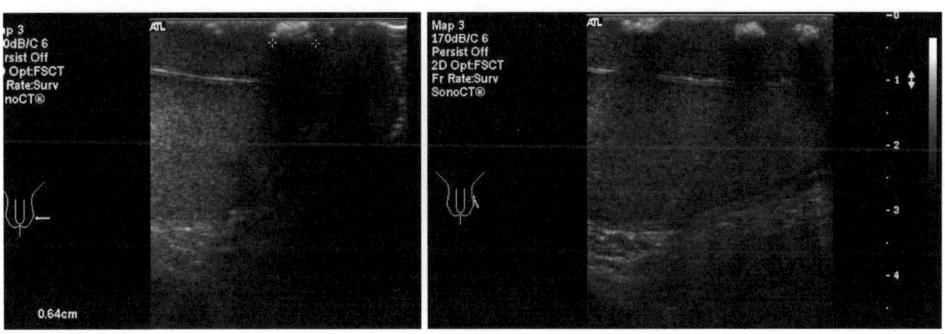

(a) (b)

Fig. 18. A 52-year-old suffered a perineal contusion 3 months previously. He presented with pain and induration over the left lower scrotum. (a) Transverse scan showed scrotal wall edematous changes, with hypoechoic areas and calcified lesions within the skin; (b) a longitudinal scan revealed similar findings that were compatible with chronic inflammatory changes

7. Conclusion

Ultrasound is convenient and important for the diagnosis of various scrotal abnormalities in clinical practice. Most notably, it is a time-saving procedure that requires only a very short time to train personnel to recognize urological emergencies. Nonetheless, a detailed medical history and physical examination should always precede the ultrasound study. Scrotal ultrasound offers clear information on whether a mass is intra- or extra-testicular, is cystic or solid, has increased or decreased focal flow, and whether the normal testicular ovoid shape is intact after a direct trauma.

A physician that performs scrotal ultrasound studies should be able to identify testicular torsion and testicular rupture in the emergency room setting, as both of these conditions require immediate surgical intervention. Lastly, although ultrasonography offers many important diagnostic clues, it is not a perfect diagnostic tool. Adjunctive diagnostic tools, such as CT or MRI scanning or surgical exploration, may be needed to make a definitive diagnosis in difficult cases.

8. Acknowledgment

We thank Dr. Sheng-Tang Wu, Dr. Feng-Ping Chuang, Dr. Chi-Wei Tsao and Dr. En-Meng (TSGH-urology) for contributing cases to this chapter. We also thank Dr. Dah-Shyong Yu (urology), Dr. Sun-Yran Chang (urology) and Dr. Ching-Jiunn Wu (radiology) for their long-term education and support with our imaging studies.

9. References

Akin, EA., Khati, NJ., Hill, MC., et al. (2004). Ultrasound of the scrotum. *Ultrasound Q*, Vol. 20, No.4, (December 2004), pp.181-200, ISSN 0894-8771

Bartolotta, TV., Midiri, M., Caruso, G. et al. (2000). Necrotizing fasciitis of the scrotum (Fournier's gangrene): ultrasound findings. *Radiol Med,* Vol. 100, No.6, (April 2001), pp. 510-512,ISSN 0033-8362

Bluth, EI., Arger, PH., Benson, CB., et al. (2001). *Ultrasonography in urology* (1st edition), Thieme, ISBN 1588900517, New York

Campbell, MF., Wein, AJ., Kavoussi, LR. (2007). *Campbell-Walsh urology* (9th edition), W.B. Saunders, ISBN 1416029664, Philadelphia

Chen, JL., Chou, YH., Tiu, CM., et al. (2010). Testicular microlithiasis: analysis of prevalence and associated testicular cancer in Taiwanese men. *J Clin Ultrasound,* Vol. 38, No.6, (July 2010), pp. 309-313.ISSN 1097-0096

Cokkinos, DD., Antypa, E., Tserotas, P., et al. (2011). Emergency ultrasound of the scrotum: a review of the commonest pathologic conditions. *Curr Probl Diagn Radiol,* Vol. 40, No.1,(January 2011),pp. 1-14, ISSN 1535-6302

Datta, V., Dhillon, G., Voci, S. (2011). Testicular torsion/detorsion. *Ultrasound Q,* Vol. 27, No.2, (June 2011), pp. 127-128, ISSN 1536-0253

de Cassio Saito, O., de Barros, N., Chammas, MC. et al. (2004). Ultrasound of tropical and infectious diseases that affect the scrotum. *Ultrasound Q,* Vol. 20, No.1, (March 2004), pp. 12-18, ISSN 0894-8771

Meng, E., Sun, GH., Wu, CJ., et al. (2004). Epidermoid cysts of the testes in Taiwanese men. *Arch Androl,* Vol. 50, No.3, (May 2004), pp. 201-205, ISSN 0148-5016

Ou, SM., Lee, SS., Tang, SH., et al. (2007). Testicular microlithiasis in Taiwanese men. *Arch Androl,* Vol. 53, No.6, (November 2007), pp. 339-344, ISSN 0148-5016

Schmitz, D., Safranek, S.(2009). Clinical inquiries. How useful is a physical exam in diagnosing testicular torsion? *J Fam Pract,* Vol. 58, No.8, (August 2009), pp.433-434, ISSN 1533-7294

3

Prostate

Ragab Hani Donkol[1] and Ahmad Al Nammi[2]
[1]*Cairo University*
[2]*Aseer Central Hospital*
[1]*Egypt*
[2]*Saudi Arabia*

1. Introduction

The value of prostatic sonography has dramatically increased in the past three decades. Transrectal ultrasound (TRUS) imaging is currently an integral part of prostate cancer diagnosis and treatment procedures, providing high-resolution anatomical detail of the prostate region. In this chapter we review the anatomy and sonographic methods in imaging of the prostate and prostatic diseases. Also we emphasize the role of new sonographic techniques, such as color and power Doppler, the use of contrast agents, 3D sonography and elastography for diagnosis of different prostate diseases especially prostate cancer. We also discuss the use of systematic and targeted sonographic-guided biopsies as gold standard for prostate cancer detection. Finally, we will elaborate the new role of ultrasound in management of prostate cancer.

2. Anatomy of the prostate

2.1 Embryology of the prostate

In the 4th week of gestation, the urogenital septum divides the cloaca into two parts: The rectum posteriorly and the primitive urogenital sinus anteriorly. In the 5th week, the distal portions of the Wolffian canal and the Mullerian canal attach to the posterior aspect of the primitive urogenital sinus (Fig. 1) to form an elevation called Mullerian tubercle. The tubercle divides the primitive urogenital sinus into vesico-urethral canal superiorly and definitive urogenital sinus inferiorly.The Wolffian canal forms the vas deferens, the ampulla of the vas and the seminal vesicle. The Mullerian canal regresses to form the utricle. Formation of the prostate begins at the 10th week of gestation by proliferation of the epithelium of the posterior urethra around the orifices of the Wolffian canal, to surround the urethral circumference. The prostatic glands formed anterior to the urethra regress and are replaced by fibromuscular stroma. The secretory function of the glands starts about the 13th week of gestation. (Brandes, 1989).

2.2 Gross anatomy of the prostate and its relations

The term "prostate" was originally derived from the Greek word "prohistani", meaning "to stand in front", and has been used to describe the organ located in front of the urinary bladder (Lowsley, 1912). The prostate is conical in shape with its long axis directed inferiorly and anteriorly. The shape and size of the prostate may vary with age. The prostate of an adult man measures 20 - 25 gms in weight. The base of the prostate is directed superiorly and in contact with the bladder base. The apex is directed inferiorly and in contact with the external sphincter above the deep fascia of the urogenital membrane. The anterior border is separated from the symphysis pubis and pubic bones by the retropubic space which contains loose areolar tissue, preprostatic venous plexus, lymphatics, nerves and puboprostatic ligament. The trapezoid area is an extraprostatic area of anatomic weakness. It may be involved by carcinoma extending through the inferior neurovascular pedicle. This area bounded by the prostate proximally, the rectourethralis muscle distally, the membranous urethra anteriorly and the rectum posteriorly (Mayers et al, 1987). Posteriorly, the prostate is related to the rectum and is separated from it by the Denoviller's fascia which extends superiorly, behind the seminal vesicles up to the peritoneal reflection. At each posterolateral aspect of the prostate, the hypogastric pelvic fascia contains the neurovascular bundle of the prostate, seminal vesicles and bladder neck (Fig. 2).

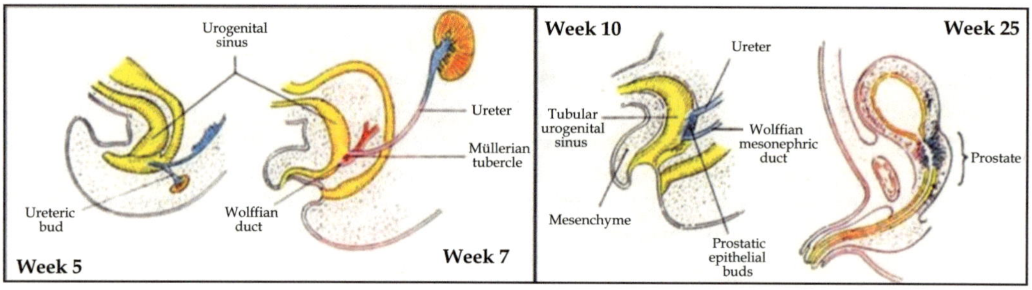

Fig. 1. The embryological origin and development of the prostatic urethra and the prostate (adapted from Delmas, 1991)

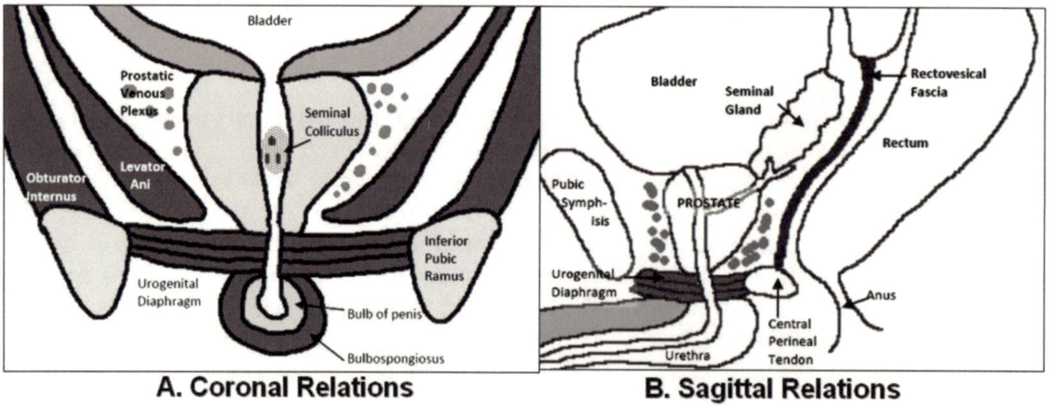

Fig. 2. Relations of the prostate in the coronal (A) and sagittal planes (B)

2.3 The distal seminal tract

It is formed of two seminal vesicles, ampullae of the vasa differentia and ejaculatory ducts. The seminal vesicle is a cystic structure, measuring about 35 mm in length and 15 mm in width. It is related anteriorly to the urinary bladder and posteriorly to the the rectum.The ampula of the vas is located medial to the seminal vesicle. The vassal ampula joins the seminal vesicle to form the ejaculatory duct. Each duct enters the base of the prostate, passes through central zone to end in the urethra below the utricle (Brandes, 1989).

2.4 Lobar concept of intraprostatic anatomy

In 1912, Lowsley demonstrated the first detailed description of the anatomy of the prostate. This traditional concept which is no longer used, divided the prostate into lobes: an anterior, posterior, middle and two lateral lobes. This method has been used to identify the prostate and prostatic disease for about 60 years. The anterior lobe was situated from the anterior margin of the gland to the level of the prostatic urethra. The middle lobe was a small area between the proximal prostatic urethra and the ejaculatory ducts. This lobe extnds form the base of the prostate to the level of verumontanum. The posterior lobe was situated posterior to the ejaculatory ducts and extends to the posterior margin of the gland. The two lateral lobes extend from the lateral margin of the gland bilaterally toward the middle part of the gland. None of these lobes has clearly defined medial margin (Lowsley, 1912).

2.5 Zonal concept of intraprostatic anatomy

The understanding of the gross and microscopic anatomy of the prostate has changed during the past few decades. Since 1965, a zonal concept of anatomy has evolved initially developed by McNeal and then modified over about three decades. The prostate is best considered to be a fusion of different glandular regions contained within a discontinuous capsule (McNeal, 1968, 1988). The prostate is composed of four glandular regions and a non-glandular region which is the anterior fibromuscular stroma (Fig. 3). The fibromuscular stroma (FMS) is the anteromedial portion of the gland is devoid of glandular tissue. This region is generally considered to be of less clinical significance. The peripheral zone (PZ) comprises the largest portion of the glandular prostate in young man (70%). The PZ is

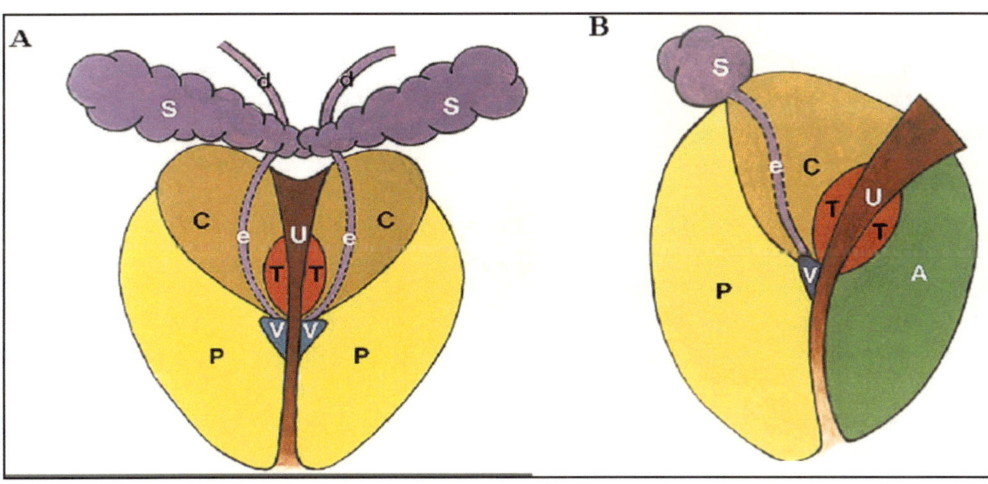

Fig. 3. Zonal anatomy of the prostate in coronal and sagittal planes showing the central zone (C), peripheral zone (P), transition zone (T) and anterior fibromuscular stroma (A). It also shows the distal seminal tract formed of the ampula of the vas deference (d) which joins the seminal vesicle (S) to form ejaculatory duct (e) which opens at vera montanium (v) (adapted from McNeal 1968)

situated posteriorly, posterolaterally and a thin layer of this tissue also extends up laterally and anterolaterally. Distal to the verumontanum, the PZ often surrounds the urethra and occupies the apical region if the prostate. The transition zone (TZ) is situated on both sides of the proximal prostatic urethra and comprises only 5 to 10% of the glandular tissue in the non hyperplastic prostate. The surgical capsule is an interface between the PZ and TZ. In the aging prostate where the TZ can show marked glandular hyperplasia and may constitute the majority of prostatic glandular elements. The periurethral glandular zone (PUG) consists of mucosal glands in the prostatic urethra itself and represents only a tiny fraction of the glandular prostate. This zone may become hyperplastic with age to form the "median lobe" which may obstruct the bladder neck. The central zone (CZ) is cone-shaped with its base forms the base of prostate, bordering the urinary bladder and seminal vesicles and its apex is at the verumontanum The CZ forms about 25% of the glandular prostatic tissue. The CZ surrounds the ejaculatory ducts throughout their entire courses in the prostate. The site where the ejaculatory ducts enter the CZ is devoid of prostatic capsule. The extraprostatic space invaginates around the ejaculatory ducts down to the verumontanum forming the "invaginated extra prostatic space". If the ejaculatory ducts are invaded by carcinoma, the tumor will have a ready "highway" to the seminal vesicles and extraprostatic space.

2.6 Correlation of the lobar and zonal concepts of anatomy of the prostate

A comparison of Lowsley lobar and McNeal zonal concepts of anatomy is possible and important to compare the clinical findings. Clinicians may still refer to lobar anatomy while radiologists use zonal anatomy. So, the anterior lobe correlates with the anterior fibro-muscular stroma. The medial lobe and the CZ are similar. The sum of the posterior and two lateral lobes correlated to a large extent with the PZ.

2.7 Correlation of the zonal anatomy and origin of prostatic diseases

With the development of cross sectional - imaging studies like transrectal ultrasound (TRUS) and magnetic resonance imaging (MRI), the zonal concept of anatomy becomes useful technique to apply because the different areas can be definite (Rifkin et al, 1990). The zonal concept of anatomy is also useful because it incorporated a clearer understanding if the development of disease. The origin of prostatic disease was poorly understood under Lowsley's concept of lobar anatomy. It was previously thought that cancer only arises in the posterior lobe and BPH develops predominantly in the lateral and, to a lesser degree in the median lobe. It is now understood that the prostate cancer develops in the acinar tissue predominantly the peripheral prostate. Although the PZ is three times larger in volume that the CZ, prostate cancer develops seven times more often in the PZ. It was shown that about 50% of cancer arises in the anterior half of the prostate, including all those cancers from the TZ (20% of the total), CZ (10%) and anteriorly situated portions of the PZ. In contrast, BPH develops exclusively from the central gland, approximately 95% from the TZ and 5% from the periurethral glandular tissue. Prostatitis (when not due to surgical manipulation) starts mainly in the PZ similar to the prostatic cancer (McNeal et al 1988).

3. Techniques and approaches of prostatic ultrasonography

Ultrasonography is firmly established diagnostic tool in prostatic imaging. Recent development in US technology has led to significant improvements in image quality, consistency and resolution. Additionally, dynamic scanners, color flow imaging and real time imaging have allowed appreciation of blood flow, reduced examination time and improved quality of the image. These advances combined with the portability, relative low cost and lack of risks of iodinated contrast media and irradiation have made US one of the most useful modality in evaluation of the prostate. Many approaches can be used to image the prostate as trans-abdominal, trans-urethral, trans-perineal and transrectal US. The common two approaches are transabdominal and transrectal ultrasound.

3.1 Trans-abdominal ultrasound

Transabdominal US of the prostate is nearly universally available and provides excellent anatomic information using the urine-filled bladder as an acoustic window. Prostate size, weight, shape and intravesical extent can be determined. Caudal angulation of the transducer to accommodate the public bone is often required. The normal prostate appears as a homogenous, round or ovoid structure with uniform low level echoes. The intraglandular zonal anatomy can not be visualized (Fig. 4). The relation between the prostate, bladder and seminal vesicles can be demonstrated (Abu-Yosef & Noryana 1982).

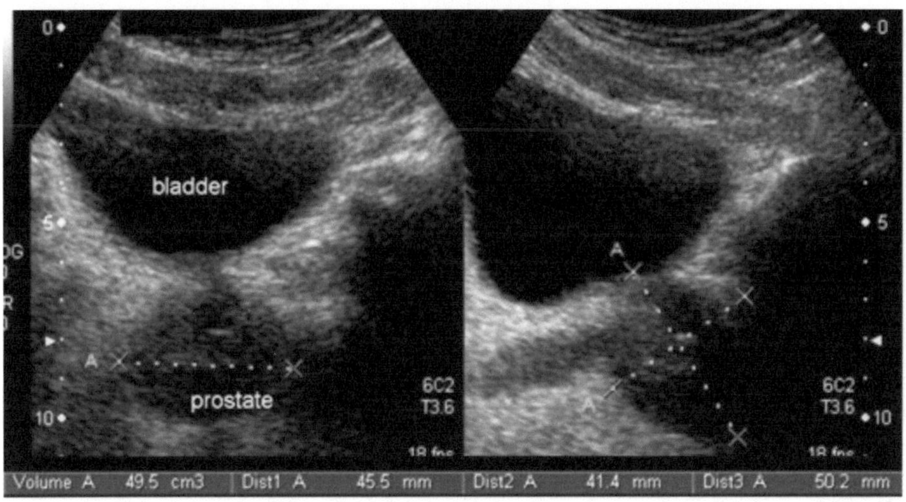

Fig. 4. Transabdonal US of a moderately enlarged prostate in axial and sagittal planes

3.2 Transrectal ultrasound (TRUS)

In 1963, Takahashi and Ouchi were the first to describe the use of TRUS to evaluate the prostate. The first clinically applicable images of the prostate obtained with TRUS were described in 1967 by Watanabe et al, they used a 3.5 MHz transducer, which at that time was considered to be state of the art, to obtain images that were clinically meaningful. As US technology has become more refined, the use of TRUS in the evaluation of prostatic disease has increased. By the mid 1980s.TRUS had become a standard diagnostic instrument of the urologists and radiologists. Most investigators today prefer equipment using hand-held transducers which are available in frequencies ranging from 3.5 MHz up to 10 MHz with the optimum frequency being around 7.0 MHz. Transrectal probes are available in different sizes and shapes with diameters ranging from 1.2 to 2 cm.

4. Sonographic anatomy of the normal prostate

Transrectal US of the prostate has revolutionized our ability to examine this organ. It provides excellent visualization of the prostate in the axial and sagittal planes.

In the axial plane, scanning usually begins at a level just above the seminal vesicles and by sequential withdrawing of the transducer in a caudal direction, the base, mid gland and the apex is visualized (Fig. 5). When scanning the most cephalad areas, the vas deferens will be visualized. They will appear as bilateral round cystic structures. Then the seminal vesicles will come into view as the vas deferens joins with them superior to the prostate. They usually appear as bow-tie configuration, but they may be rounded, lobulated or flattened. At the level of the base of the prostate, the prostate appears as a symmetrical crescent-shaped with triangular postero-lateral margin. The normal prostate will appear hyperechoic to the sminal vesicles and will have a homogenous echopattern. The CZ and TZ cannot be individually distinguished by their echogenicity. However the PZ appears more echogenic with homogenous echotexture. At the level of mid gland, the prostate becomes ovoid in shape. The anterior fibromuscular tissue is seem and has an echogenicity equal to or less than that of the glandular areas. The hypoechoic periurethral glandular tissue is demonstrated as hypoechoic area in the midline. Posterior and lateral to the PUG tissue, the PZ appears more echogenic and homogenous. The apex of the prostate appears more rounded. The obturator internus and levator anu muscles appear as hyperechoic structures lateral to the prostate apex. The prostate is surrounded by hyperegenic layer comprising the prostatic capsule and surrounding fat and fascia. The normal prostatic urethra is rarely visualized. The advantages of axial scanning include visualization of the left-right symmetry and echotexture,visualization of the anterior lateral portions of the PZ in a single view and assessment the lateral extracapsular spread of carcinoma (Rifkin, 1997).

In the sagittal plane scanning starts in the midline where the entire prostate can be visualized in one image. The seminal vesicle will be superior and posterior to the base of the prostate, and the vas deferens will be seen anterior to the seminal vesicles. The seminal vesicles will be less echogenic than the prostate and will appear rounded in shape. In the midline sagittal plane, the hypoechoic periurethral tissue will be seen and may be difficult to differentiate form the anterior fibromuscular stroma. The rest of the prostate will be homogenous in echogenicity with the PZ slightly more echogenic than the CZ and TZ (fig. 6). By tilting the transducer slightly to the right or the left of midline, the lateral aspects of the prostate and seminal vesicles will be visualized. The lateral aspects of the prostate are normally more rounded and homogenous in ehcogenicity. The ejaculatory ducts can be identified as hypoechoic lines structures between two parallel echogenic lines as the course from the seminal vesicles through the CZ into prostatic urethra. The advantages of sagittal scanning include evaluation of the base and apex of the prostate in a single view, accurate measurement of the cranio-caudal diameter of the prostate or of a lesion within the prostate and better demonstration of the prostatic urethra and ejaculatory ducts ((Rifkin, 1997)

Estimation of prostate volume may be useful in a variety of clinical settings. In cases of BPH, most urologists prefer to perform transurethral resections for glands under 60 grams, while open prostatectomy is preferred for glands over 60 grams (Narayan & Foster 1991). Other potential users include the comparison of the prostate volume with levels of PSA for early detection of the prostatic cancer. PSA density is an index calculated by dividing PSA by the volume of the prostate measured by TRUS. In absence of cancer, prostatic volume is directly

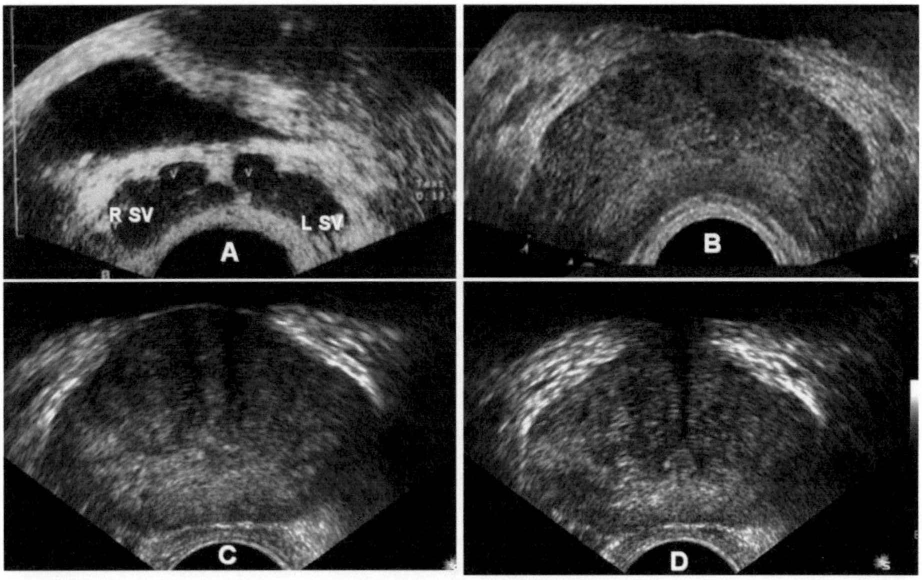

Fig. 5. TRUS axial images. (A) the level of distal seminal tract; showing seminal vesicle (SV) and vasl ampulla (V), (B) level of prostate base, (C) level of mid gland and (D) level of vera montanum showing its appearance as tour Eiffel

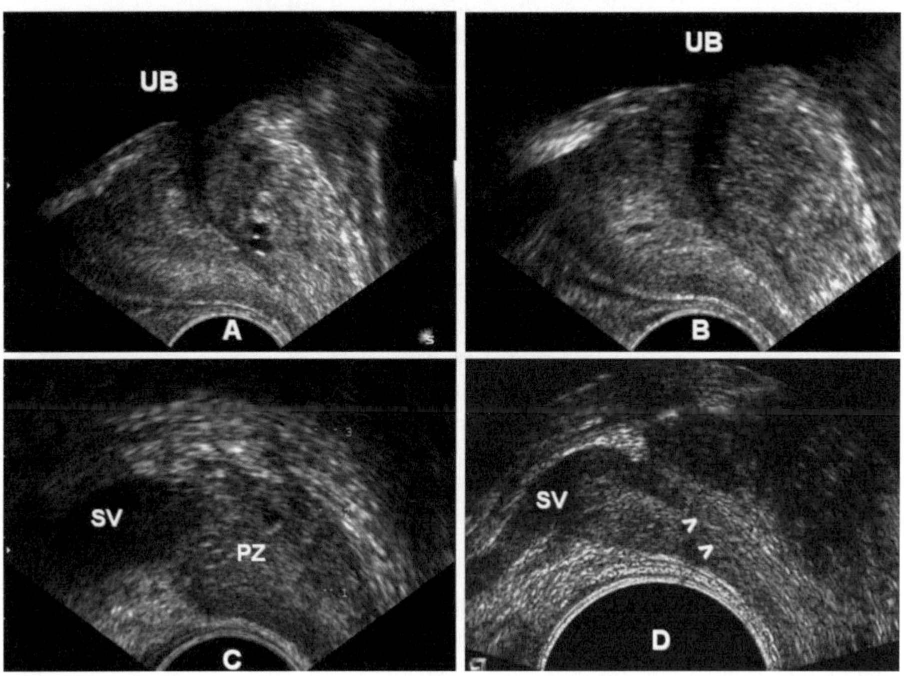

Fig. 6. TRUS sagittal images; (A) in midline; (B) in paramedical region; (C) peripheral part of the gland which is formed mainly of peripheral zone (PZ) and above it the body of seminal vesicle (SV) and (D) shows the confluence of vas and seminal vesicle (SV) to form the ejaculatory duct (arrowhead)

proportional to circulating serum PSA (Benson et al., 1992). Benign prostatic hyperplasia is associated with, on average, only 0.26 ng/mL PSA per gram of tissue, whereas cancer results in a density 10-fold higher (Hammerer et al., 1995). Any PSA value greater than that predicted by gland volume should raise a suspicion of prostate cancer. Also, the pre-treatment estimation of the volume of prostate cancer can provide important prognostic information after hormonal or radiation therapy. (Terris & Stamey 1991). The commonly used method in measuring prostate volume is the elliptical method. This formula can be transformed into volume = 0.523 x d_1 x d_2 x d_3. Maximal width and height diameters are obtained at the largest appearing mid gland axial image section. The length dimension can be obtained on midline sagittal plane (Fig. 9). This method is widely used because it is easy and fast method. The fact that it is slightly less accurate than other methods is not documented (Terris & Stamey,1990).

5. Diseases of the prostate and their sonographic appearance

5.1 Cysts of the prostate

Cysts of the prostate are confusing abnormalities because they are uncommon and their origin is uncertain. Small cysts are asymptomatic while large cysts may present with symptoms of urinary tract irritation, obstruction or hypofertility. The cysts may be complicated by infection, and stone formation. They may be turned malignant in about 3% of cases (Litirup et al., 1988). The cysts are usually unilocular, sharply defined, thin walled and anechoic. They vary size from 0.5 cm to 3.0 cm in diameters (Fig. 7). Prostatic cysts are either midline prostatic cysts like utricle cyst and Mullerian duct cyst or lateral prostatic cysts as cysts of the ejaculatory ducts or acquired cysts which are associated with prostate cancer, PBH, and prostatic abscess (Patel et al., 2002). Utricle cysts are dilatation of the prostatic utricle which may be congenital (megautricle) or acquired due to obstruction of its orifice by inflammation (utriclocele). The utricle cysts are small intraprostatic midline cysts.. Mullerian duct cysts are remnants of Mullerian duct. These cysts are relatively large, extends superiorly and inferiorly from the level of the verumontanum even outside the prostate. Ejaculatory ducts cysts are present along the course of the ejaculatory ducts within the CZ. They are usually paramedian and unilateral. They are complex cysts with solid and cystic components.They containing spermatozoa. Extra-prostatic cysts are either cysts of the seminal vesicles or the ampulae of the vas. They are congenital in origin and associated with urinary tract anomalies. Some patients are manifested by obstructive azospermia and TRUS can classify the patients without cysts where TRUS-guided aspiration and seminal vesiculography can be performed and patients with cyst where TRUS-guided cyst aspiration and opacification can be performed (Donkol, 2010).

5.2 Inflammatory diseases the prostate

Acute prostatitis is acute bacterial inflammation of the prostate. The clinical diagnosis usually is not difficult. The patient has fever, perineal and low back pain; pain with defecation of after ejaculation; urethral discharge associated with dysuria, urgency, frequency, or retention. On examination, the prostate is swollen, boggy and tender. Griffiths and associates in 1984 described three characteristic sonographic features seen in a group of 40 patients with an acute inflammation of the prostate as a periurethral echo-poor halo, a prominent periprostatic venous plexus and hypoechoic areas within the prostate, predominantly in the peripheral zone (Griffiths et al., 1984).

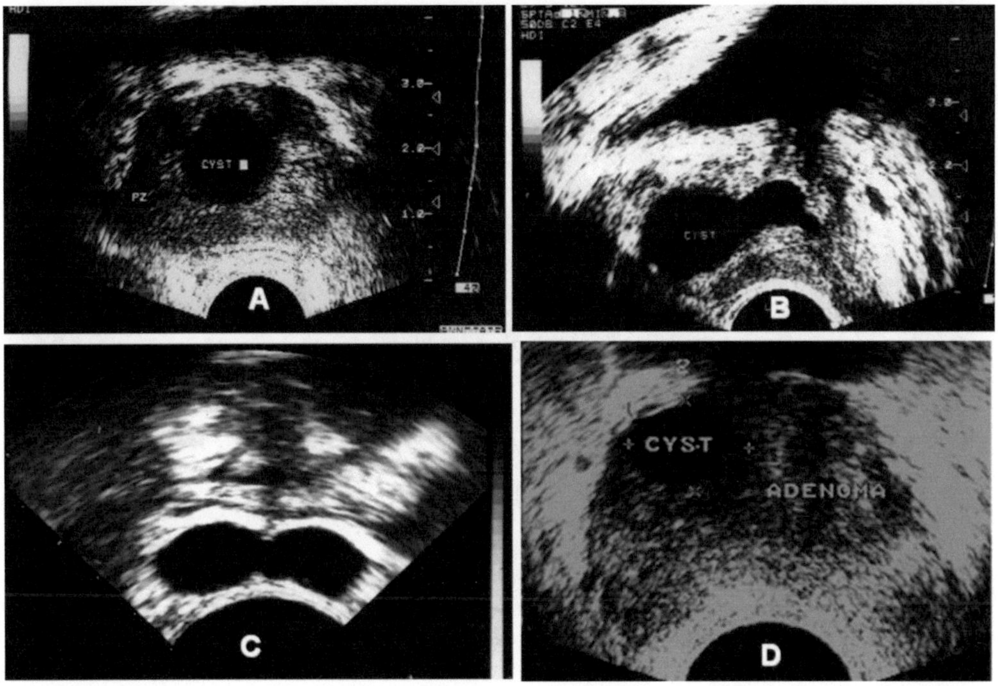

Fig. 7. TRUS of different prostatic cysts. (A) Axial TRUS of a utricle cyst; the cyst is midline and intraprostatic. (B) Sagittal TRUS of Mullerian duct cyst; the cyst is midline is midline with supraprostatic extension. (C) Axial TRUS of bilateral seminal vesicles cysts in a patient with obstructive azospermia. (D) Axial TRUS shows an acquired intraprostatic cyst in the in the right part of adenoma of benign prostatic hypertrophy

Chronic prostatitis may be infective as a complication of acute prostatitis or noninfective secondary to congestion of the prostate or urinary reflux into the prostate resulting in inflammatory or fibrotic reaction or both within the prostate. Chronic prostatitis has varied sympthomatology and lack of physical signs. The diagnosis currently rests on the finding of excessive leukocytes in prostatic secretions. Sonographic findings include high density echoes, mid range echoes, echo-lucent zones, ejaculatory duct calcifications, capsular irregularity, capsular thickening and periurethral zone irregularity (Fig. 8 A&B). The sensitivity and specificity of these signs are low (Doble & Carter, 1989)

Prostatic abscesses have been reported in an older age group due bladder outlet obstruction and urinary tract infection. Iatrogenic prostatic abscess have been reported after biopsy or instrumentation. Half of the patients presenting in acute retention and half presenting with irritative voiding symptoms. Of the patients 40% have fever, 25% have associated epididymo-orchitis. On examination, the majority showed enlarged prostate but only 20% present with the classic signs of prostatic fluctuance and tenderness on DRE (Sohlberg et al., 1991). Abscess can be identified as irregular hypoechoic area containing diffuse mid-range echoes within an enlarged gland (Fig. 8 C). Once identified, the lesions may be aspirated transperineally under ultrasound control (Doble & Carter, 1989).

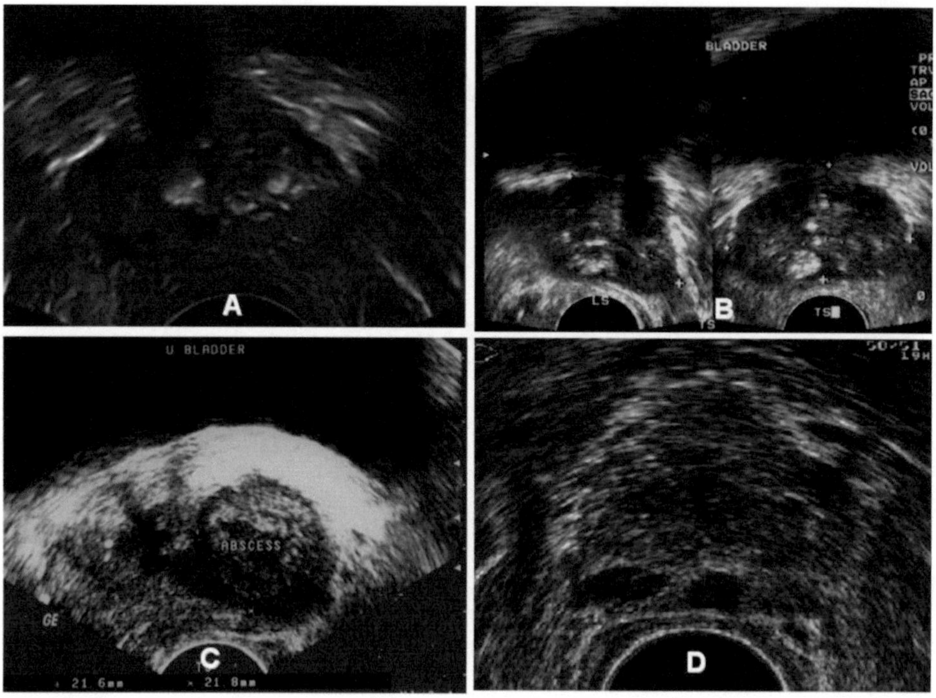

Fig. 8. (A) TRUS of a patient with chronic prostatitis shows calcification of periurethral tissue. (B) TRUS of another patient with chronic prostatitis shows calcification of peripheral zone. (C) TRUS of a case of prostatic abscess with a relatively thick wall and echogenic fluid content. (D) TRUS of a patient with granulomatous prostatitis shows multifocal hypoechoic lesions in the peripheral zone mimicking prostatic cancer

The exact aetiology of granulomatous prostatitis remains undetermined. It is thought to be due to ductal obstruction and ectasia with subsequently extravasation of luminal contents into the glandular stroma. In most patients, these changes are thought to be idiopathic but in others, it can be also linked with specific infecting agents (tuberculosis, schistosomiasis, and fungi). In patients with granulomatous prostatitis, the prostate is usually firm, nodular or indurated on DRE, PSA may be elevated. Patients may present with symptoms of outflow tract obstruction, acute retention or urinary infection. Sonographic findings are single or multiple areas of low echogenicity in the peripheral zone (Fig. 8 D) or heterogeneous echotexture of the gland. The hypoechoic areas are indistinguishable from carcinoma and diagnosis must be established by biopsy (Clements et al., 1993).

5.3 Prostatic calcifications and calculi

Primary prostatic calculi develop in the prostatic ducts and acini. They are usually multiple and small (1-5mms). Secondary dystrophic calcifications are associated with infection, obstruction, necrosis in a prostatic adenoma or radiation therapy. They are usually larger and more irregular than primary calculi. It needs to be emphasized that dystrophic prostatic calculi are not precancerous (Hricak, 1990). Sonographically calcifications appear as bright echogenic foci with or without posterior acoustic shadowing. Calculi can be seen within the seminal vesicles, vassal ampulae or ejaculatory ducts (Fig. 9).

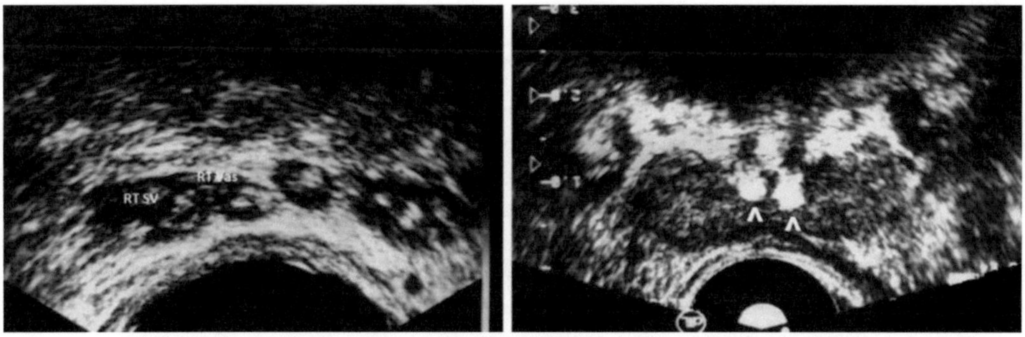

Fig. 9. (A) TRUS shows multiple flecks of calcifications seen in both seminal vesicles (SV) and vassal ampulae. (B) TRUS shows bilateral ejaculatory ducts calculi (arrow heads) in a patient with obstructive azospermia

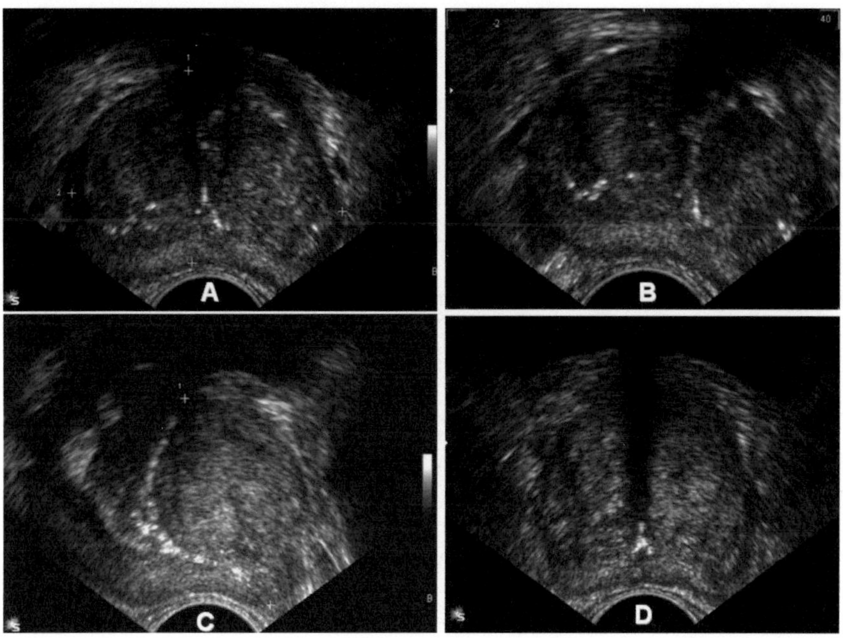

Fig. 10. (A) & (B) TRUS of BPH shows bilobed adenoma causing compression and flattening of the PZ. (C) TRUS of another case of BPH shows calcified surgical capsule separating the adenoma from the PZ. (D) TRUS of another patient with BPH shows large bilobed adenoma separating from the flattened PZ by hypoechoic surgical capsule

5.4 Benign prostatic hyperplasia

Benign prostatic hyperplasia (BPH) is rarely seen in males less than 40 years of age. It affects 50 to 70% of men older than 60, and 80 to 85% of men older than 80 years. BPH begins in the inner region of the prostate adjacent to the urethra. BPH may be diffuse or focal; forming prostatic adenoma. The normal prostatic tissue is displayed caudally and posteriorly to form the surgical capsule (Mc Neal, 1983). Ultrasound is the primary imaging modality for evaluation of the aging men with known or suspected BPH. By transabdominal US prostatic size, weight, shape and intravesical extent can be determined. Uncomplicated BPH usually produce a diffusely – altered inhomogenous echotexture, but distinct nodular enlargement cannot be differentiated from the surrounding gland (Fig. 5). Residual urine and bladder volume can be measured by the same formula used for estimating prostatic size (volume=0.52 x d1 x d2 X d3. Upper tract changes secondary to BPH are best evaluated using abdominal US. TRUS provides the best cross-sectional anatomy of the prostate and it is more accurate than transabdominal US to assess volume of the prostate and adenoma. BPH has a varied echotexture but is usually homogenous solitary or multiple adenomas (hyperplastic nodules) may be imaged, confined or extending outwards from the central gland often compressing the peripheral zone (Fig. 10). Although symmetry is the rule asymmetrical increase in size, especially near the bladder neck are common. Cysts, calcifications, prostatitis, infarctions and carcinoma may be coincident with BPH. The thick surgical capsule interposed between the central and peripheral gland can be appreciated. (Naryan & Foster, 1991).

5.5 Prostatic cancer

Carcinoma of the prostate is the most common human cancer, found at autopsy in 30% of men at age 50, 60% of men at age 80 – 90 up to 100% in those over age 90. It is now the second most common cancer in men. Pathological evidence of prostate cancer is found in 10-20% of patients undergoing surgery for BPH. 68% of prostatic carcinomas originate in the PZ, 24% in the TZ, and 8% in the CZ. Carcinoma of the prostate is often adenocarcinoma with varying grades of differentiation in 95% (Mc Neal, 1983). Unlike lung and colon cancer, prostatic cancer is predominantly latent. The patient may present with the symptoms and signs of prostatism and occasionally haematuria. It has been speculated that prostatic cancer disseminates first by invading into the periprostatic tissues, then by lymphatic embolization, and finally by hematogenous dissemination. Prostatic cancer can also spread by direct local invasion and through vascular and lymphatic channels. Seminal vesicle invasion almost always results from direct spread of the tumor into the ejaculatory duct while crossing inside and prostate. The primary field of lymphatic drainage of the prostate includes the perivesical, hypogastric, obturator, presacral and preciatic lymph nodes. The obturator nodes are the commonest site of involvement (Mc Laughlin et al., 1976). Osseous metastases are present in about 85 percent of patients dying of prostatic cancer. Osseous metastases involve the cancellous bone, altering the normal internal architecture with proliferating osteoblasts and new bone formation. The commonest sites for visceral metastases from prostatic cancer lung, liver and adrenal gland, but virtually any organ may be involved. Pulmonary metastases, occurring in 25 to 38 percent of patients dying of prostatic cancer. Metastases to the central nervous system usually occur in the meninges and may be clinically silent. Other neurogenic manifestations of prostatic cancer include organic brain syndrome, raduculopathy, and paraneoplastic syndromes (Jacobs, 1983).

5.5.1 Detection of prostate cancer

TRUS is useful for early detection of prostate cancer, guided biopsy, local staging, and follow up after treatment. Its role in screening of asymptomatic men is still controversial. (Clements et al., 1993).The first step in any sonographic examination of the prostate should be to gain an overall impression of the gland's shape and size. An irregular asymmetric gland often signals malignancy even in the absence of the identifiable lesion. Even small prostatic cancer often alters the shape of the prostate. Distortion or bulging of the posterior boundary of the prostate is suggestive of the presence of cancer. Lateral distortion is of less significance because hyperplastic nodules of the TZ cause considerable asymmetric bulging. In advanced cancer, discontinuity of the capsule or seminal vesicles irregularity often can be seen (Shinohara et al.., 1989).

Prostate cancer has different echotexture; it may be hypoechoic, isoechpic or hyperechoic (Fig. 11). Most cancers consist of a dense mass of cells which destroys the normal glandular structure. The malignant tissue contains few sonographically detectable interfaces and therefore appears hyperechoic region in relation to the adjacent normal tissue. The most common feature of all visible cancer is a central hypoechoic region relative to the peripheral zone of the normal prostate. The margins of the tumor all ill defined as the malignant cells invade between normal prostatic acini (Shinohara et al., 1989). The hypoechoic tumors represent 70-75% of prostate tumors (Hamper & Sheth, 1993). Approximately 30-35% of clinically detected prostate cancer cannot be distinguished from the normal surrounding prostatic tissue and is termed isoechoic. Several features may contribute to cancer being undetectable by US: tumor size, grade, location, and stage, technique of the study, equipment used and the experience of the operator. Absence of the normal margin between the PZ and TZ in a rounded prostate should alert the sonographer to the possibility of a large infiltrating tumor. Also, a palpable abnormality in the presence of an apparently normal US scan should be biopsied to avoid missing an isoechoic cancer (Shabsigh et al., 1989). In case of presence of large adenoma of BPH, the PZ is compressed. So, it is less easy to detect a PZ cancer (Shinohara et al., 1989). Hyperechoic tumors are rare. Prostatic calculi that have been engulfed by cancer may account for a mixed echogenic pattern. Hyperechoic foci within the tumor correspond pathologically to comedonecrosis and calcification within highly undifferentiated anaplastic tumors or unusual deposits of intraluminal crystalloid secretions.

The sonographic appearance of early prostate cancer is not specific. The positive predictive value for a hypoechoic focal lesion to be cancer has ranged from 0% to 50%. Overall, the incidence of malignancy in US suspicious lesion is 20% to 255 (Hamper & Sheth, 1993). Information from US-guided biopsy of the prostate has shown that many suspicious areas seen on TRUS do not correspond to cancer: negative biopsy rated of 58 to 70.8% has been reported (Shabsigh et al., 1989). There is a big list of differential diagnosis of intraprostatic hypoechoic lesions. First anatomic structures as periurethral tissue, ejaculatory duct complex, periprostatic veins and neuovascular bundles. Second are benign prostatic diseases as hyperplastic nodule (stromal types), prostatitis, abscess, cysts and hematoma. Lastly sonographic artifacts as inappropriate use of the focal range of transducer, acoustic shadowing, reverberation artifacts and edge effect (Shinhara et al., 1989). Mc Neal and associates have emphasized the importance of measurement of the volume of prostate cancer as a determinant of pathologic stage and prognosis. They described a strong association between tumor volume and the incidence of extracapsular extension and lymph node metastases (Mc Neal et al., 1986). Estimation of tumor volume by TRUS is often inaccurate for two reasons. Tumor size is usually underestimated, as the tumor tends to infiltrate invade between normal prostatic tissues. So, the margin of the tumor may therefore be indistinguishable from normal prostate. Second is prostate cancer is often multifocal. So, U.S underestimates the maximum diameter of a focus of cancer by an average of 4.2 mm (Shinohara et al., 1989).

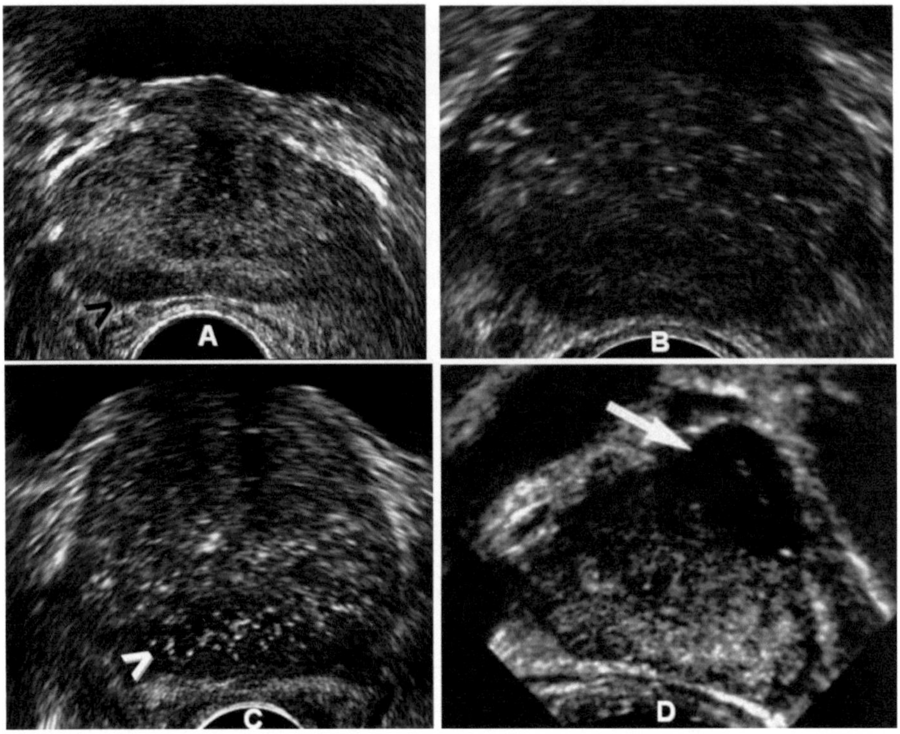

Fig. 11. TRUS of four different patients with prostate cancer. The carcinoma appears as focal hypoechoic area (arrow head) in the right PZ (A), diffuse hypoechogenicity of the whole gland (B), focal hyperechoic area (arrow head) in the posterior PZ (C) and focal hypoechoic area (arrow) in the central gland (D)

5.5.2 Extra capsular extension of prostate cancer

Prostate cancer spreads locally through pathways of least resistance. The areas of local spread include the invaginated extraprostatic area around the ejaculatory duct to the seminal vesicles, at the apex where the capsule is deficient, areas of capsule penetration by superior and inferior neurovascular bundles. The prostatic capsule usually cannot be distinguished sonographically from the prostatic parenchyma. Consequently, the continuos hyperechoic border around the normal prostate, (usually referred as the "capsule"), is actually represents the acoustic interface between the prostate and the periprostatic fat (Scardino et al., 1989). Sonographic signs of capsular penetration include bulge or irregularity of the prostate contour and disruption or discontinuity of the echogenic periprostatic boundary echo (Hamper & Sheth, 1993). Spread of the cancer to the neurovascular bundle is suspected if the tumor is close to the posterolateral aspect of the prostate with irregularity of the contour at this region as well as interruption of the echogenic periprostatic boundary echo. TRUS is able to detect neurovascular involvement with sensitivity of 66% and specificity of 78% (Fig. 12 and 13).

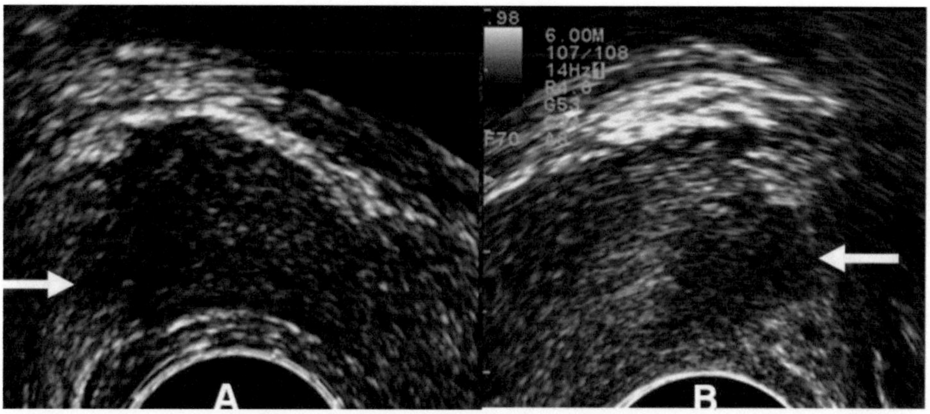

Fig. 12. Two different patients with right and left lateral extracapsular extension (arrows)

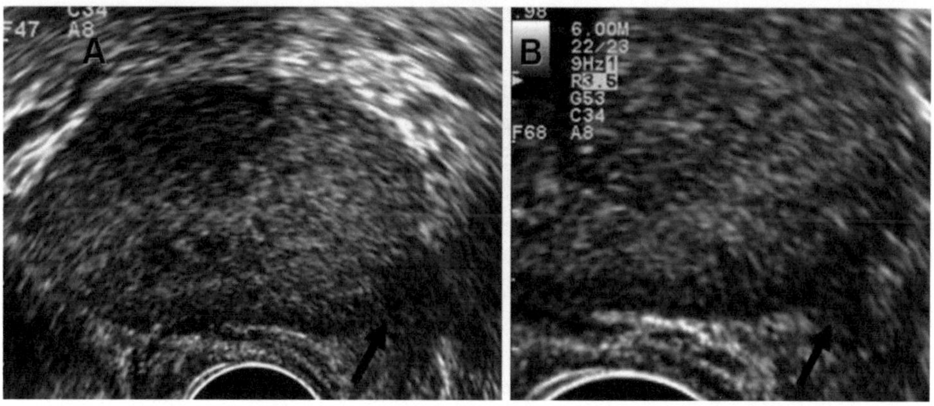

Fig. 13. A case of prostate cancer with left posterolateral extension through the neurovascular bundle (arrows)

The pattern and extent of seminal vesicle invasion vary widely. Type I is the most common pattern. It shows invasion along the ejaculatory ducts into the seminal vesicle. Type II is the second most common pattern. The invasion of seminal vesicle occurs from a tumor that penetrates the capsule and invades the seminal vesicles in continuity. Type III is the least common pattern, where small isolated foci of tumor in the seminal vesicles. The sonographic criteria for seminal vesicles invasion have traditionally been described as asymmetry in size, irregularity in outline, atrophy and distension, but the validity of these signs has rarely been substantiated by surgical or pathological staging (Shinohora et al., 1988). The accuracy of detection seminal vesicle invasion using sonography is 86% (Terries et al., 1990). The apex of the prostate must be carefully assessed sonographically to detect involvement of the rhamoboid area. This area bounded by the prostate proximally, the rectourethralis muscle distally, the membranous urethra anteriorly and the rectum posteriorly. It is best demonstrated by TRUS on the sagittal view. TRUS has no role in nodal staging. Also, it had limited role in detection of invasion of neighboring tissue, e.g. bladder, rectum and muscles of the pelvic side wall. These disadvantages of TRUS can be explained by its limited field of view (Scardino et al., 1989).

5.5.3 Response to treatment of prostate cancer

After treatment by ochidectomy and hormonal therapy, the gland becomes smaller and assumes a more circular shape. Most of the decrease in volume occurred within the first three months. A variable series of changes in the US appearance of the gland may be seen. In some patients, the area of abnormal echogenicity may persist. In others, it disappears. The integrity of the capsule may appear to be resorted in patients with previous capsule breech. It may be extremely difficult to demonstrate U.S whether the active cancer is still present or not (Clements et al., 1989). Following radiotherapy for cancer, the prostate becomes small and echogenic. Anechoic or hypoechoic lesions following radiotherapy frequently represent persistent cancer and the positive predictive value of such lesions for cancer is 91%. Most foci of cancer with marked radiation effect tend to be isoechoic. The non malignant prostate tissue generally retains its normal echogenic appearance after irradiation. Lesions over 5mm in the diameter persisting for 12 months following radiotherapy are suspicious of malignancy and should be biopsied (Egawa et al., 1991). A decrease in total prostate volume is not a reliable indicator of prognosis as normal and malignant prostatic tissue will shrink in response to radiotherapy. Measuring PSA is probably more useful in the follow up of the prostate cancer (Richards, 1992). After radical retropubic prostatectomy (for clinically non invasive prostatic cancer), the patients are routinely followed up at periodic interval with DRE and measuring PSA. Elevation of PSA above the female range indicates either local progression, recurrence of distant metastases. Post-operative mature fibrotic tissue at the site of operation is difficult of distinguish form recurrent tumors by means of TRUS. The main value of TRUS in case of presence of post operative palapable mass may be in accurate positioning of the biopsy needle about the vesico-urethral anastomosis (Wasserman et., 1992).

6. Ultrasound guided prostatic biopsy

The most important role for TRUS is to provide visual guidance for biopsy. Approximately 25% to 30% of cancers are isoechoic, random biopsies of the PZ, in addition to sampling all suspicious lesions should be done. In the technique of random prostatic biopsies, multiple samples are taken from different parts of the gland mainly apex, mid gland and base bilaterally (Hamper & Sheth 1993). In general, TRUS guided prostate needle biopsy should be performed in men with an abnormal DRE, an elevated PSA (>4.0 ng/ml) or PSA velocity (rate of PSA change) >0.4 to 0.75ng/ml/yr. Also, men who were diagnosed with high-grade prostatic intraepithelial neoplasia (PIN) or atypia on a previous prostate needle biopsy should undergo a repeat biopsy 3 to 12 months later. Less commonly agreed upon recommendations for TRUS guided prostate needle biopsy include, age-specifi c PSA elevation, low percentage free PSA (< 22% to 25%), and prostate specifi c antigen density (PSAD) > 0.15, which is a measure of the amount of PSA relative to the overall prostatic volume (Hamper & Sheth 1993).US- guided prostate biopsies can be performed either transperineally or transrectally.

Transperineal approach is the first way described for US-guided prostate biopsy in 1981. The probe is fixed to a stabilizing biopsy stand. The perineum should be infiltrated local anesthetic. The entire gland is inspected and once a suspected area is identified, the biopsy needle is inserted and the track of the needle is monitored on the viewing screen. When the needle tip approaches the area to be biopsied, the needle is positioned so that the cutting section can be passed through the abnormal area under visual guidance (Muldoon & Resnick, 1989). The drawbacks of transperineal U.S guided biopsy are difficult needle due to relatively long transperineal needle path, it is time consuming procedure, and patients tolerate the procedure poorly because of perineal pain and side effects of local anaesthesia. (Clements et al., 1993). Transperineal approach is preferable if prostate abscess or inflammatory disease is suspected.

Transrecta approach was first described in 1987, since then, this technique has been described as a superior method of performing a core biopsy of the prostate (Weaver et al., 1991). The transrectal approach offers the advantage of a shorter needle with easier needle placement, and quicker and relatively painless procedure. Local anesthesia is not required and it is done on an out-patients basic (Clements et al,. 1993). Hodge et al reported that systematic sampling of the prostate guided by TRUS improved the detection rate of prostate cancer over merely sampling hypoechoic or other lesions. By taking sextant biopsies from the mid lobe (parasagittal) of each side of the prostate at the apex, middle, and base (Fig. 14), the cancer detection rate was superior to lesion-directed biopsies (Hodge et al., 1989). This technique was accepted over the time as the standard of care and helped to emphasize that TRUS was more useful for biopsy than for imaging. In the current PSA era, though, most men who are undergoing prostate biopsy do not have palpable abnormalities or hypoechoic lesions This has lead investigators to question the sampling adequacy of the standard sextant prostate biopsy template and to propose alternate "extended pattern" biopsy schemes to improve prostate cancer detection. The alternate prostate biopsy templates aim to improve sampling of the prostate by either increasing the number of core biopsies taken and/or by directing the biopsies more laterally to better sample the anterior horn (Chen et al, 1999, Naughton et al., 2000). During biopsy, the puncture path is shown on the monitor as electric dotted line. The probe should be positioned so that the puncture path passes through the designated area. Without moving the probe, the needle is introduced through the needle guide and the needle tip is positioned proximal to the suspicious area. A trigger action biopsy gun is used to obtain a core specimen in an instance once the biopsy needle in place. The biopsies performed while the biopsy needle is directed parallel to the transducer in the sagittal plane so the needle seen as an echogenic linear structure approaching the suspicious area, instead of an echogenic dot in the axial plane (Lee et al., 1988).

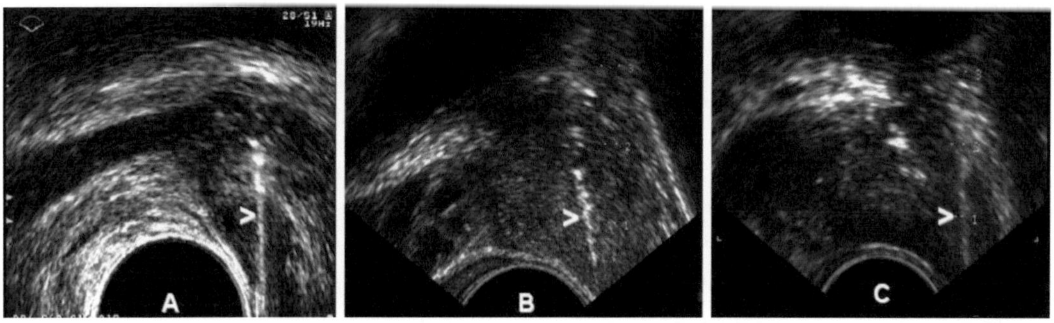

Fig. 14. Systematic TRUS -guided biopsy of the upper (A), middle (B) and lower (C) parts of the lateral regions peripheral zone (arrowheads)

7. Role of new ultrasound techniques in diagnosis of prostate cancer

Conventional gray-scale US has low sensitivity and specificity and is mainly used for guiding systematic prostate biopsies. With the development of new US techniques, such as three dimensional US color and power Doppler US, the use of US contrast agents and elastography, the role of US for prostate cancer detection has dramatically improved.

7.1 Three dimensional (3D) US of the prostate

It gives views of the prostate in the 3 orthogonal planes; sagital, transverse and coronal and in any other oblique planes (Fig. 15). The detection rates of prostate cancer were significantly improved with 3D- TRUS. Also it may improve the biopsy yield by determining appropriate sites for target and systematic biopsies (Cool et al., 2008, Shen et al., 2008). With 3D imaging, spatial relationships much clearer, so radiologist/urologist can better assess the extent of disease. It may make it easier to determine whether the "prostate capsule" has been penetrated to detect possible extra-capsular tumor extension which is a key factor in staging of prostate cancer. It provides valuable information to plan for alternative therapies, like radiotherapy of the prostate and robotic prostatectomy. The 3D images are saved and they can be reviewed as many times as needed. Diagnosis can be achieved by retrieving the saved images which is most convenient for the operator and patient, leading to faster patient turnaround (Liang et al., 2010, Bax et al., 2008).

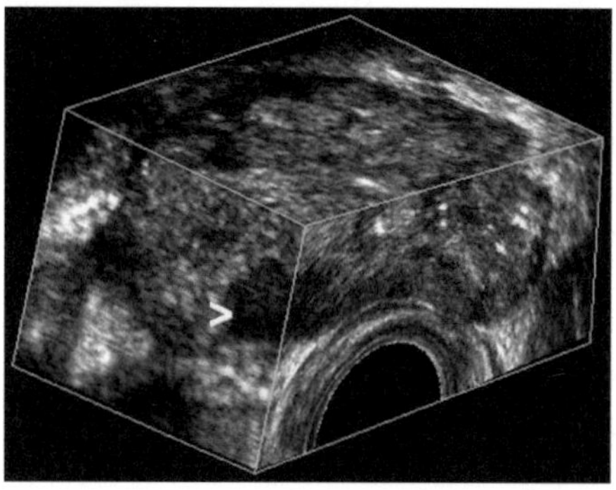

Fig. 15. 3D images of a prostate with cancer. The image has been 'sliced' to reveal a hypoechoic lesion in the right side of the PZ (arrowhead) proved to be a cancer

7.2 Color Doppler sonography of the prostate

Color Doppler TRUS (CD-TRUS) has been applied to evaluate the vascularity within the prostate and the surrounding structures. Preliminary studies demonstrated increased flow within or surrounding prostate neoplasm, whereas prostatitis and BPH showed a diffusely abnormal flow.However, the flow of focal prostatitis was not significantly different from cancer. By using objective measures, as resistive indices, no statistically significant difference was found between cancer and benign conditions (Rifkin et al, 1993). CD-TRUS may help in determining the site of biopsy. If the level of PSA is elevated with DRE normal in one patient, the presence of hypervascular focal lesion in PZ makes the lesion the target of the biopsy. But, if the nodule is hypovascular, we have to biopsy the anterior part of the gland to detect carcinoma of the TZ. (Cornud et al., 1993). Early results have suggested that up to 85% of men with prostate cancers greater than 5 mm in size have visibly increased flow in the area of tumor involvement. In addition, hypervascularity may be seen in patients with more difficult to identify, isoechoic and hyperechoic lesions (Fig. 16). Unfortunately, subsequent studies suggested that some prostate cancers are hypovascular. Many studies prove the benefits of CD-TRUS for the evaluation of prostatic disease, especially carcinoma. The motivation behind the application of color Doppler US is to detect tumor neovascularity. Cancerous tissue generally grows more rapidly than normal tissue and demonstrates increased blood flow; as compared to normal tissue and benign lesions. Color Doppler US may demonstrate an increased number of visualized vessels, as well as an increase in flow rate, size and irregularity of vessels within prostate cancer (Newman et al., 1995 Littrup et al., 1995, Ismail et al., 1997)

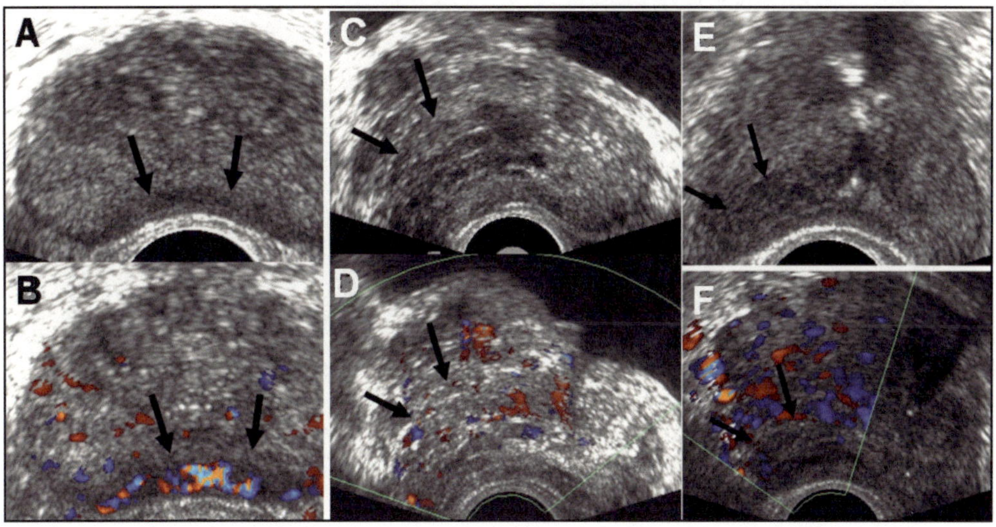

Fig. 16. (A) TRUS shows hypoechoic areas proved to be cancer (arrows). (B) Color-Doppler shows the same area to be of high vascularity (arrows). (C) TRUS of another patient with prostate cancer appears as hypoechoic area (arrows). (D) The same area appears with normal vascularity in color Doppler. (E) TRUS of a third patient with hypoechoic lesion of prostate cancer appears as hypoechoic (arrows). (F) The same lesion appears of low vascularity in color Doppler

7.3 Power Doppler sonography of the prostate

Power Doppler US is an amplitude-based technique for the detection of flow. It is more sensitive to slow flow and is less angle-dependent than color Doppler US. This technique has been less commonly applied to the assessment of prostate tumor vascularity, and there are few papers addressing its use. Some studies showed that prostate cancer are hypervascular by power Doppler (Fig. 17) so it may be useful in detection of prostate cancer (Inahara et al., 2004). Halpern et al assessed the value of gray-scale, color and power Doppler US for detection of prostatic cancer. They investigated 251 patients prior to biopsy and they hey concluded that power Doppler may be useful for targeted biopsies when the number of biopsy passes must be limited but that there is no substantial advantage of power Doppler over color Doppler (Halpern et al., 2000).

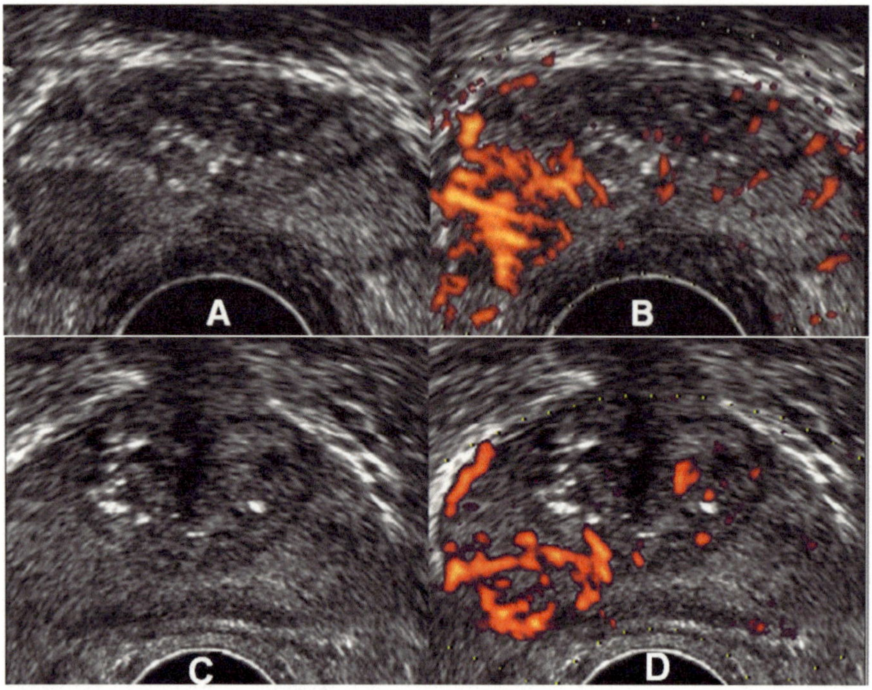

Fig. 17. (A) TRUS show a hypoechoic lesion in the right posterolateral aspect of the peripheral zone proved to be cancer. (B) The same area is hypervascular in power Doppler (C) TRUS in another patient with prostate cancer shows no evident focal lesion in grey scale US. (D) Power Doppler of the same patient show focal area of increased vascularity in the right side of the peripheral zone proved to be carcinoma by targeted biopsy

7.4 Contrast enhanced ultrasound imaging

Recently developed US contrast agents can improve the detection of low-volume blood flow by increasing the signal-to-noise ratio. Unlike radiographic contrast media, which diffuse into the tissue and may obscure smaller vessels, microbubble echo-enhancing agents are confined to the vascular lumen, where they persist until they dissolve. They have two important acoustic properties, first, they are many times more reflective than blood, thus improving flow detection. Second, their vibrations generate higher harmonics to a much greater degree than surrounding tissues (Forsberg et al, 1998). Bree RL and De Dreu SE showed that contrast enhanced color Doppler US had a sensitivity of 53%, specificity of 72%, and a positive predictive value of 70% in distinguishing prostate cancer from benign lesions in 72 patients identified by PSA screening (Bree RL & DeDreeu SE,1998). Most investigators showed increased sensitivity in detection of prostate cancer after the use of contrast enhanced US (Fig. 20). In the study of Bogers et al, they showed that sensitivity of enhanced images was 85% (specificity 80%) compared with 38% for unenhanced images (specificity 80%) and 77% for conventional gray-scale transrectal US (specificity 60%) (Bogers et al., 1999). Frauscher et al reported the value of contrast enhanced color Doppler in a prospective study in 90, and 230 male screening volunteers (Frauscher et al., 2001, 2002). They found that targeted biopsies based on contrast enhanced color Doppler detected as many cancers as systematic biopsies, with fewer than half the number of biopsy cores. Halpern et al, in their prospective study of contrast-enhanced transrectal US in 60 patients who underwent sextant biopsy of the prostate concluded that the sensitivity increased from 38% at baseline to 65% after contrast injection (Fig. 18). However there was no significant change of specificity between baseline study (83%) and during contrast aging (80%) in the same study (Halpern et al., 2001).

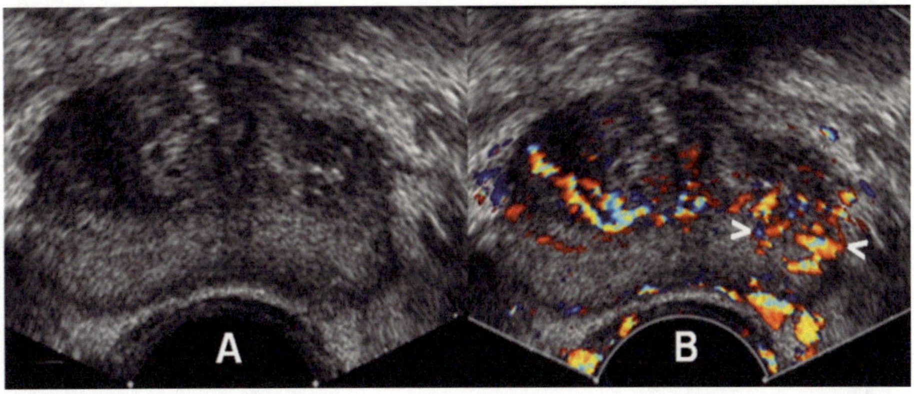

Fig. 18. (A) TRUS of a patient with prostate cancer show no evident focal lesions in grey scale US. (B) Contrast enhanced TRUS shows focal area of hypervascularity in the left side of the peripheral zone (arrowheads) proved to be carcinoma by targeted biopsy

7.5 Elastography of the prostate

Elastography or strain imaging was first described in 1991 (Ophir et al., 1991). This technique can be used to detect degree of stiffness of the tissues. In a pilot study done by Klauser et al, patients with clinically localized prostate cancer who underwent radical prostatectomy were examined prospectively. They found that elastography detected 28 of 32 cancer foci (sensitivity 88%) and they concluded that elastography is a sensitive new imaging modality for the detection of prostate cancer (Klauser et al., 2003). Konig et al. evaluated elastography for biopsy guidance for prostate cancer detection in 404 men underwent systematic sextant biopsy. They found that in 127 of the cancer proved 151 cases (84.1%), prostate cancer was detected using elastography as an additional diagnostic feature. They concluded that it is possible to detect prostate cancer with a high degree of sensitivity using real-time elastography in conjunction with conventional diagnostic methods for guided prostate biopsies (Konig et al., 2005). Supersonic shear imaging (SSI) is a new US-based technique for real-time visualization of soft tissue elastographic properties. Using ultrasonic focused beams, it is possible to remotely generate mechanical vibration sources radiating low-frequency, shear waves inside tissues (Bercoff et al., 2004). Athanasiou et al studied quantitative ultrasonographic elastography of breast lesions in 46 women. They concluded that SSI provides quantitative elasticity measurements, thus adding complementary information that potentially could help in breast lesion characterization with B-mode US (Athanasiou et al., 2010). Recently a preliminary study by Correas et al done to evaluated the feasibility of TRUS quantitative Shear Wave Elastography (SWE) for prostate cancer evaluation in 21 patients presenting with increased PSA values (Fig. 19). Elasticity measurements and ratios between nodules and adjacent parenchyma were calculated. They found that signals were obtained in both the peripheral and the transition zones with good correlation to anatomical areas, macro-calcifications exhibited very high stiffness values and prostate cancer nodules exhibited a high stiffness than the adjacent peripheral gland. Also they noticed that peripheral adenomatous hyperplasia and focal prostatitis exhibited a significantly lower stiffness. They concluded that TRUS quantitative SWE is a feasible technique for prostate cancer evaluation. It provides additional information about stiffness of nodules localized in the peripheral zone (Correas et al., 2011). These preliminary results are encouraging but a larger multicentric evaluation remains necessary.

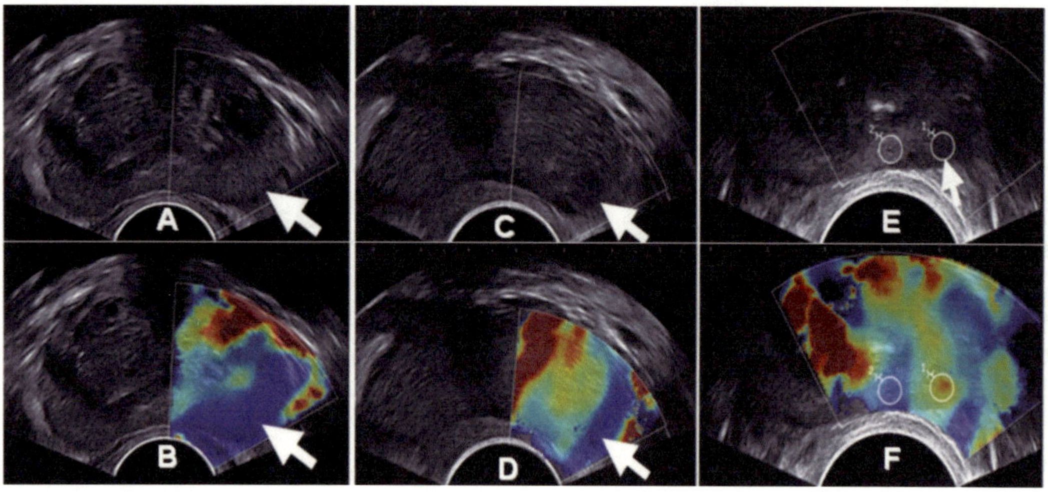

Fig. 19. (A) TRUS of a normal homogeneous PZ. (B).TRUS-SWE shows homogeneous blue coding of PZ (arrow) indicating its soft texture. (B) TRUS of another patient shows a hypoechoic area in left PZ proved to be carcinoma (atypical pattern). (D) TRUS-SWE of the same patient shows the focal area has blue coding (arrow) indicating its soft texture. (E) TRUS of another patient with a hypoechoic nodule in the left PZ proved to be carcinoma (arrow). (F) TRUS-SWE of the same patient shows a strong increase in stiffness values of the focal area (red) with a ratio of 2.8 compared to the surrounding PZ (typical pattern) (adapted from Correas et al 2011)

8. Role of ultrasound in prostate cancer treatment

Recent interest in focal therapy for localized prostate cancer has been driven by downward stage migration, improved biopsy and imaging techniques. Several techniques have potential for focal ablation of prostate cancer.

8.1 TRUS-guided cryotherapy for prostate cancer

Cryotherapy is tissue ablation by local induction of extremely cold temperatures. The first use cryoablation in urological disorders started in the 1960s for management of benign prostatic hyperplastic tissue (Gonder et al., 1966). This was followed shortly thereafter by the treatment of prostate cancer via an open perineal approach (Fig. 20). The major impediment to early acceptance of the modality, however, was the inability to accurately monitor cryoprobe placement and ice-ball formation. Major advances in the past 20 years, which have reinvigorated investigation into the use of cryotherapy for prostate cancer, have included the use of TRUS monitoring of probe placement and freezing (Onil et al,1993). A significant recent development was the introduction of cryotherapy probes that use argon gas rather than liquid nitrogen (De La Taille et al., 2000). Outcomes have now been reported as late as 7 years following treatment of prostate cancer and seem to compare favorably with contemporary series of patients who receive radiation therapy (Bahn et al., 2002). Marberger et al reported that cryotherapy has been used for some time as a form of first-line therapy for complete ablation of the prostate or and as a second-line therapy for local recurrence after radiotherapy (Marberger et al., 2008).

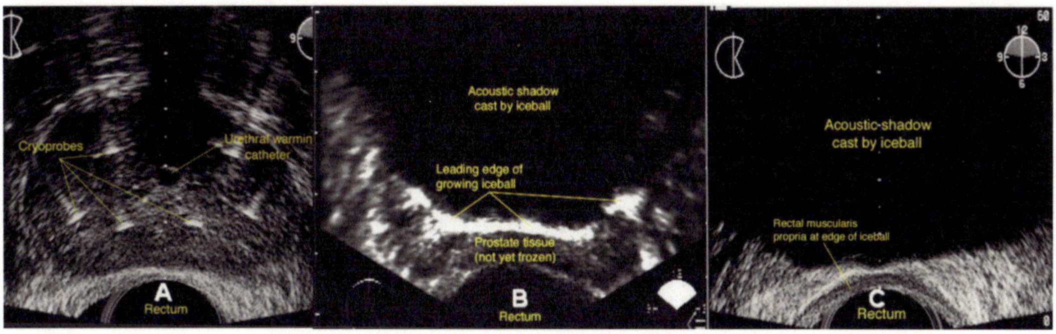

Fig. 20. (A) TRUS of the prostate illustrating placement of the cryoprobes and urethral-warming catheter. (B) TRUS of the prostate during cryoablation showing the ice ball, growing posteriorly, is echodense and casts a dark acoustic shadow. (C) The ice ball extends posteriorly to include the whole prostate tissue. Transrectal sonogram of the prostate illustrating placement of the cryoprobes and urethral-warming catheter

8.2 High-intensity focused ultrasound (HIFU)

HIFU is one of the newer methods that have been developed to treat early stage prostate cancers. High energy is delivered to the affected area by ultrasound, this result in the targeted cancerous cells heating up and being destroyed. Using extracorporeal HIFU, temperatures of greater than 60°C can be achieved in the target tissue. The prostate can be easily treated with this modality via a transrectal probe. Gelet et al pioneered the use of transrectal HIFU in the treatment of localized prostate cancer. Prostates smaller than 40 mL or those with an anteroposterior diameter of less than 5 cm are best suited for this treatment. During the procedure, the whole gland is treated. They reported that 78% of low-risk patients were disease-free and had negative biopsy results at an actuarial 5-year follow-up (Gelet et al., 2004). Some of the advantages of HIFU are that it is able to be repeated if cancer reappears; it can destroy cancer in targeted areas of the prostate without destroying other areas of the prostate; and it can be given to patients who may not be able to take other forms of prostate treatment such as brachytherapy. Marberger et al reported that HIFU has been used widely in Europe for complete ablation of the prostate, especially in elderly men who are unwilling or unable to undergo radical therapy. For low- or intermediate-risk cancer, the short- and intermediate-term results have been acceptable. Focal use of HIFU should reduce the adverse sexual and urinary side effects of whole gland ablation (Marberger et al., 2008).

8.3 Vascular-targeted photodynamic therapy (VTFT)

VTFP is a minimally invasive ablative treatment for localized prostate cancer and may represent a preferred option for men with low-risk disease who want to balance the risks and benefits of treatment. (Lepor, 2008). VTPT has been used for whole gland ablation of locally recurrent cancer after radiotherapy and for focal ablation of previously untreated cancer. In combination with a new, systemically administered photodynamic agent, laser light is delivered through fibers introduced into the prostate under TRUS. This technique does not heat the prostate but destroys the endothelial cells and cancer by activating the photodynamic agent. Damage to surrounding structures appears to be limited and can be controlled by the duration and intensity of the light. (Marberger et al., 2008).

8.4 TRUS-guided prostate brachytherapy

Brachytherapy is an effective treatment for localized prostate cancer with high patient tolerability and acceptable morbidity outcome data. It delivers a high dose of radiation to a small target volume of tissue, minimizing radiation side-effects to adjacent structures. Brachytherapy is an alternative to radical surgery and external beam radiotherapy and can be delivered in two different ways: permanent seed implants using iodine or palladium seeds or using temporary removable implants with iridium wires. TRUS is essential for accurate imaging guidance to place the radioactive sources into the prostate (Fig. 21). Prostate brachytherapy data has now matured as a treatment with consistent results reported from major centers in the US and Europe (Henry et al., 2010, Battermann et al., 2008).

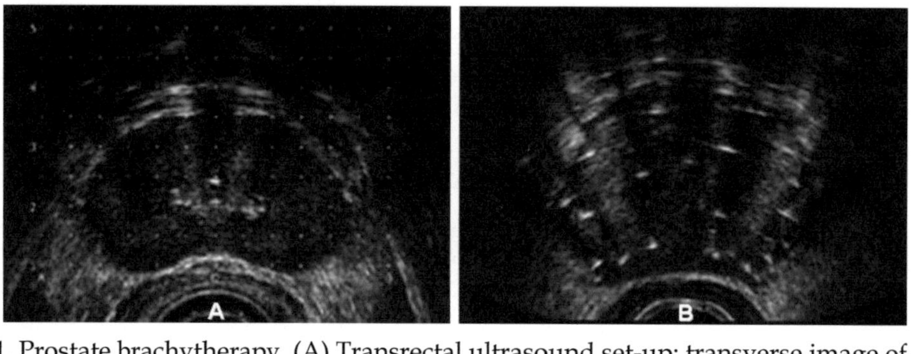

Fig. 21. Prostate brachytherapy. (A) Transrectal ultrasound set-up: transverse image of the prostate with 5mm template overlay. (B) Transverse image of the prostate after seed implant (echogenic areas)

9. Conclusion

One of the major advances that have greatly improved our understanding of prostatic diseases is the development of sonography especially TRUS. It is considered the first imaging modality in diagnosis of prostate diseases. Improvement of the application of the new advances in US for the detection and clinical staging of prostate cancer is promising. TRUS-guided procedures are now widely used in diagnosis and treatment of prostate cancer. Radiologists and urologists should be well trained in the application of these new US techniques and should therefore play an important role in the management of prostate cancer in the future.

10. References

Abou Yousef M M and Naryana AS (1982). Tran rectal ultrasound in the evaluation of the prostatic size. J. Clin ultrasound. 10: 275-278.

Athanasiou A, Tardivon A, Tanter M, Sigal-Zafrani B, Bercoff J, Deffieux T, Gennisson JL, Fink M, Neuenschwander S (2010). Breast lesions: quantitative elastography with supersonic shear imaging--preliminary results. Radiology. Jul; 256(1):297-303.

Babaian RJ, Toi A, Kamoi K, Troncoso P, Sweet J, Evans R, Johnston D, Chen M. (2000). A comparative analysis of sextant and an extended 11-core multisite directed biopsy strategy. J Urol; 163:152-157.

Bahn DK, Lee F, Badalament R, Kumar A, Greski J, Chernick M (2002). Targeted cryoablation of the prostate: 7-year outcomes in the primary treatment of prostate cancer. Urology Aug; 60(2 Suppl 1):3-11.

Battermann J, Boon T, Moerland M (2004). Results of permanent prostate brachytherapy, 13 years of experience at a single institution Radiother Oncol; 71:23-28

Benson MC, Whang IS, Pantuck A, Ring K, Kaplan SA, Olsson CA, et al (1992). Prostate specific antigen density: a means of distinguishing benign prostatic hypertrophy and prostate cancer. J Urol; 147:815-9.

Bax J, Cool D, Gardi L, Knight K, Smith D, Montreuil J, Sherebrin S, Romagnoli C, Fenster A (2008). Mechanically assisted 3D ultrasound guided prostate biopsy system. Med Phys. Dec ;35(12):5397-410.

Bercoff J, Tanter M, Fink M (2004). Supersonic shear imaging: a new technique for soft tissue elasticity mapping. IEEE Trans Ultrason Ferroelectr Freq Control. Apr;51(4):396-409

Bogers HA, Sedelaar JP, Beerlage HP, de la Rosette JJ, Debruyne FM, Wijkstra H, Aarnink RG (1999). Contrast enhanced three-dimensional power Doppler angiography of the human prostate: correlation with biopsy outcome. Urology; 54: 97–104.

Brandes D. (1984) prostate gland embryology, anatomy and histology. In: G. Hills. Uropathology. Chirchill, Livingstone, New York; 1165-1180.

Bree RL, De Dreu SE (1998). Contrast enhanced color Doppler of the prostate as an adjunct to gray-scale identification of cancer prior to biopsy. Radiology; 209: 418.

Correas1 J.-M., KHAIROUNE A., Tissier A.-M, Vassiliu V., EISS D., Hélénon O (2011). Trans-rectal quantitative Shear Wave Elastrography: application to prostate cancer - A feasibility study.Poster No.: C-1748 Congress: ECR 2011.

Chen ME, Troncoso P, Tang K, Babaian RJ, Johnston D (1999). Comparison of prostate biopsy schemes by computer simulation. Urology; 53:951-960.

Clements R, Gower TK, Griffeth GT, Peeling WB (1993) Transrectal ultrasound appearance of granulomatous prostatitis. Clinc. Radiol; 47: 174-176.

Gonder MJ, Soanes WA, Shulman S (1966). Cryosurgical treatment of the prostate. Invest Urol. Jan; 3(4):372-8

Cool D, Sherebrin S, Izawa J, Chin J, Fenster A (2008). Design and evaluation of a 3D transrectal ultrasound prostate biopsy system. Med Phys. Oct; 35(10):4695-707.

Cornud F, Belin X, Fromont G. (1993). Prostate normale. In: Imaging de la prostate, H. Nahum ed. Medecine - Sciences Flammavior, Paris; 3-18.

Delmas V, Dauge MC (1991). Embryology of the prostate- current state of knowledge. In: Khoury S CC, Murphy G, Denis L, ed. Prostate cancer in questions. Edinburgh, UK: ICI publications;16-17.

De La Taille A, Benson MC, Bagiella E, Burchardt M, Shabsigh A, Olsson CA, et al (2000). Cryoablation for clinically localized prostate cancer using an argon-based system: complication rates and biochemical recurrence. BJU Int. Feb; 85(3):281-6.

Doble A, Carter SS. (1989) Ultrasonographic findings in prostatitis. Urol Clinc. North Am; 18, 4.

Donkol, RH (2010). Imaging in male-factor obstructive infertility.World J Radiol 2(5):172-179.

Egawa S, Wheeler TM, Scardino PT (1991). The sonographic appearances of irradiated prostate cancer. Brit J. Urol; 172-177.

Forsberg F, Merton DA, Liu JB et al (1998). Clinical applications of ultrasound contrast agents. Ultrasonics; 36: 695–701.

Frauscher F, Klauser A, Halpern EJ, Horninger W, Bartsch G (2001). Detection of prostate cancer with a microbubble ultrasound contrast agent. Lancet; 357: 1849–50.

Frauscher F, Klauser A, Volgger H,Halpern EJ, Pallwein L, Steiner H, Schuster A, Horninger W, Rogatsch H, Bartsch G (2002). Comparison of contrast enhanced color Doppler targeted biopsy with conventional systematic biopsy: impact on prostate cancer detection. J Urol; 167: 1648–52.

Gelet A, Chapelon JY, Poissonnier L, Bouvier R, Rouvière O, Curiel L (2004). Local recurrence of prostate cancer after external beam radiotherapy: early experience of salvage therapy using high-intensity focused ultrasonography. Urology.Apr;63 (4):625-629.

Giffiths GJ, Grooks AJR, Roberts EE, Evans KT, Buck AC, Thomas PJ, Peeling WB (1984) Ultrasonic appearance associated with prostatic inflammation: a preliminary study. Clinc Radiol., 35 : 343- 345.

Hammerer PG, McNeal JE, Stamey TA (1995). Correlation between serum prostate specific antigen levels and the volume of the individual glandular zones of the human prostate. J Urol ;153:111- 114.

Halpern EJ, Rosenberg M, Gomolla LG (2001). Contrast enhanced sonography of the prostate. Radiology; 219: 219–25.

Hamper UM, Sheth S (1993). Prostate ultrasonography. Semin roentg; 28, 1: 57 – 73.

Henry AM, Al-Qaisieh B, Gould K, Bownes P, Smith J, Carey B, Bottomley D, Ash D (2010). Outcomes following iodine-125 monotherapy for localized prostate cancer: the results of leeds 10-year single-center brachytherapy experience. Int J Radiat Oncol Biol Phys. Jan 1; 76(1):50-56.

Hodge KK, McNeal JE, Terris MK, Stamey TA (1989). Random systematic versus directed ultrasound guided transrectal core biopsies of the prostate. J Urol ;142:71-75.

Hricak H (1990). The prostate gland. In: Hricak H, Carrington BM (eds.). MRI of the pelvis. A text atlas. California Martin Dunitz:

Inahara M, Suzuki H, Nakamachi H, Kamiya N, Shimbo M, Komiya A, Ueda T, Ichikawa T, Akakura K, Ito H (2004). Clinical evaluation of transrectal power doppler imaging in the detection of prostate cancer. Int Urol Nephrol ;36(2):175-80.

Ismail M, Petersen RO, Alexander AA, Newschaffer C, Gomella LG (1997). Color Doppler imaging in predicting the biologic behavior of prostate cancer: correlation with disease-free survival. Urology; 50: 906–12.

Jacobs S, C (1983). Spread of prostatic cancer to bone. Urology 21 : 337.

Klauser A, Koppelstaetter F, Berger AP, Horninger W,Lorenz A, Frauscher F (2003). Real-time elastography for prostate cancer detection: preliminary experience. Radiology; 229 (Suppl): 1395

Konig K, Scheipers U, Pesavento A, Lorenz A, Ermert H,Senge T (2005). Initial experiences with real-time elastography guided biopsies of the prostate. J Urol; 174: 115–17.

Lee F, Littrup PJ, Torp-Pedersen ST, Mettlin C, McHugh TA, Gray JM, Kumasaka GH, McLeary RD (1988) Prostate cancer: Comparison of transrectal US and digital rectal examination for screening. Radiology; 168 : 389- 394.

Lepor H (2008).Vascular targeted photodynamic therapy for localized prostate cancer.Rev Urol. fall; 10(4): 254–261.

Liang K, Rogers AJ, Light ED, Von Allmen D, Smith SW (2010). Simulation of autonomous robotic multiple-core biopsy by 3D ultrasound guidance. Ultrason Imaging. Apr; 32(2):118-27.

Littrup PJ, Klein RM, Gross ML, Sparschu RA, Segel MC, Zingas AP (1995). Color Doppler of the prostate: histologic and racial correlations. Radiology; 197: 365

Lowsley OS (1912). The development of human prostate gland with reference to the development of other structures of the neck of the urinary bladder. Am J Anat, 13: 299-349.

Marberger M, Carroll PR, Zelefsky MJ, Coleman JA, Hricak H, Scardino PT, Abenhaim LL (2008). New treatments for localized prostate cancer. Urology. Dec;72(6 Suppl):S36-43.

Mc Langhin AP, Saltzstein SL McCullough, DL and Gittes RF (1976) prostatic carcinoma: Incidence location of unsuspected lymphatic metastasis. J. Urol. 115 - 89.

Mc Neal JE (1968). Regional morphology and pathology of the prostate. Am J Clinc Pathol, 49: 347 - 357.

Mc Neal JE (1983). The prostate gland; morphology and pathology. Monogr. Urol., 4: 5 -13.

Mc Neal JE (1988). Normal anatomy of the prostate and changes in benign prostatic hypertrophy and carcinoma. Semin US CT, MRI, 9: 329 -334.

Muldoon L and Resnick Ml. Result of ultrasonography of the prostate (1989). Urol Clinc North Am, 16, 4: 693 - 701.

Myers RP, Geollner JR, Cahil DR (1987) Prostate shape, external striated urethral sphincter and radical prostatectomy: The apical dissection. J Urol, 138: 543-548.

Naughton CK, Miller DC, Mager DE, Ornstein DK, Catalona WJ (2000). A prospective randomized trial comparing 6 versus 12 prostate biopsy cores: impact on cancer detection. J Urol.; 164:388-392.

Naryan P, Foster L (1991). The rule of intravenous urography and magnetic resonance imaging in the evaluation of men with symptomatic benign prostatic hyperplasia. Probl urol, 5, 3: 369 379.

Newman JS, Bree RL, Rubin JM (1995). Prostate cancer: diagnosis with color Doppler sonography with histologic correlation of each biopsy site. Radiology; 195: 86–90.

Ophir J, Cespedes I, Ponnekanti H, Yazdi Y, Li X (1991). Elastography: a quantitative method for imaging the elasticity of biological tissues. Ultrason Imaging; 13:111–34.

Onik GM, Cohen JK, Reyes GD, Rubinsky B, Chang Z, Baust J (1993). Transrectal ultrasound-guided percutaneous radical cryosurgical ablation of the prostate. Cancer. Aug 15; 72(4):1291-9.

Patel U, Rickards D (2002). Handbook of Transrectal Ultrasound and Biopsy of the Prostate. Martin.Dunitz Ltd, London.

Richards D (1992). Transrectal ultrasound, 1992. Brit J Urol; 69, 449-465.

Rifkin MD, Dahnert W, Kurtz AB (1990). State of the art: endorectal sonography of the prostate gland. AJR; 154:691-700

Rifkin MD (1997). Ultrasound of the Prostate. 2nd edn.Philadelphia, PA: Lippincott-Raven.

Rifkin MD, Sudakoff GS, Alexander AA (1993). Prostate: techniques, results, and potential applications of color Doppler US scanning. Radiology; 186: 509–13.

Scardino PT, Shinohara K, Wheeler TM, Carter SS (1989). Staging of prostate cancer: Value of ultrasonography. Urol Clinc North AM; 16, 713-733.

Shabsigh R, Kadmon D, Fishman IJ (1989). Ultrasonographically guided transperineal prostate biopsy in patients with suspicious glands and previously negative digitally guided biopsies. J. Endourol., 3: 185.

Shen F, Shinohara K, Kumar D, Khemka A, Simoneau AR, Werahera PN, Li L, Guo Y, Narayanan R, Wei L, et al (2008). Three-dimensional sonography with needle tracking: role in diagnosis and treatment of prostate cancer. J Ultrasound Med. Jun; 27(6):895-905.

Shinohara K, Scardino PT, Carter ST, Wheeler TM (1989). Pathological basis of the sonographic appearance of the normal and malignant prostate. Urol Clinc North AM; 16, 4: 675-691.

Sohlberg OE, Chetner M, Ploch N, Brawer MK (1991). Prostatic abscess after transrectal ultrasound guided biopsy. J Urol; 146, 420-422.

Takahashi H, Ouchi T. The ultrasonic diagnosis in the field of urology (1963). Proc Jap Soc Ultrasonics Med; 3:7.

Terris MK, McNeal JE, Stamey TA (1990). Invasion of the seminal vesicles by prostatic cancer: Detection by transrctal sonography. AJR; 155; 811-815.

Terris MK, and Stamey TA (1991). Determination of prostatic volume by transrectal ultrasound. J Urol, 145: 984-987.

Wasserman NF, Kapoor DA, Hildebrandt WC, et al (1992) Transrectal ultrasound in evalaaution of patients after radical prostatectomy.Radiology; 185; 361-372.

Watanabe H, Igari D, Tanahasi Y, Harada K, Saito M. Development and application of new equipment for transrectal ultrasonography. J Clin Ultrasound. 1974; 2:91-98.

Weaver RP, Noble MJ, Weigle JW (1991). Correlation of ultrasound guided and digitally directed transrectal biopsies of palpable prostatic abnormalities. J Urol.; 145:516-518.

4

Advances in Breast Ultrasound

Heino Hille
Office for Obstetrics and Gynecology, Hamburg, Germany

1. Introduction

Breast ultrasound was introduced as a clinical method in breast imaging in the seventies of the 20th century (Jellins, 1971; Kobayashi, 1974). In the Anglo-Saxon countries breast ultrasound was employed mainly by radiologists, by gynecologists predominantly in Germany.

In the early period the indication for breast ultrasound was the differentiation between the cystic or solid nature of palpable lumps (Figs. 1, 2). To make this distinction is easier in ultrasound than in mammography. On this way ultrasound became an accepted method as an adjunct to mammography for further analysis of equivocal mammographic lesions.

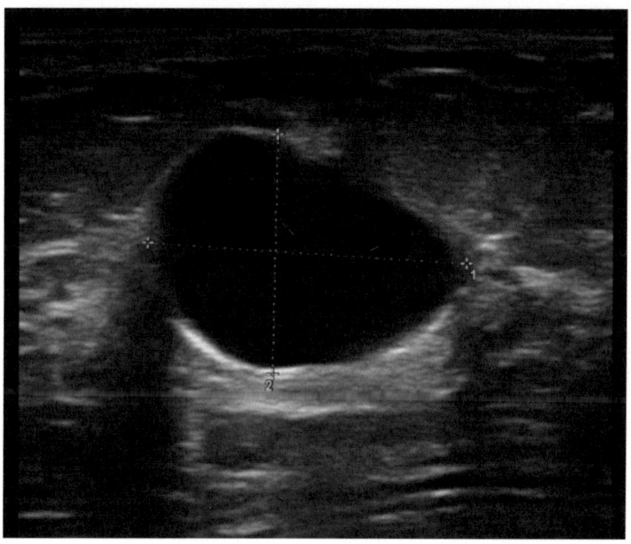

Fig. 1. Typical cyst: anechoic with distinct and smooth margins, benign

Though till now in guide lines of early detection of breast carcinoma indications for breast ultrasound are restricted in this sense, already in the eighties of the 20th century, the capability of breast ultrasound went far beyond this limits (Hackelöer et al., 1986). In contrast to mammography ultrasound is able to generate a detailed map of the anatomic structure of the breast. Because of this ability sonography is qualified to diagnose many benign and malign diseases of the breast by its own (Teboul & Halliwell, 1995).

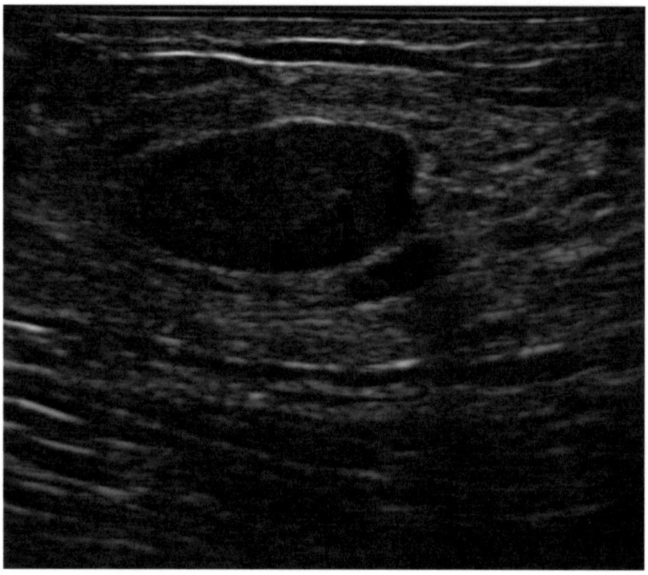

Fig. 2. Typical fibroadenoma: solid, isodens, distinct and smooth margins (pseudocapsule), benign

2. Contemporary principles of breast ultrasound

Breast ultrasound is a dynamic (live) examination, the diagnostic procedure is performed by scanning systematically the whole breast in perpendicular planes. Though not unusual in Anglo-Saxon countries, it´s not sufficient to make a diagnosis on the basis mainly of printed or frozen digital pictures like in mammography. It is necessary to scan both whole breasts in real time. Only in this way is it possible to get a true impression of the architecture of the individual breast. Only with this background structural and architectural distortions as well as differences in the architecture of both sides will be remarkable. To classify the margins of a lesion in detail the dynamic examination is basically as well.

During whole breast scanning there are several steps to absolve:

What kind of breast parenchyma exists in respect of density (that is the relation of glandular to fatty tissue), echogenicity, homogeneus or inhomogeneous structure?

Are there any distinct lesions or masses?

In case of a lesion: the sophisticated description of the lesion related to standardized terms with final submission in BI-RADS categories with recommendation which way to follow up, is mandatory (ACR, 2003; Madjar et al. 2006).

Are there non mass like structural distortions requesting further analysis or complementary imaging modalities?

Principles of the description and the classifying of a discovered lesion are described in known textbooks and publications of breast ultrasound (Madjar & Mendelson, 2008; Stavros, 2004).

Examples and illustrations of cases with *typical sonographic appearance*, see below (Fig. 3, 4, 5, 6).

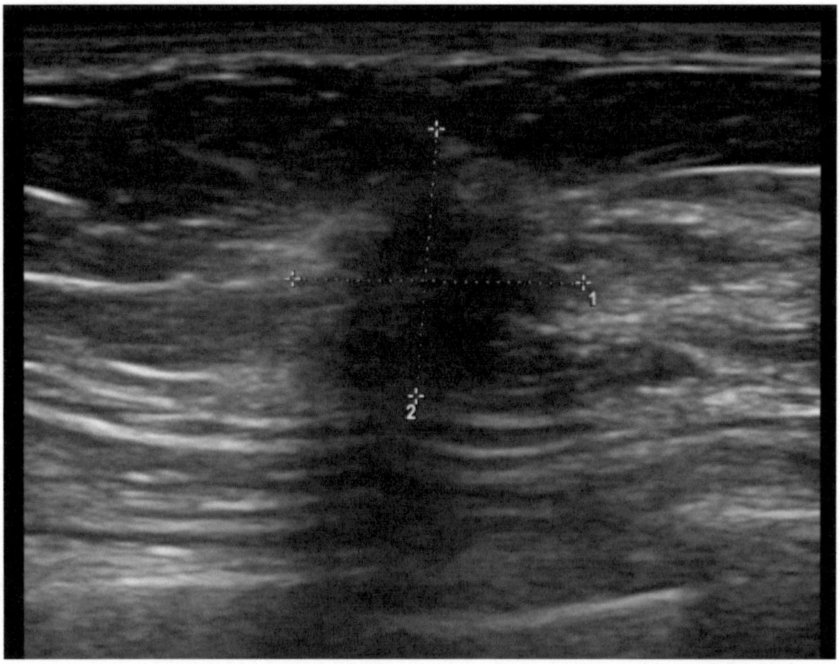

Fig. 3. Typical carcinoma: Architectural distortion, hypoechoic and echoinhomogeneous, margins ill-defined with echogenic halo, spiculae, acoustic shadow, vertical orientation

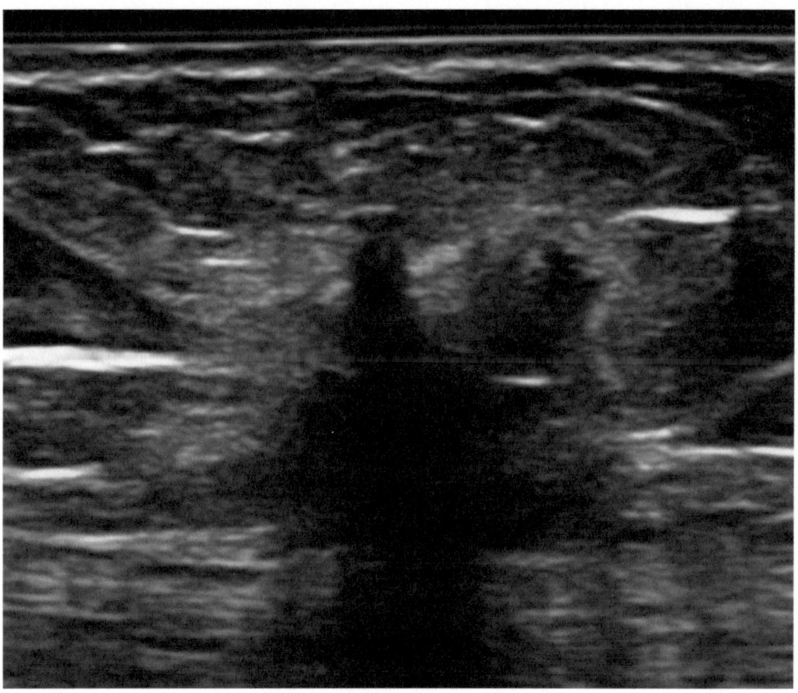

Fig. 4. Another carcinoma with typical architectural distortion, hypoechoic, acoustic shadow, desmoplastic reaction (echogenic halo)

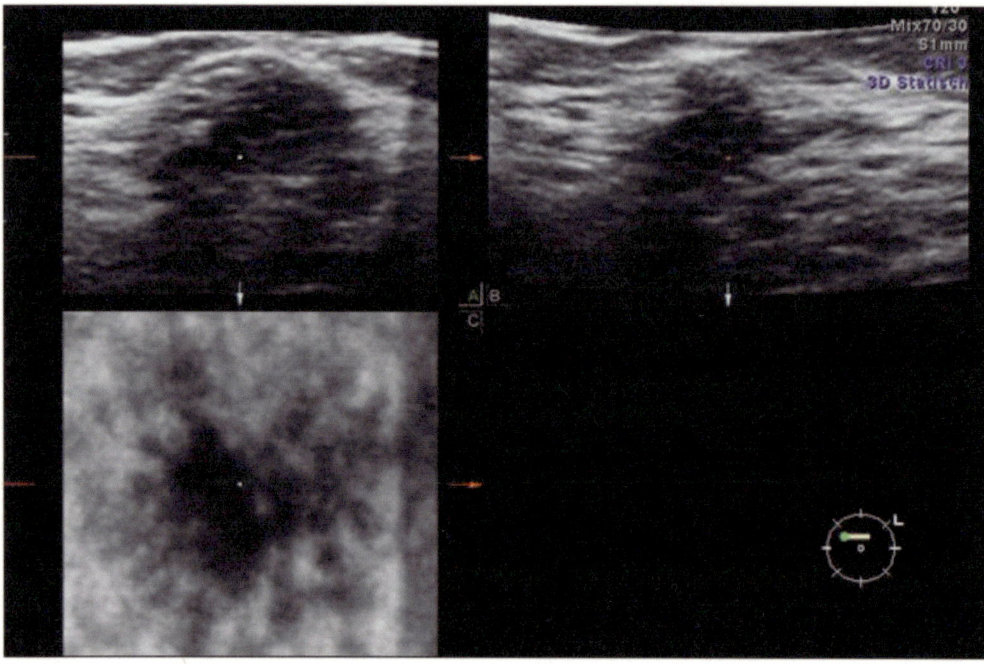

Fig. 5. Palpable lump: DCIS (ductal-in-situ-carcinoma): hypoechoic with indistinct margins, retraction pattern in the C-plane

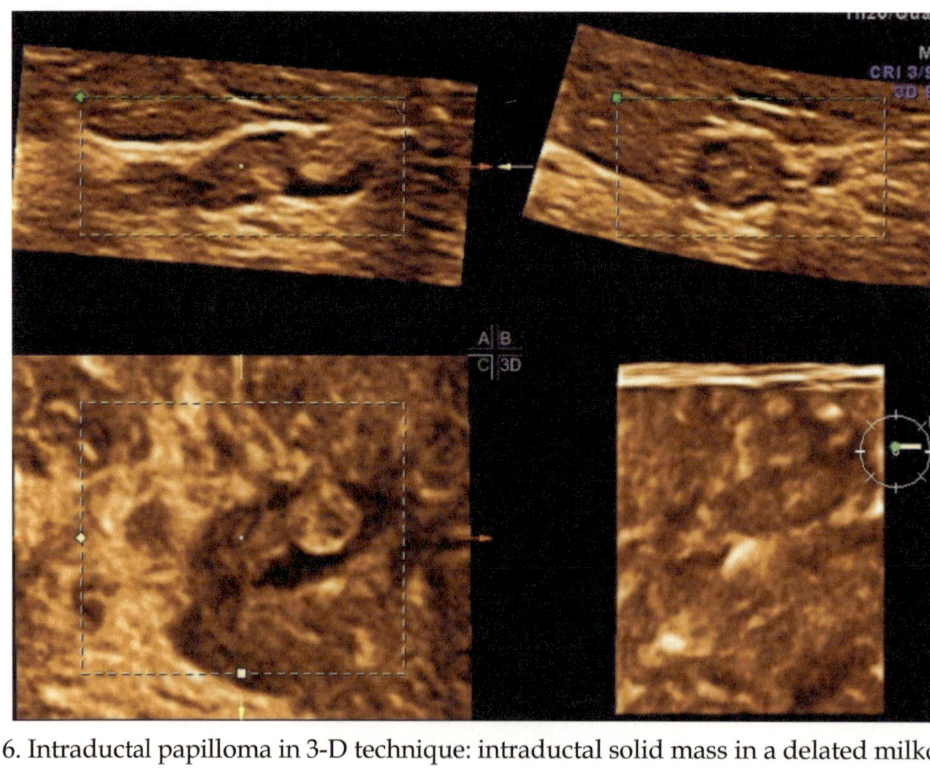

Fig. 6. Intraductal papilloma in 3-D technique: intraductal solid mass in a delated milkduct

3. New insights in breast ultrasound

To make the distinction between a benign and a malign or between a probably benign and a probably malign lesion, the differentiation of the margins and the echogenicity is essential. But with developing technology and experience some classical criteria like sound transmissing - shadowing versus enhancement - and the direction of growing - horizontal versus vertical - lose relevance. Enhancement is no longer a distinguishing marker for a benign lesion nor is this the horizontal growing pattern. By use of contemporary technology (Compound Scanning, Tissue Harmonic) enhancement can be observed in malign lesions as well and the growing pattern of ductal carcinomas often starts horizontal. Figs. 7, 8, 9 demonstrate not well known, but not rare characteristics of malign breast lesions.

With progress in resolution of the machines not smooth and not distinct circumscribed margins of fibroadenomas become more visible. Especially in the C-plane of the 3-D mode often fingerlike continuities are remarkable. That means that the finding of non smooth oval or round margins alone is no longer conclusive to submit this lesion to BI-RADS 4 (suspect) (Fig. 10, 11, 12).

On the other hand circumscribed margins are not rare - not only in special forms of carcinoma like medullary or mucinous carcinoma - but even in ductal carcinoma (Figs. 8, 15).

In this sense breast ultrasound with contemporary high definition ultrasound has become not easier, but more sophisticated.

Additional technical modules like color Doppler and 3-D therefore gain on relevance.

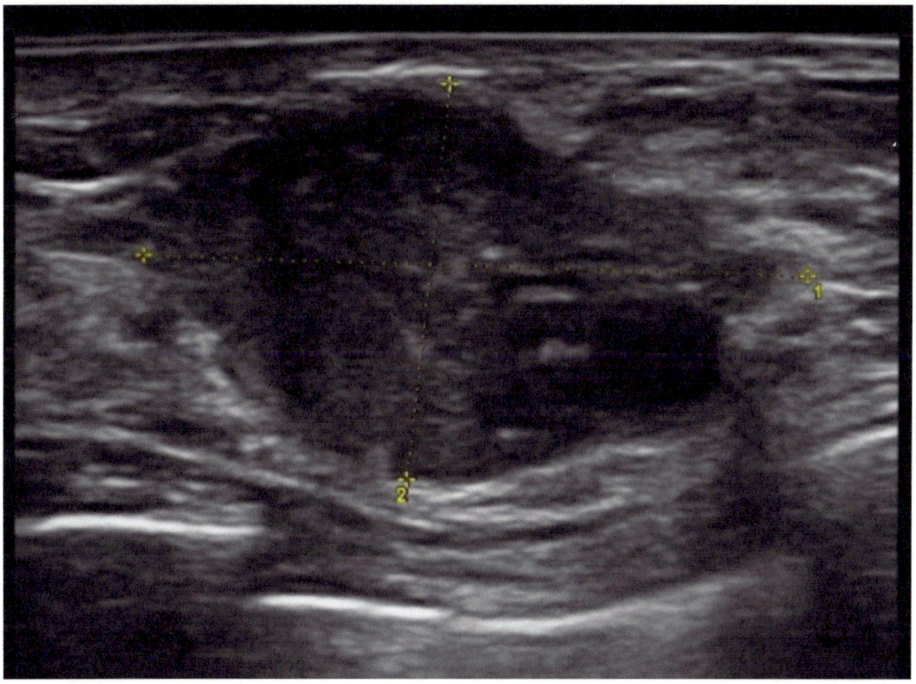

Fig. 7. A more horizontal orientation of a carcinoma, sound transmission attenuated only marginal, but predominantly enhanced

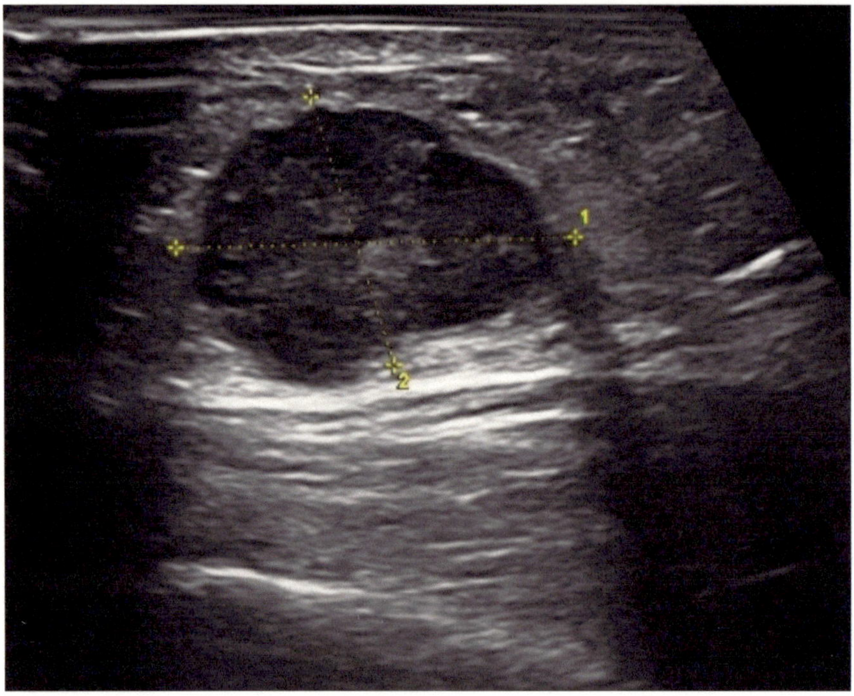

Fig. 8. Ductal carcinoma, smooth surrounded with sound - enhancement

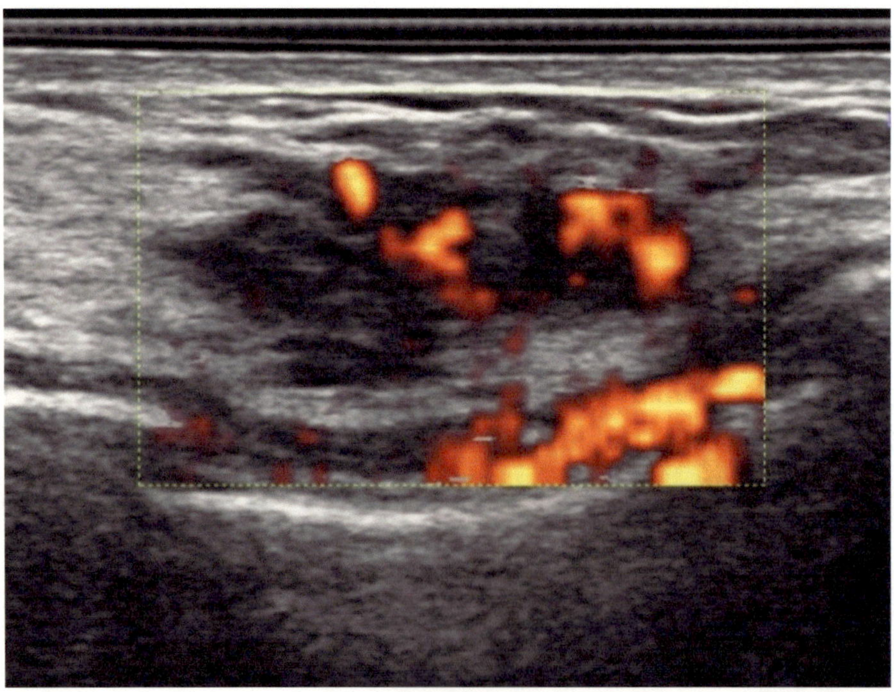

Fig. 9. DCIS: Horizontal growing pattern of a DCIS with microinvasion, clear vascularization in color Doppler

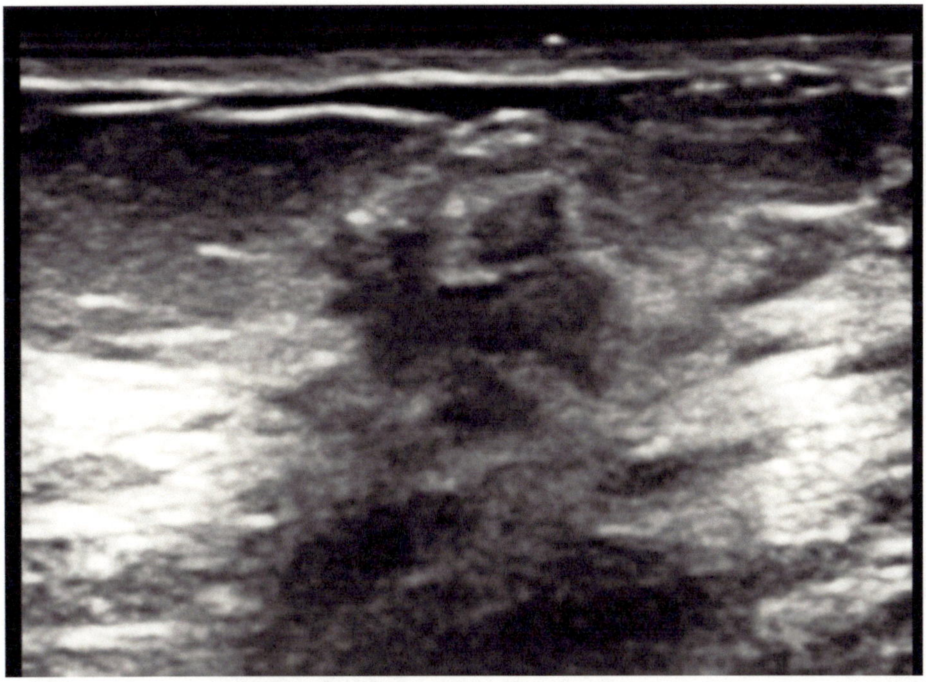

Fig. 10. Fibroadenoma: indistinct and not smooth margins (by this way not distinguishable from a carcinoma)

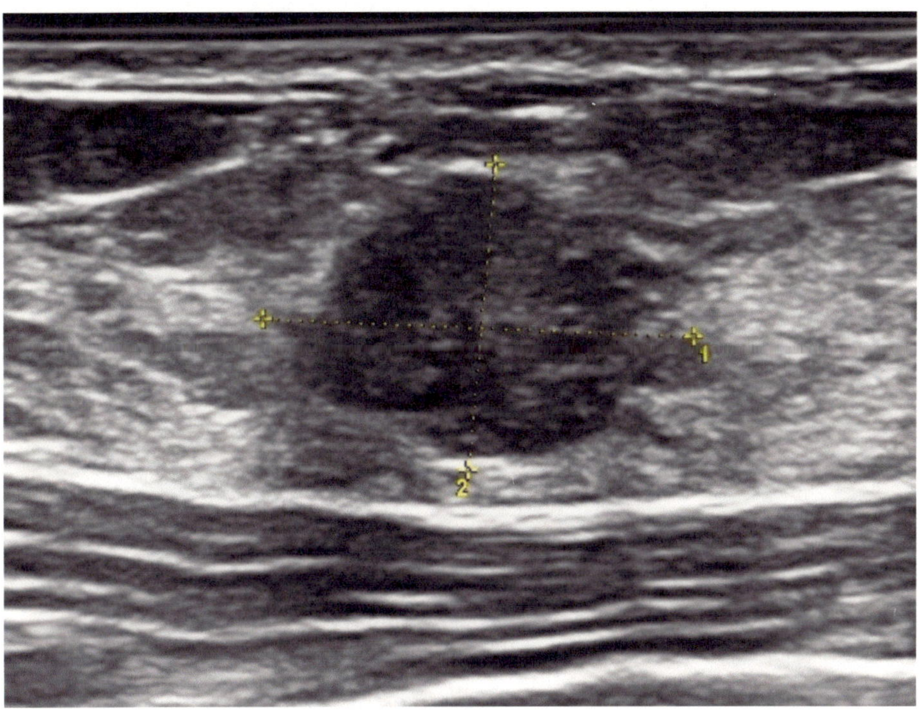

Fig. 11. Fibroadenoma: fingerlike continuities (not rare)

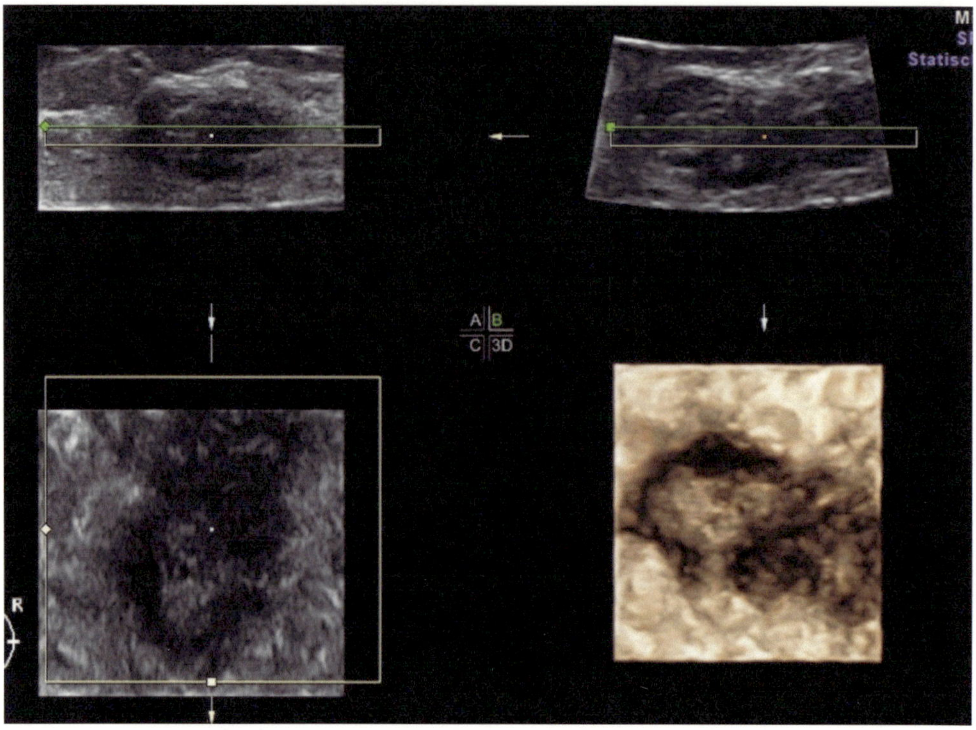

Fig. 12. The same lesion of Fig. 11 in 3-D mode

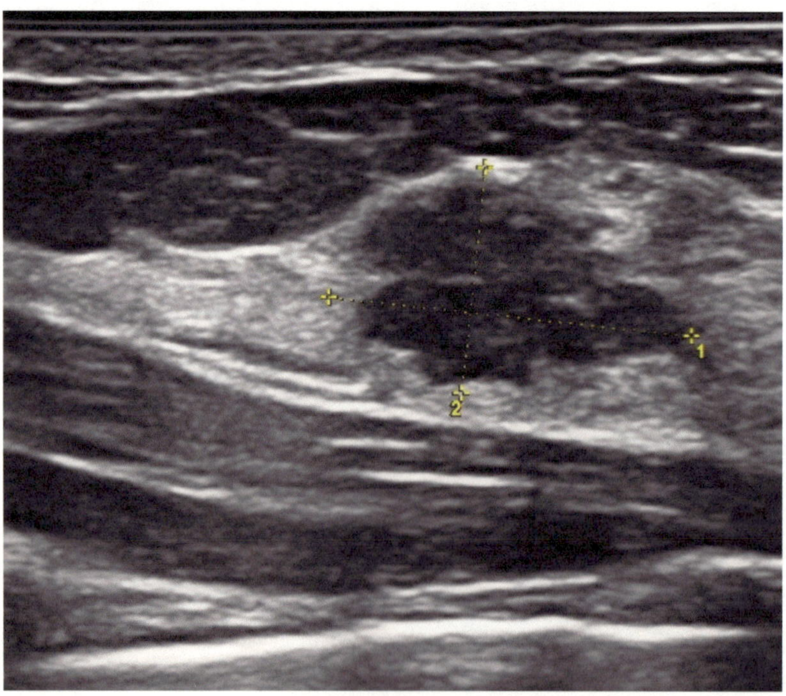

Fig. 13. Fibroadenoma with not smooth margins

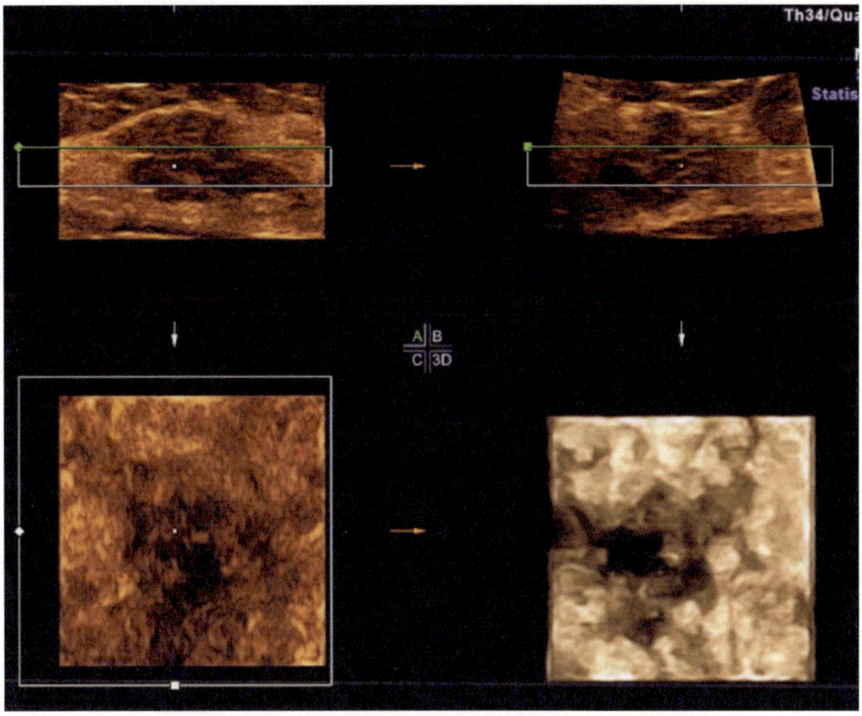

Fig. 14. Fibroadenoma of Figure 12 in 3-D mode with a canyon-like impression

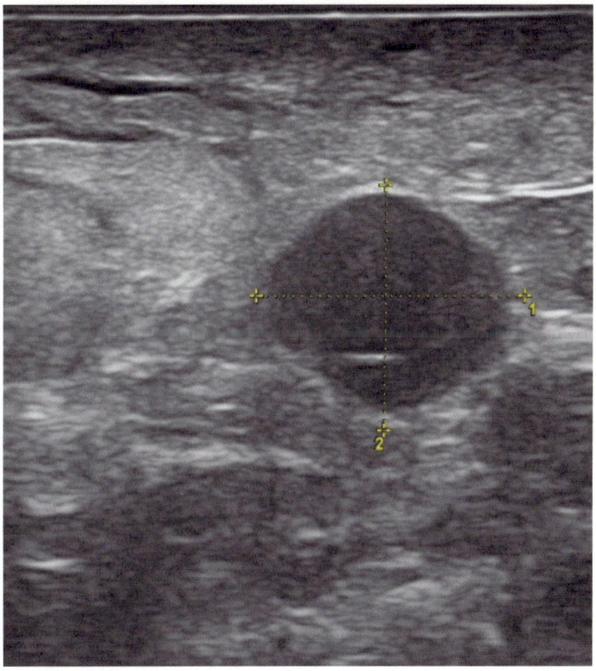

Fig. 15. Inflammatory, invasive ductal carcinoma with smooth and distinct margins, at first misinterpreted as mastitis

4. Color Doppler

Though color Doppler is not routinely used in all institutions performing breast ultrasound, in our view color Doppler is fundamental as an additional criterion in discriminating malign from benign lesions (Weismann, 2006). But as it is with other marker: the fact of a proven vascularity generates not for itself a definite submission to a suspect cluster. It is important to observe the type of vascularization: color signals running straight into the lesion are a hint of malignancy, whereas angiogenesis round the border of a lesion is not. Of course the degree of vascularization is relevant. Vascularization within the lesion stresses suspicion of malignancy, but is not a verification of malignancy. The missing of vascularization on the other hand is not a proof of benignancy (Figs. 16, 17).

The detection of significant vascularization within a lesion shifts an otherwise benign looking lesion from BI-RADS 3 (probably benign) to BI-RADS 4 (suspect), proposing it to core biopsy.

Quantitative spectral Doppler has not proven to be of relevance.

5. 3-D ultrasound

3-D technique, now available in breast ultrasound by different manufacturer, is a valuable tool to obtain a detailed impression of the margins and the surroundings of a lesion in a view from above (the so called C-plane). Necessary is a special probe with automated acquisition of different planes. The option of Volume Rendering strengthens the spacious impression of the lesion with its relationship to the neighborhood. By use of 3-D technique additional criteria for lesion submission could be applied. Pattern of retraction or compression in the near surroundings of a lesion are of importance. Star-like retraction

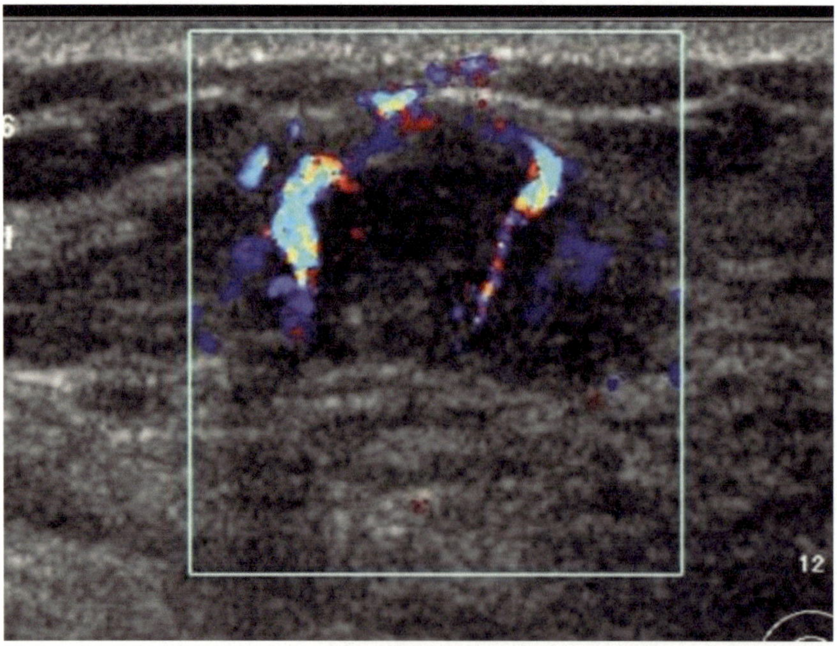

Fig. 16. DCIS (in pregnancy) with powerful vascularization

pattern is a hard marker for malignancy, whereas a compression pattern hints to benignancy (Fig. 19). With retraction pattern in the C-plane otherwise (in the A- and B-Plane) benign looking lesions are to subordinate to BI-RADS 4 (suspect) (Figs. 5, 17, 18).

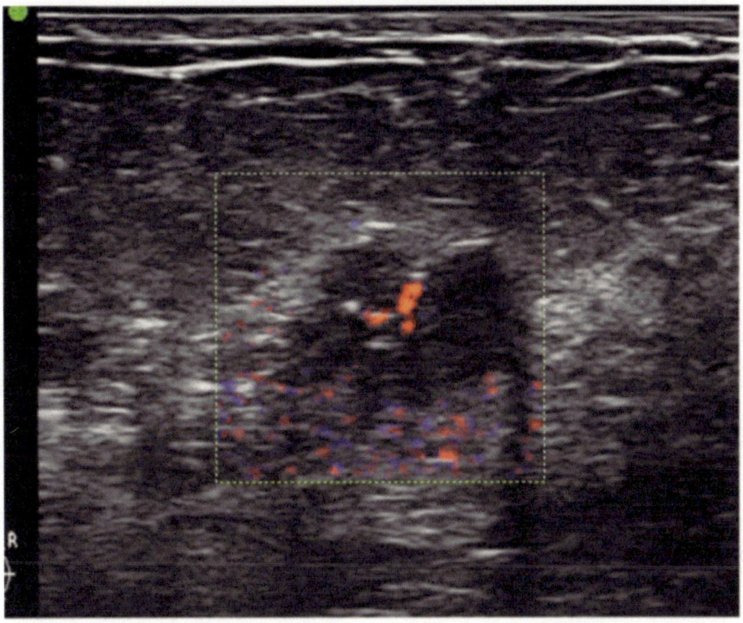

Fig. 17. Carcinoma: not easy detectable. Suspicion was strengthened by color Doppler

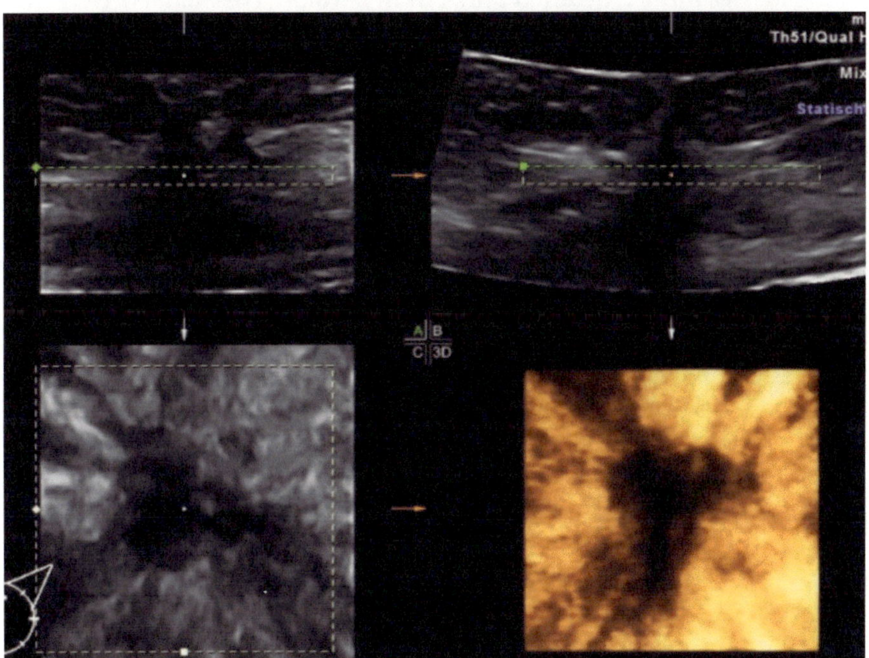

Fig. 18. Carcinoma of Fig. 17 in 3-D mode: suspicious retraction pattern

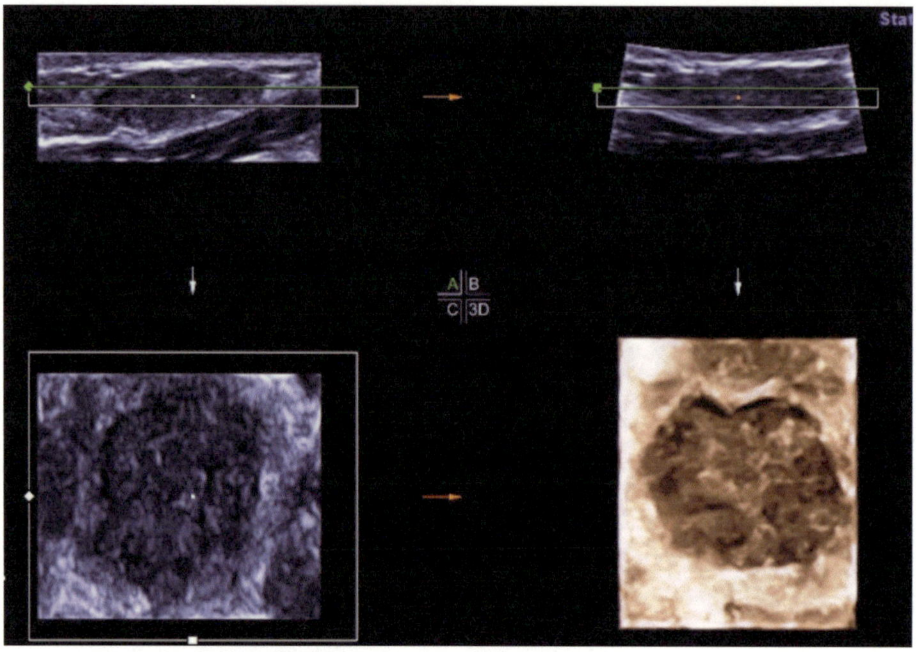

Fig. 19. Compression pattern of a benign fibroadenoma

However, carcinomas often may show indeterminate surrounding in the C-plane (not definite retraction phenomenon) as well. 3-D seems to be of similar value to color Doppler in differentiating masses further, detected previous in B-Mode (Weismann & Hergan, 2007).

The basic principle of sonographic diagnosis in breast ultrasound is to put all criteria in a synopsis or a mosaic, not to make a scarce diagnosis on one or two single signs.

6. Architectural distortion and structural disturbance

Architectural distortion is a term primary used in mammography and then became familiar in breast ultrasound too. In breast ultrasound it describes a well known hard marker for a malign lesion: the continuity of the glandular structure of the parenchyma is interrupted by an anechoic or hypoechoic irregular surrounded lesion (Figs. 3, 4).

What here is called "structural disturbance" is a far less obviously and more diffuse change in the echotexture of the gland of different extension. Echogenicity in local disturbances is somewhat more sonolucent, surroundings are not striking but poorly defined. It may correspond to a local discreet irregular course of the milk ducts. Such regions may represent only local mastopathic changes or preinvasive lesions like DCIS or so called "radial scars". In other cases even invasive carcinomas, i.e. triple negative (often mammographic occult) carcinomas may be present (Figs. 20, 21, 22, 23, 25).

To discover local "structural disturbances" whole breast scanning of each side is mandatory. It is necessary to take notice of the difference of a local disturbed region to the normal structure and echotexture of the individual breast and the difference to the other side. Specificity of breast ultrasound of such a lesion is not high, but this corresponds to the complexity of breast parenchyma in the sense of an extreme variable biological substrate.

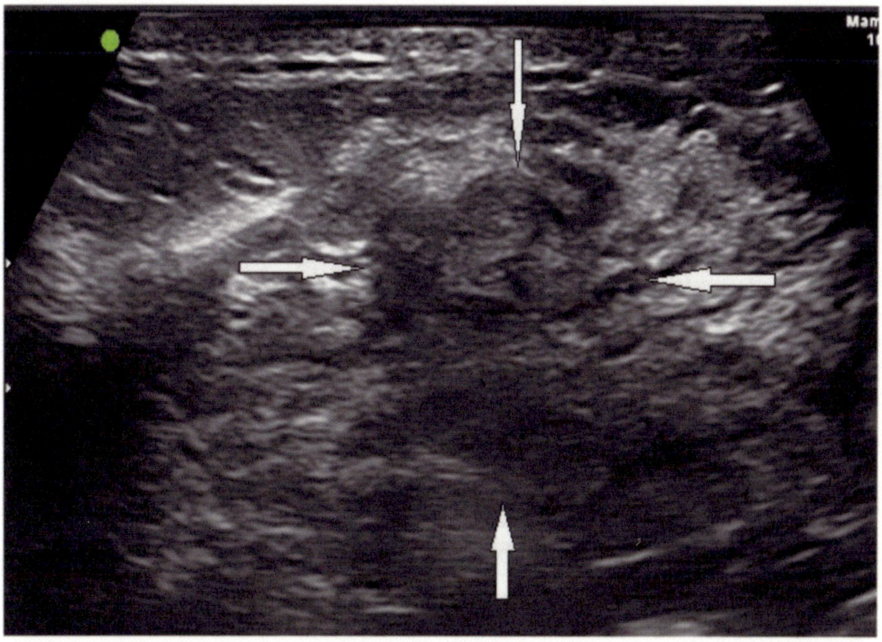

Fig. 20. Structural distortion: indistinct and ill defined, discreet sonolucent region in the center of the gland. The regular architecture of the gland-parenchyma is somewhat disturbed, but not disrupted: DCIS, in a dynamic examination better detectable than in a frozen picture

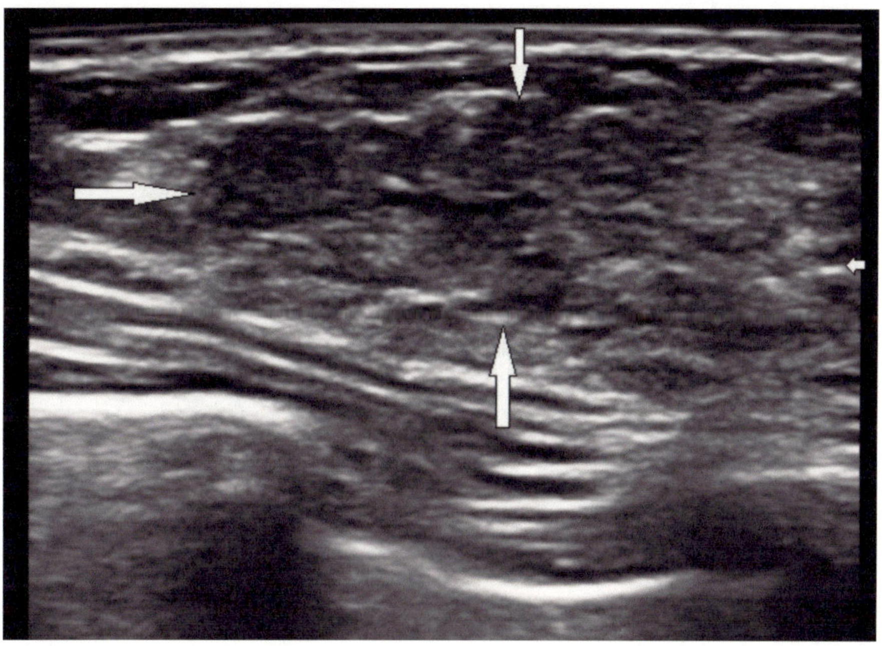

Fig. 21. DCIS in the outer upper region of the breast: not well defined extended region with lobulation and disturbed architecture

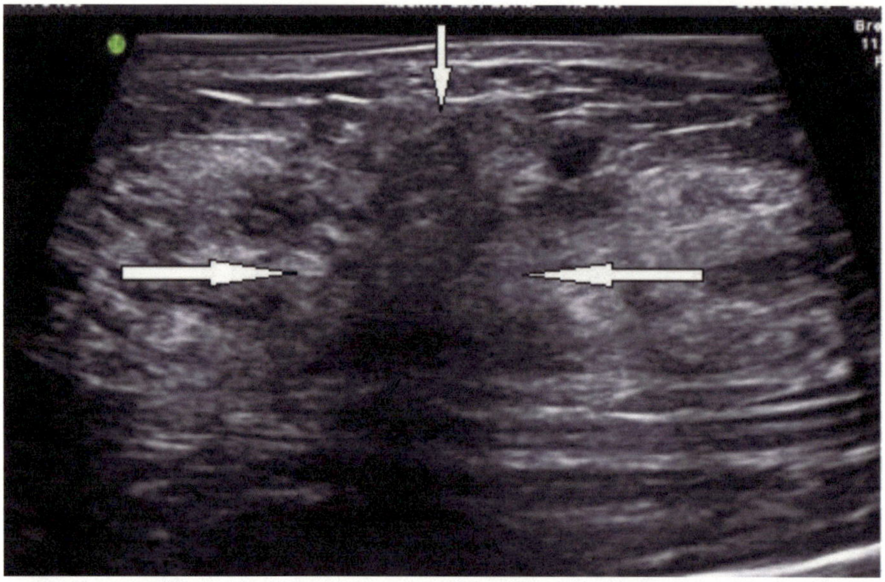

Fig. 22. A region with sonolucent structural disturbance

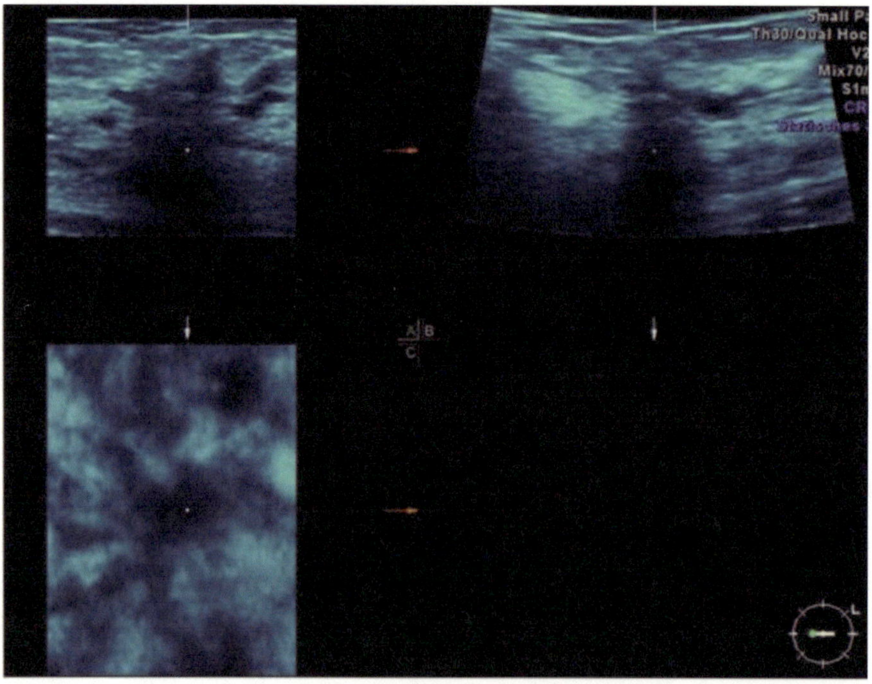

Fig. 23. Same lesion like Fig. 22: Suspicious retraction pattern in 3-D: "radial scar" with DCIS

Diagnosing and describing such local disturbances requires best technological equipment and some years of experience. However, this seems to be the most important field of progress in breast ultrasound: to become able to distinguish fine differences in the echotexture, not only to detect distinct striking masses.

It may be difficult and controversial to submit "structural disturbances" in BI-RADS 3 (probably benign) or 4 (suspect). At minimum such regions are to expose to complementary image modalities, i.e. mammography, perhaps MRI too and they are recommended for follow up. In more striking cases and high risk patients core biopsy should be preferred.

There is a need for further evaluation of the relevance of this type of ultrasound findings.

7. Ultrasound and DCIS (ductal carcinoma in situ)

In general ultrasound is thought to be not competent in detecting DCIS in comparison to mammography. That this is not true in some regards has been shown in the last decade. Breast ultrasound is especial important in detecting DCIS without microcalcifications. Today we do not know the real biological proportion of DCIS with and without microcalcifications (Hille et al., 2007).

The second entity is DCIS as a palpable lump, i.e. symptomatic DCIS. It could be shown that sonography is superior to mammography in detecting theses lesions (Yang et al., 2004), (Figs. 5, 16, 21).

Revealing "structural disturbances" seems to be of relevance to remove shortages of breast ultrasound in respect of diagnosing DCIS and to discover lesions that are otherwise, i.e. in mammography, occult (Figs. 9, 20, 22).

In a study evaluating the diagnostic competence of imaging methods in respect of breast carcinomas, which were operated, the sensitivity of sonography for DCIS was not far behind mammography (Berg et al., 2004)

Nevertheless, microcalcifications as a hint for DCIS is not reliable seen in ultrasound, when presenting without a mass (that means without sonolucent surroundings). This is the reason that - especially in a screening setting – sonography does not match mammography in diagnosing DCIS (Fig. 24).

8. Is breast ultrasound a screening tool?

The most controversial debate is going on about this topic. Most radiologists accept breast ultrasound mainly as an adjunct to mammography: mammography always first and then after - in cases of mammographical equivocal lesions or very dense breasts - ultrasound complementary. But that seems a traditional point of view and connected to specific interests. Ultrasound is time consuming, when performed by the physician in comparison to other modalities and is not well granted by insurances.

Under scientific and healthcare aspects the main point should be: What is the capacity of breast ultrasound in detecting early breast carcinoma in asymptomatic women? What we can say now: Breast ultrasound performed with high technology and in experienced hands at least has an equal, probably higher sensitivity for invasive carcinomas in comparison to mammography (Benson et al., 2004; Berg et al., 2008; Kolb et al., 2002) In respect to DCIS sensitivity is lower in published studies, but in this field there is evolvement, see above. Breast ultrasound can play an important role in detecting aggressive breast carcinoma not presenting microcalcifications like cases of "triple negative" types, often arising in younger women in dense breasts (Fig. 25). Recently investigations discovered that these cancers represent an important proportion of so called "interval cancers" in mammographic screening (Haakinson et al., 2010).

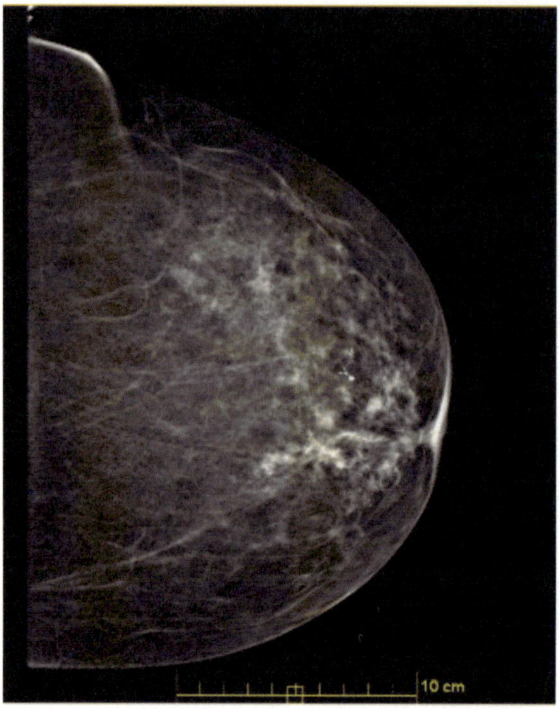

Fig. 24. Extended DCIS with microcalcifications in mammography, not visible in ultrasound

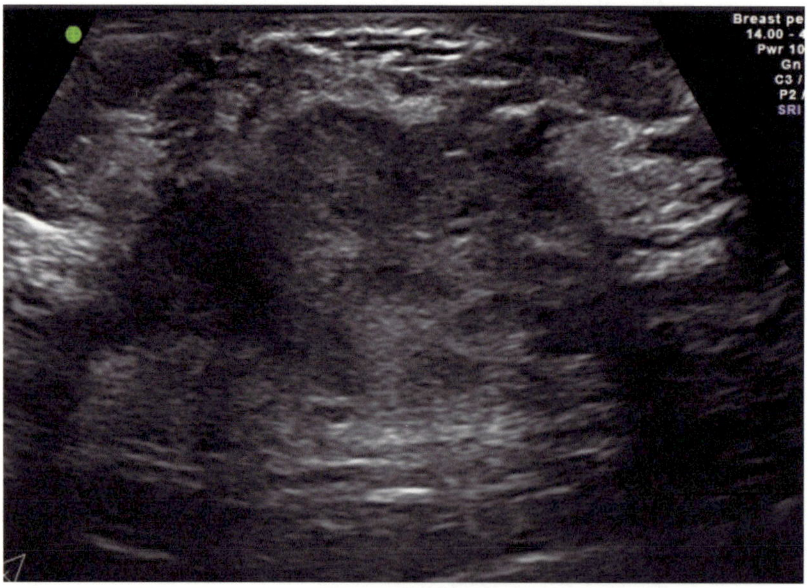

Fig. 25. "Triple-negative" carcinoma: extended, but not so obvious and with discreet structural changes

One important advantage of breast ultrasound is the absence of ionization. Sonography could be repeated without restriction.

Compared to mammography and MRI, ultrasound-machines are cheap. Special laboratories and assistants are not necessary.

But there are open questions and disadvantages of breast ultrasound. First, breast ultrasound is extremely dependant on the expertise of the physician and on the used technology. Second, handheld breast ultrasound does not produces an image document of the whole breast, that could be examined outside the laboratory. Therefore problems of quality control exist. New technologies of automated aquired 3-D volumes may remove these shortages in future. Third, there is a lack of randomizised trials comparing ultrasound versus other modalities.

Recently published studies demonstrate the feasibility of breast ultrasound as a preventive medical check-up in gynecological offices (Lenz, 2011; Madjar et al., 2010).

9. Areas of progress in breast ultrasound

9.1 Contrast- enhanced breast ultrasound

Contrast agents, intravenous applied, to improve sensitivity and specificity in breast ultrasound in detecting vascularization had been researched over a decade. Till now this - in sonography of the liver established - expanded procedure has not become a method of standard in breast ultrasound. The main reasons may be, that the procedure is more expensive and time consuming and is not suitable for breast-screening. A lesion which is to examine further with contrast agents is to detect in conventional B-Mode first. But there might be clinical indications for contrast agents instead of radioactive agents in future to test sentinel lymph nodes (Goldberg et al., 2011; Sever et al., 2011).

9.2 Elastography

At time manufacturer are equipping machines with elastography modules and some study groups are researching the potential role of this method. In conventional B-mode detected lesions were additionally examined in respect of the characteristics of stiffness. Different techniques, color coded or shear-wave techniques are used (Figs. 26a,b). Elastography is

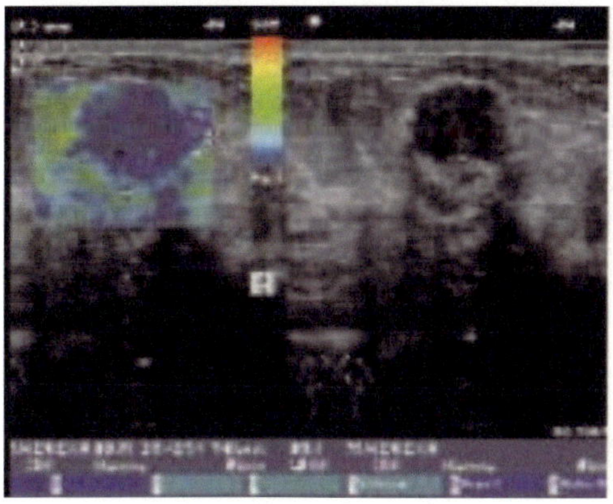

(a)

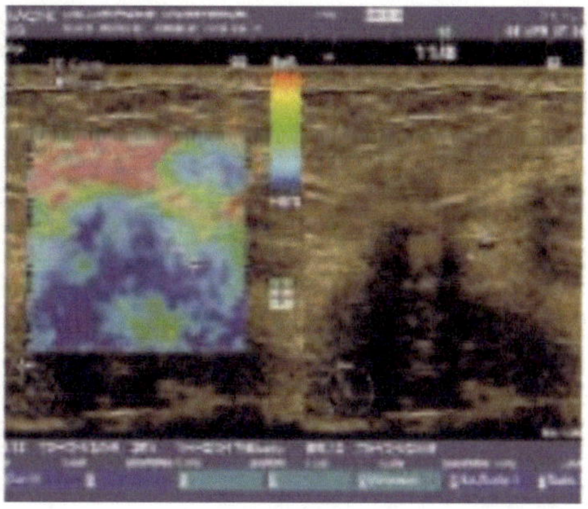

(b)

Fig. 26. (a) (b) Elastography of carcinoma, coded in blue. (Figures by courtesy of R. Ohlinger, center of breast diseases, university of Greifswald, Germany) extremely observer dependent in applying pressure by the handheld probe. Results are different and today it remains unclear, if specificity of breast ultrasound in discriminating benign from malign lesions can increase with elastography in a reliable way, so that invasive biopsies could be spared (Baldwin, 2011).

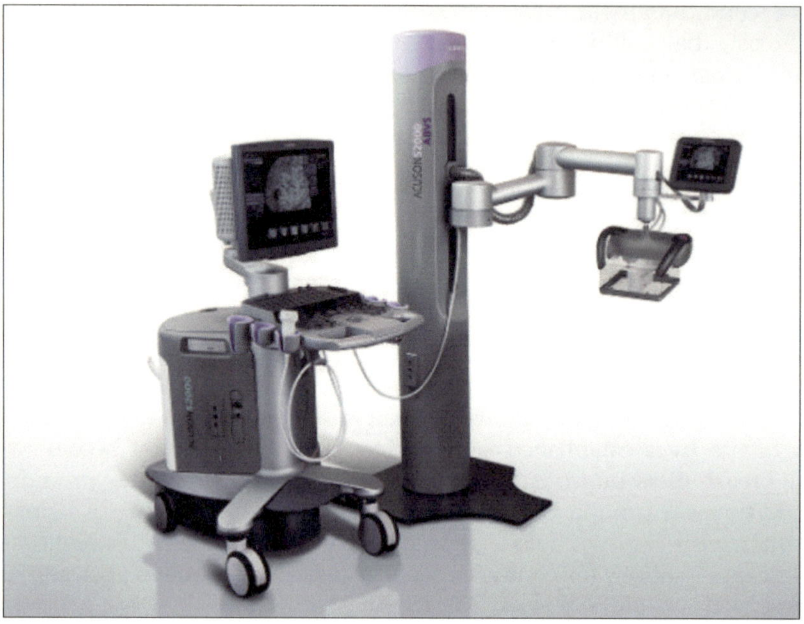

Fig. 27. Automated 3-D system (ABVS), figure with license by courtesy of SIEMENS AG

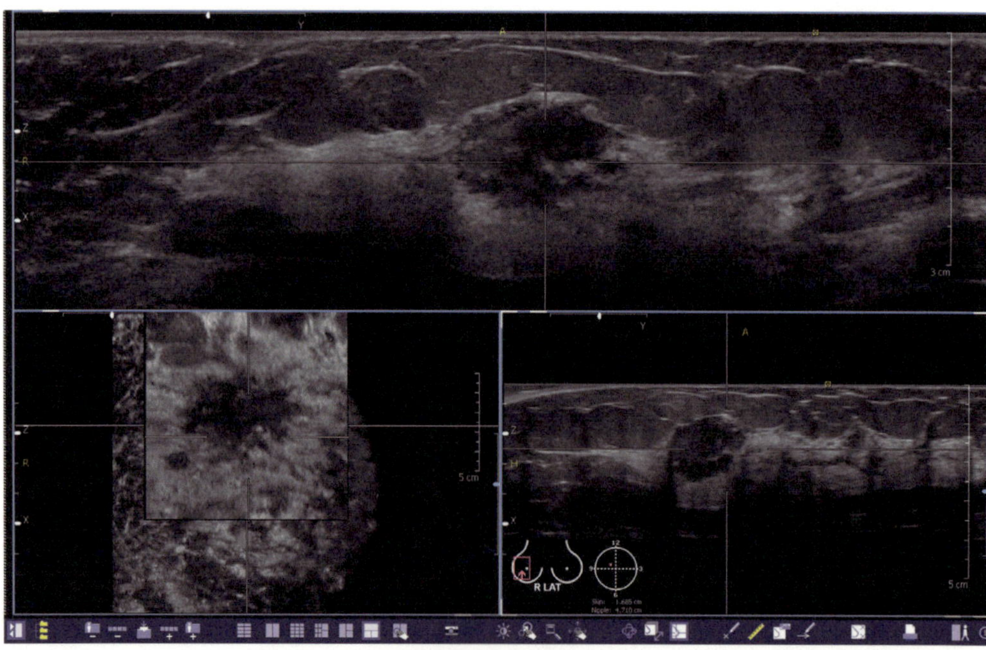

Fig. 28. Carcinoma in 3 planes bei ABVS, with license by courtesy of SIEMENS AG

9.3 Automated 3-D

Today a system is available, which acquires 3-D volumes of the whole breast (Fig. 27, 28). The resolution of the system is sufficient. The volume of the breast is acquired from different directions with a special probe by means of a large contact area. Than after the observer has to go through the whole volume to detect suspicious regions at the computer. The rendered C-Plane and the A- and B-plane could be presented in parallel on the screen. In future this step may be done by help of CAD (Computer Aided Detection). The acquisition itself could be done by assistant persons (sonographers).

Till now it is unclear, if an automated system can match traditional handheld breast ultrasound in accuracy performed by an expert and if the duration of the examination could be reduced. If suspect findings in the acquired volume are to check in handheld ultrasound afterwards, additional examination time would be required. There is a need for bigger trials (Chang et al., 2011; Moon et al., 2011)).

Advantages are the repeatability and the independence of the diagnostic procedure from patient´s presence. In aspects of a possible ultrasound screening this advantage may be helpful.

10. Conclusion

Breast ultrasound is a valuable tool for diagnosing breast carcinoma as well as benign diseases of the breast. Breast ultrasound could not only used as an adjunct to mammography and in symptomatic cases, but could probably used as a screening tool in asymptomatic women. Especially in women with dense breasts sonography will overcome mammography with a higher detection rate for invasive carcinomas.

Of special importance will be the capacity for detecting local "structural disturbances" as a hint for hidden malignancies.

Color Doppler and 3-D mode had proven to be of importance. Elastography has to demonstrate this in future.

A high technological standard and a very good experience of the examiner are prerequisites.

11. References

American College of Radiology (ACR) (2003). *ACR-BI-RADS® - Breast Imaging Reporting and Data System (BI-RADS™)*. Breast Imaging Atlas. 3rd ed. Reston (VA): ©America College of Radiology

Baldwin, P. (2011). Breast ultrasound elastography. *Radiologic Technology*, 82: 347M-365M

Benson S.R.; Blue J.; Judd K.; et al. (2004) Ultrasound is now better than mammography in detection of invasive breast cancer. *Am J Surg*, 188: 381-385

Berg, W.A.; Gutierrez, L.; Ness Aiver, M.S.; Carter, W.B.; Bhargavan, M.; Lewis, R.S.; Ioffe, O.B. (2004). Diagnostic accuracy of mammography, clinical examination, US, and MR imaging in preoperative assessment of breast cancer. *Radiology*, 233: 830-849

Berg, W.A.; Blume, J.D.; Cormack, J.B. et al. (2008). Combined screening with ultrasound and mammography vs. mammography alone in women at elevated risk of breast cancer. *JAMA*, 299: 2151-2163

Chang, J., M.; Moon, W., K.; Cho, N.; Park, J., S.; Kim, S. J. (2011). Breast cancers initially detected by hand-held ultrasound: detection performance of radiologists using automated breast ultrasound data. *Acta Radiol,* 52: 8-14

Goldberg, B., B.; Merton, D., A.; Liu, J., B.; Forsberg, F.; Zhang, K.; Thakur, M.; Schulz, S.; Schanche, R.; Murphy, G.,F.; Waldman, S., A. (2011). Contrast-enhanced ultrasound imaging of sentinel lymph nodes after peritumal administration of Sonazoid in a melanoma tumor animal model. *J Ultrasound Med,* 30: 441-453

Haakinson D., J.; Stucky, C., C.; Dueck, A., C.; Gray, R. J.; Wasif, N.; Apsey, H., A.; Pockaj, B. (2010). A significant number of women present with palpable breast cancer even with a normal mammogram within 1 year. *Am J Surg,* 200: 712-717

Hackelöer, B.J., Duda V. & Lauth G. (1986). *Ultraschall-Mammographie.* Springer, ISBN 3-540-16233-X, Berlin

Hille, H.; Vetter, M.; Hackelöer, B., J. (2007). The Suitability of High-Resolution Ultrasound for the Detection of DCIS. *Ultraschall in Med,* 28: 307-312

Jellins, J.; Kossof, G.; Buddee F.,W.; Reeve T., S. (1971). Ultrasonic visualization of the breast. *Med Journ of Australia,* 1: 305-307

Kobayashi, T. (1974). Clinical evaluation of Ultrasound techniques in breast tumors and malignant abdominal tumors. *Excerpta medica,* 191-198

Kolb, T.; M.; Lichy, J.; Jeffrey, H. (2002). Comparison of the performance of screening mammography, physical examination, and breast ultrasound and evaluation of factors that influence them: An analysis of 27.825 patient evaluations. *Radiology,* 225: 165-175

Lenz, S. (2011). Breast ultrasound in office gynecology –Ten years of experience. *Ultraschall in Med,* 32: S3-S7

Madjar, H.; Ohlinger, R.; Mundinger, A.; Watermann, D.; Frenz, J. P.; Bader, W.; Schulz-Wendtland, R.; Degenhardt, F. (2006). BI-RADS-Analogue DEGUM Criteria for Findings in Breast Ultrasound - Consensus of the DEGUM Committee on Breast Ultrasound. *Ultraschall in Med* 27: 374-379

Madjar H., Mendelson E., B. (2008). *The practice of breast ultrasound.* 2nd revised edition. Thieme, ISBN 10-313124342, Stuttgart

Madjar, H.; Becker, S.; Doubek, K.; Horchler, T.; Mendoza, M.; Moisidis-Tesch, C.; Näther, B.; Niebling, K.; Pröls, U.; Schardt, A.-R.; Ulrich, S.; Zahn, U. (2010). Impact of Breast Ultrasound Screening in Gynecological Practice. *Ultraschall in Med,* 31: 289-295

Moon, W., K.; Shen, Y., W.; Huang, C., S.; Chiang, L., R.; Chang, R., F. (2011). Computer-aided diagnosis for the classification of breast masses in automated whole breast ultrasound images. *Ultrasound Med Biol,* 376: 539-548

Sever, A., R.; Mills, P.; Jones, S., E.; Cox, K.; Weeks, J.; Fish, D.; Jones, P., A. (2011). Preoperative sentinel node identification with ultrasound using microbubbles in patients with breast cancer. *AJR,* 2: 251-256

Stavros A., T. (2004). *Breast ultrasound.* Lippincott, Williams & Wilkins. ISBN 0-397-51624-X, Philadelphia

Teboul, M.; Halliwell, M. (1995). *Atlas of ultrasound and ductal echography of the breast.* Blackwell, ISBN 0-632-03329-0, London

Weismann C. (2006). Role of colour Doppler ultrasound in breast imaging. *EJC Supplements,* 4:41-42

Weismann C., Hergan K. (2007). Current status of 3D/4D volume ultrasound of the breast. *Ultraschall in Med* 28: 273-282

Yang, W.T.; Tse, G.M.K. (2004). Sonographic, mammographic and histopathologic correlation of symptomatic ductal carcinoma in situ. *AJR,* 182: 101-110

5

The Accuracy of Ultrasound in the Pre-Operative Localisation of Parathyroid Lesions in Primary Hyperparathyroidism: A Review of the Literature

S. Alford[1], W. Barber[1], G. Cheung[2] and K. Thoirs[1]
[1]*School of Health Sciences, University of South Australia*
[2]*Flinders Medical Centre, Bedford Park, South Australia*
Australia

1. Introduction

Primary hyperparathyroidism (PHPT) is caused by excessive autonomous secretion of parathormone (PTH), usually as a result of a parathyroid adenoma (80-85%), and less frequently due to parathyroid gland hyperplasia (15%-20%) or carcinoma (1%) (Kaplan et al.1991). Patients often suffer from mild subjective symptoms such as weakness and tiredness, but if untreated, symptoms progess to include dementia, depression, peptic ulcer disease, pancreatitis, constipation, renal calculi, and diffuse bone and joint pain (Clark 2003).

PHPT can be diagnosed by detecting elevated PTH and blood calcium levels (Carlier et al. 2008). The most effective treatment or cure for PHPT is parathyroidectomy, the surgical removal of the affected parathyroid glands. Surgery has traditionally been performed using a traditional bilateral neck exploration (BNE), but in recent times, minimally invasive parathyroidectomy (MIP) has replaced this approach as a first line surgical choice in the United States, Australia, and mainland Europe (Palazzo 2004). MIP compared to BNE neck exploration has comparable clinical outcomes and complications, but can reduce length of hospital stays and operating times by 50% (Udelsman 1999). Successful cure for PHPT using MIP depends on consistently reliable methods for localizing parathyroid lesions, so the surgeon can direct the dissection to the site of the abnormal parathyroid gland (Johnson et al. 2007). The success of the resection can be assessed by means of intraoperative intact parathyroid hormone (IOPTH) assay (Quiros et al. 2004). Surgeons experienced in MIP can explore both the upper and lower glands on the same side of the neck from a slightly enlarged incision if the localization study has not identified the lesion correctly, and in cases where preoperative localization has failed to identify a gland on the contralateral side, the surgeon may proceed to BNE.

The Nuclear Medicine (NM) Technetium 99m (Tc^{99m}) sestamibi examination is a common imaging choice to preoperatively localize diseased parathyroid glands (Levy et al. 2011). The Tc^{99m} sestamibi examination involves the injection of a radiopharmaceutical, made up of a radioisotope (Tc^{99m}) and a pharmaceutical tracing agent (sestamibi). A dual phased technique is used, where a gamma camera detects the radiation emitted from within the patient in an early phase at 15–30 minutes (Figure 1) and in a late phase at 2–4 hours (Figure 2) after intravenous administration of the radioisotope. Diseased parathyroid glands are detected based on the time-related differential washout of radioactivity between the thyroid gland and a parathyroid lesion. In diseased parathyroids there is a retention of Tc-99m sestamibi within the parathyroid in the second phase (Nguyen 1999). The disadvantages of NM localization examinations include that they use ionizing radiation, require an injection to the patient of a radiopharmaceutical (Levy et al. 2011) which carries a slight risk of adverse reactions (Mujtaba et al. 2007). NM studies also require a high level of patient cooperation to remain still for extended periods, which may be difficult in elderly, ill or confused patients. This is particularly important when integrated single-photon-emission computed tomography and computed tomography (SPECT/CT) systems (Figure 3), which are prone to misregistration errors due to patient movement (Bybel et al. 2008) are used to improve sensitivity.

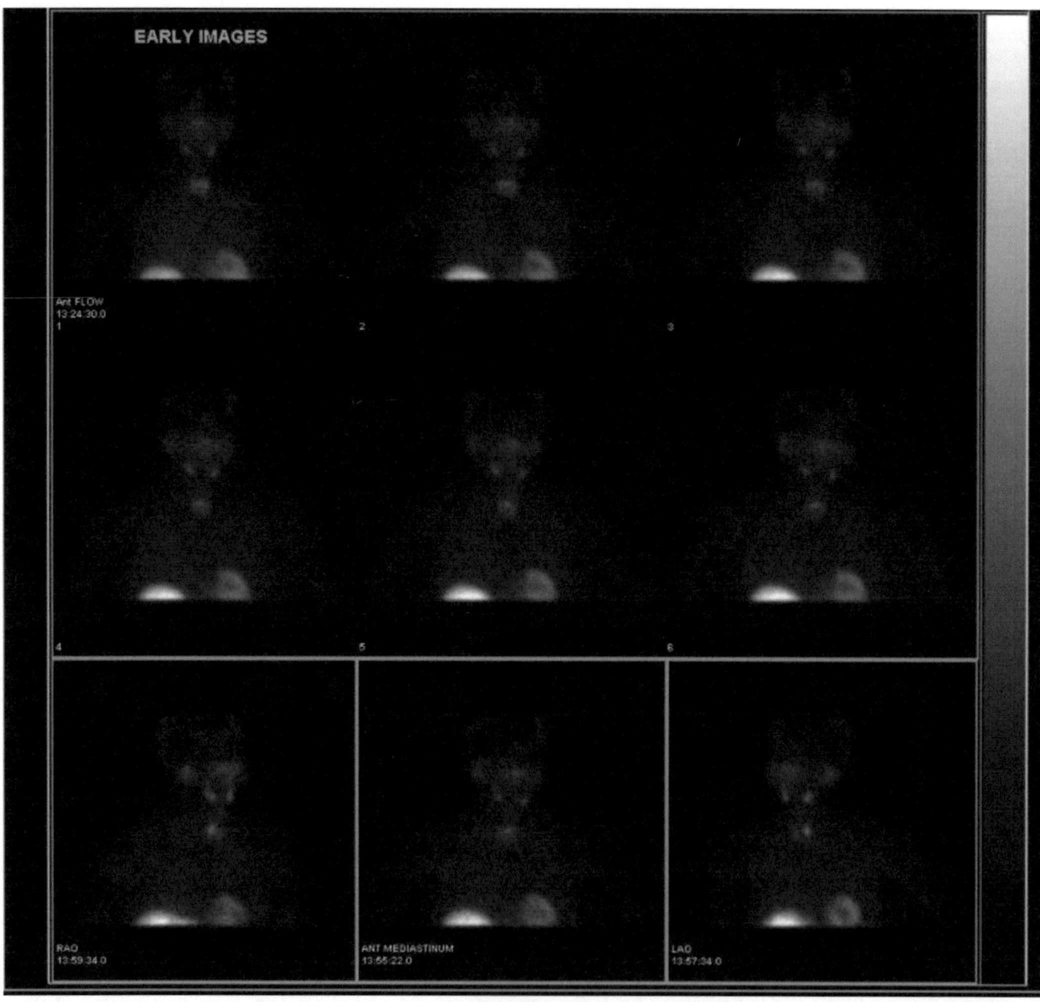

Fig. 1. Early phase parathyroid Nuclear Medicine scan. Image courtesy of Royal Adelaide Hospital, Department of Nuclear Medicine, PET & Bone Densitometry

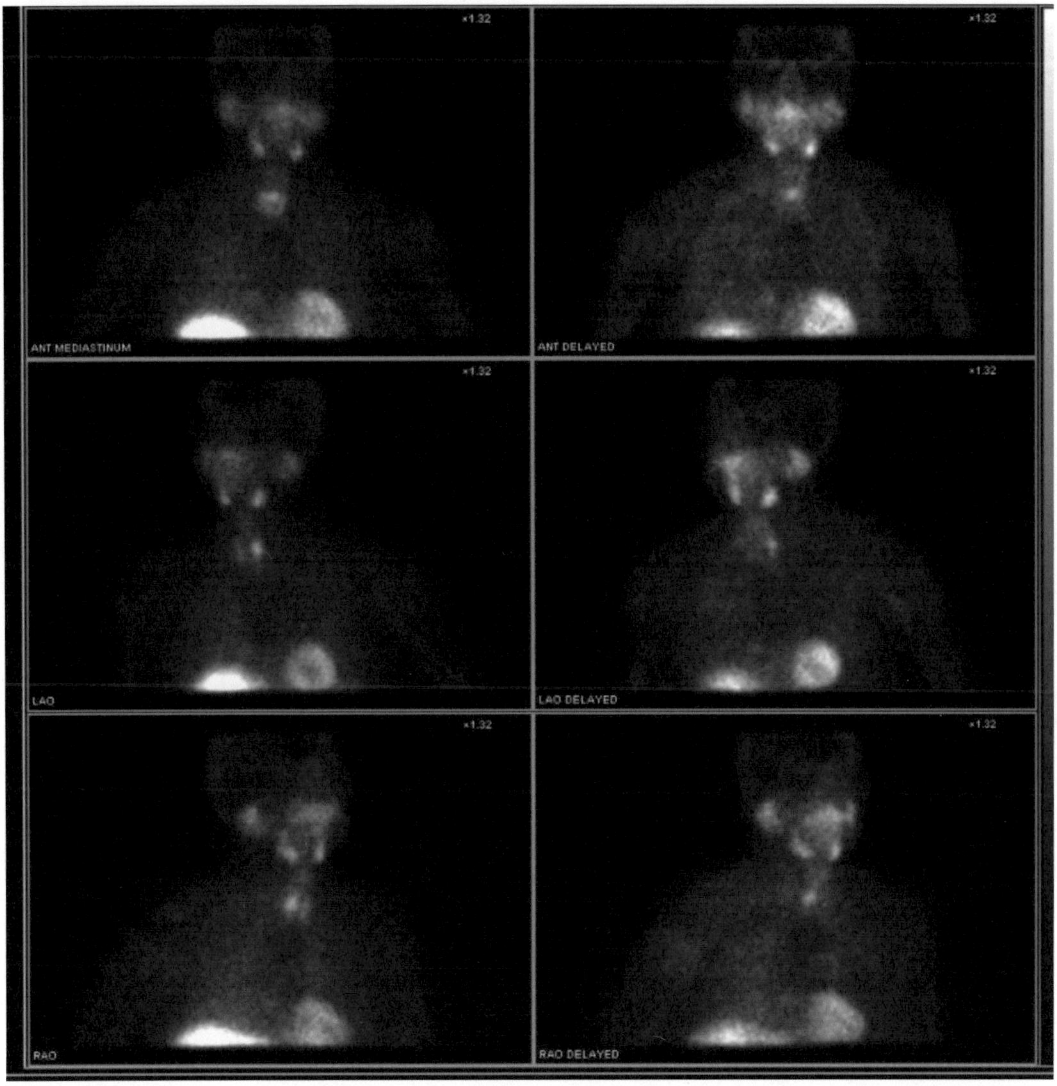

Fig. 2. Late phase parathyroid Nuclear Medicine scan demonstrating parathyroid lesion in superior mediastinum. Image courtesy of Royal Adelaide Hospital, Department of Nuclear Medicine, PET & Bone Densitometry

Parathyroid ultrasound (US) has emerged as an alternative or complementary localization procedure to NM techniques because it does not use ionizing radiation or an injection to the patient (Levy et al. 2011), and has greater tolerance for patient movement. US is considered to be one of the most cost-effective, quick and easy imaging modalities, but it has demonstrated variable performance over time and between varying clinical environments (Whiting et al. 2003; Mihai et al. 2009) when localizing parathyroid lesions. Older studies, such as those by Liou et al. (1996) have shown US to have sensitivities and specificities up to 75 per cent and 95 per cent respectively, compared to Tc^{99m} sestamibi which showed 87.5 per cent sensitivity and 100 per cent specificity.

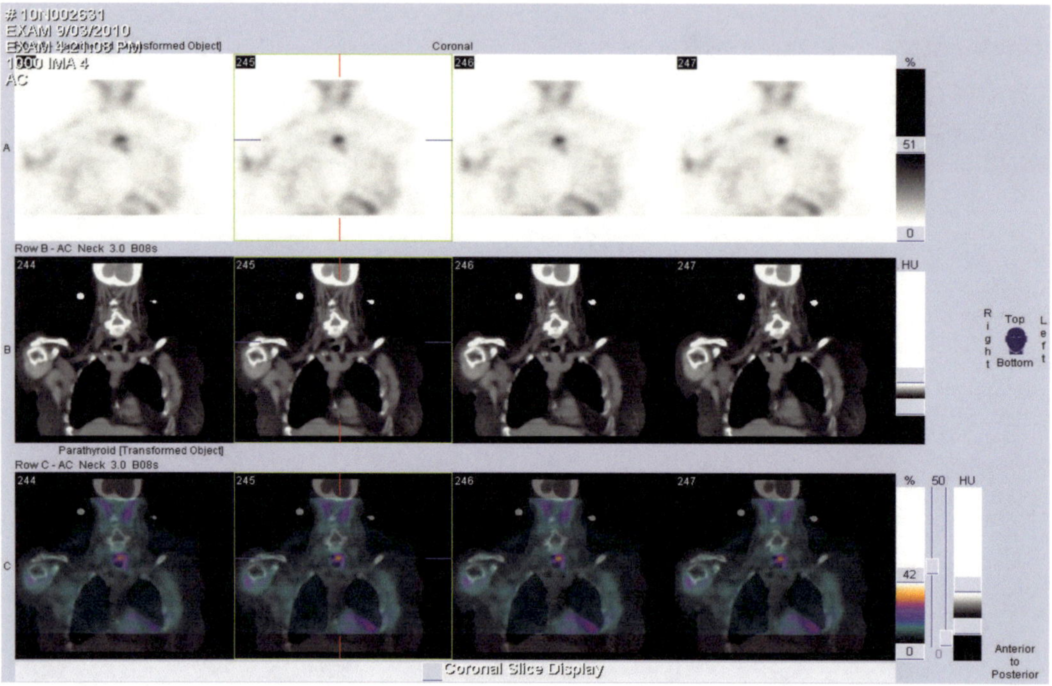

Fig. 3. SPECT/CT parathyroid Nuclear Medicine scan demonstrating parathyroid lesion in superior mediastinum. Image courtesy of Royal Adelaide Hospital, Department of Nuclear Medicine, PET & Bone Densitometry

Variability in the performance of US to localize parathyroid lesion may be due to the variability of the anatomical location of the glands themselves. The possibility of ectopic glands and variation in the number of glands presents challenges for US (Yeh et al. 2006), as the field of view in each image is small and requires a careful and thorough scanning technique. Ectopic glands may be obscured in US examinations by bony and air filled structures that impede US penetration. For example, retro-sternal, retro-oesphageal and retro-tracheal glands are difficult to localize with US. Intra-thyroid lesions (Figure 4), which are rare, may also be difficult to localize because they are difficult to differentiate from thyroid nodules (Kobayashi et al. 1999).

The US equipment and sonographer expertise and protocols also have the potential to influence the accuracy of the ultrasound examination (Mihai et al. 2009). US requires comprehensive and reproducible protocols as it is very operator-dependent, and localization accuracy may vary according to the level of experience of the sonographer (Yeh et al. 2006). The size of diseased glands may be very small and therefore the successful localization of very small structures with US may be constrained by the resolution of the ultrasound system (Lo et al. 2007). Older US units can be compromised by image quality compared to modern equipment, and this may have contributed to the lower rates of accuracy reported in older studies (Levy et al. 2011). The use of colour Doppler (Figure 6) to identify enlarged feeding arteries to parathyroid adenomas has also been reported to increase detection rates (Reeder et al. 2002).

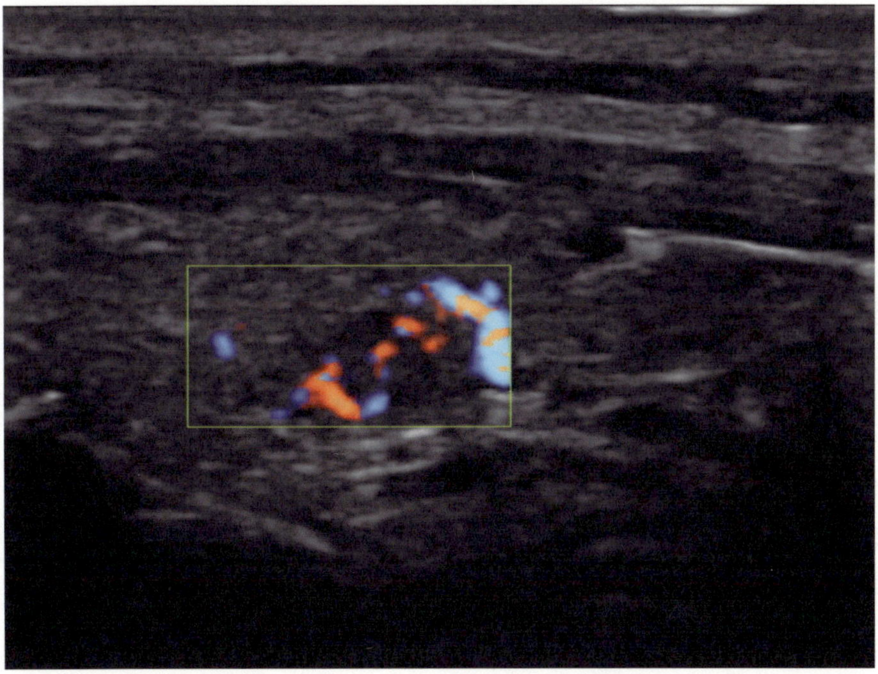

Fig. 4. Intra-thyroid parathyroid adenoma demonstrated on ultrasound image. Image courtesy of Division of Medical Imaging, Flinders Medical Centre

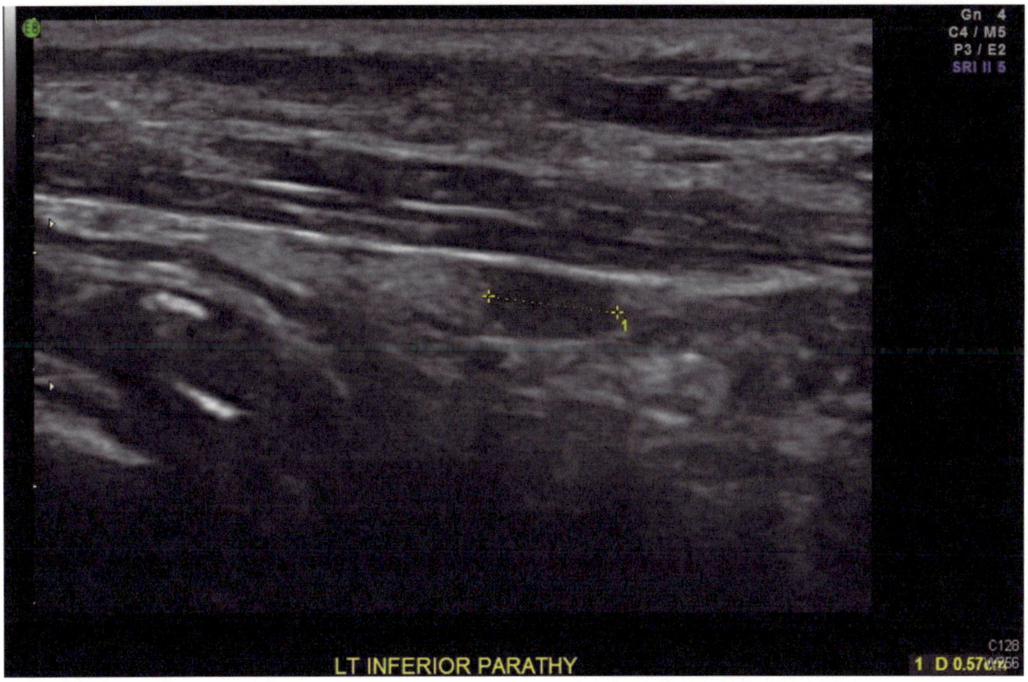

Fig. 5. Small inferior parathyroid adenoma demonstrated on ultrasound image. Image courtesy of Division of Medical Imaging, Flinders Medical Centre

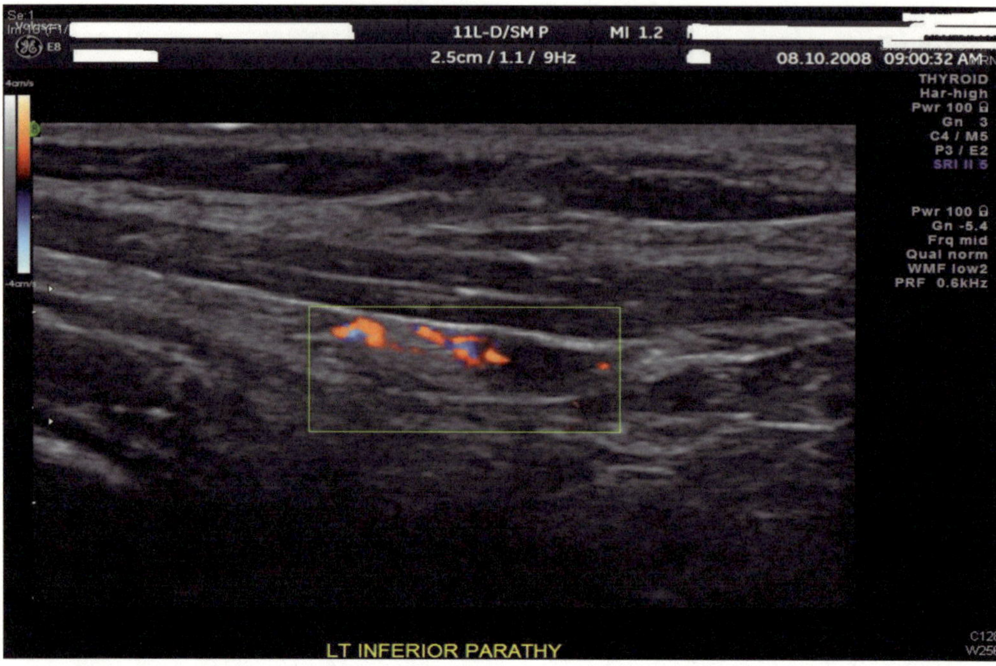

Fig. 6. Small inferior parathyroid adenoma demonstrated on ultrasound image. A feeding artery is demonstrated with the application of Colour Doppler. Image courtesy of Division of Medical Imaging, Flinders Medical Centre

Many medical imaging/radiology departments offer both NM and US studies to localize parathyroid lesions preoperatively. Imaging departments should periodically assess their performance through audits for quality assurance purposes. Benchmark performance levels can be identified through critical review and synthesis of the literature. With this in mind we performed a systematic review of the recent literature to determine the current performance of preoperative parathyroid US localizing parathyroid lesions in PHPT. We included an assessment of NM localization studies as a comparison.

2. Systematic review

2.1 Search strategy

A search of the literature was performed on 25 May, 2011 using Medline via Ovid, EMBASE via Ovid, ScienceDirect and Scopus databases (Table 1). Five groups of terms were searched using the Boolean-phrase methodology.

Category	Search terms
Population	parathyroid* or hyperparathyroid*
Intervention	ultraso* or sonograph*
Intervention	efficacy or effective* or accura* or precis* or sensitiv* or specific*
Outcome	localis* or localis* or locat* or identif*
Population/Assessment	preoperative or pre-operative or pre operative

Table 1. Search strategy

2.2 Inclusion and exclusion criteria

We included prospective studies published after 2003 in English, which focused on the performance of preoperative US and NM localization of parathyroid lesions in PHPT. In order to be included the studies must have described a randomized or consecutive sampling strategy, cases must have been selected based on suspicion or diagnosis of PHPT and all cases must have undergone US, NM and parathyroidectomy. The results of both US and NM must have been compared to surgical findings, with or without postoperative hormone assays. Studies were excluded if they were not available in English. The review excluded all articles reporting on case studies, literature reviews, paediatric focused studies, animals and retrospective study designs. Studies which focused on intra-operative or endoscopic ultrasound were also excluded.

2.3 Search results

The search returned a total of 1205 articles (Table 2), of which 313 duplicates were removed. Twenty-seven articles in languages other than English were excluded. Based on titles alone, 798 studies were excluded after application of the selection criteria. Two authors both reviewed the abstracts of the remaining 67 articles and analyzed them using the inclusion and exclusion criteria. Seven articles were selected to be included in the review (Figure 7).

Database	Limitations applied	Results
Medline via OvidSP	English language, journal article, 2002 to 25 May 2011, human subjects	150
EMBASE via OvidSP	English language, article, 2002 to 25 May 2011, human subjects	155
ScienceDirect	Journal article, 2002 to 25 May 2011	556
Scopus	English language, article, 2002 to 25 May 2011, human or humans	344

Table 2. Search results

All the studies identified from the search were well-designed non-experimental descriptive studies, with no identified randomized clinical trials. The methodological quality of the articles was assessed using an adapted QUADAS checklist (Whiting et al. 2003) (Table 3) by two independent reviewers, with discrepancies between reviewers resolved by consensus. The articles were all of similar methodological quality.

All seven studies examined populations of patients who had a diagnosis of PHPT which was established by elevated PTH and calcium levels in the blood. In all studies, diagnosis was confirmed by successful surgical removal of parathyroid pathology with or without post surgical follow up histology and blood assays. Five studies additionally confirmed surgical success with follow up assays (Bhansali et al. 2006; Carlier et al. 2008; Lo et al. 2007; Prasannan et al. 2007; Shaheen et al. 2008), and three studies confirmed the nature of the excised lesion(s) with histology (Mihai et al. 2006; Lo et al. 2007; Carlier et al. 2008).

The US and NM localization examinations were always performed prior to surgery, therefore bias was minimized due to blinding to the surgical results. All studies, except two,

(Mihai et al. 2009, Prasannan et al. 2007) stated that the US was interpreted without knowledge of the results of the NM scan. While, this approach limits risk of contamination between the two localization studies and provides an independent assessment of the localization study's performance, it does not mirror usual clinical practice. In clinical practice each test is often treated as complementary to the other, and is not interpreted in isolation with the alternate test. The combination of the findings from both US and NM has been proven to increase the overall sensitivity in identifying and localizing parathyroid lesions (Bhansali et al. 2006; Lo et al. 2007; Sugg et al. 2004).

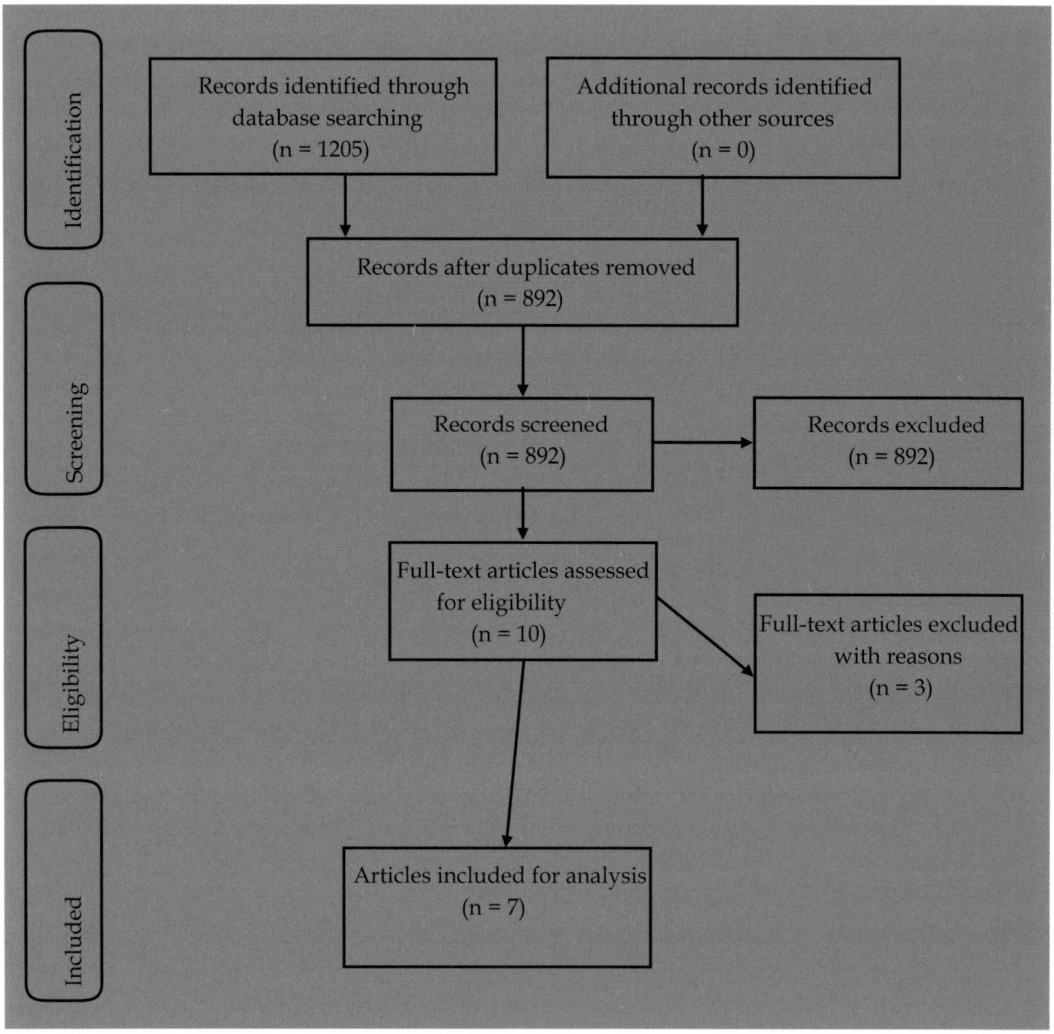

Fig. 7. Flow chart of article selection process

All studies, excepting two, described the ultrasound equipment and the experience or credentials of the operator, the type of NM technique used, the type of surgical technique and cut off values of normal for post- and pre-operative blood assays. This information is important when interpreting and transferring the findings to other settings, especially when

Item	Bhansali et al. (2006)	Carlier et al. (2008)	Lo et al. (2007)	Mihai et al. (2006)	Prasannan et al. (2007)	Shaheen et al. (2008)	Sugg et al. (2004)
1 Was the spectrum of patients representative of the patients who will receive the test in practice?	Yes	Yes	Yes	Yes	Yes	Yes	Yes
2 Were selection criteria clearly described?	No	No	No	No	No	No	No
3 Is the reference standard likely to correctly classify the target condition?	Yes	Yes	Yes	Yes	Yes	Yes	Yes
4 Is the time period between reference standard and index test short enough to be reasonably sure that the target condition did not change between the two tests?	Unclear	Unclear	Unclear	Unclear	Unclear	Unclear	Unclear
5 Did the whole sample or a random selection of the sample, receive verification using a reference standard of diagnosis?	Yes	Yes	Yes	Yes	Yes	Yes	Yes
6 Did patients receive the same reference standard regardless of the index test result?	Yes	No	No	No	No	Yes	No
7 Was the reference standard independent of the index test (i.e. the index test did not form part of the reference standard?)	Yes	Yes	Yes	Yes	Yes	Yes	Yes
8 Was the execution of the index test described in sufficient detail to permit replication of the test?	Yes	Yes	Yes	Yes	No	No	Yes
9 Was the execution of the reference standard described in sufficient detail to permit its replication?	No	No	No	Yes	Yes	Yes	Yes
10 Were the index test results interpreted without knowledge of the results of the reference standard?	Yes	Yes	Yes	Yes	Yes	Yes	Yes
11 Were the reference standard results interpreted without knowledge of the results of the index test?	Unclear	No	No	No	No	Unclear	Unclear
12 Were the same clinical data available when test results were interpreted as would be available when the test is used in practice?	Unclear	Unclear	Unclear	Unclear	Unclear	Unclear	Unclear
13 Were uninterpretable/ intermediate test results reported?	No	No	No	No	No	No	No
14 Were withdrawals from the study explained?	Unclear	Unclear	Yes	Unclear	Unclear	Unclear	Unclear

Legend: Cells shaded white = Yes; Cells shaded grey = Unclear; Cells shaded black = No.

Table 3. Methodologic quality of articles

tests and procedures are complex and variable. The exceptions were Prasannan et al. (2007) who provided no information on the execution of the Tc^{99m} sestamibi scan, and Shaheen et al. (2008) who provided no information on the experience or credentials of the operator(s). Whilst most studies used pre-operative or post-operative hormone assays, only three studies (Bhansali et al. 2006; Prasannan et al. 2007; Sugg et al. 2004) provided clear cut-off values for normal or abnormal assays.

Only two studies in this review, applied a standardized surgical approach for all patients (Bhansali et al. 2006; Shaheen et al. 2008), with a trend in the studies to mirror current clinical practice, and adjust the surgical approach (MIP or BNE), based on the results of the localization studies (Quiros et al.2004). Common surgical practice is to still to use BNE in cases of suspected multiglandular disease and those with equivocal pre-operative localization (Johnson et al. 2007). The potential bias arising from using more than one approach to confirm the presence and location of lesions is probably minimal because there were few cases reported across the studies where parathyroid lesions were not found at surgery.

All studies appeared to be undertaken under clinical conditions where patients were undergoing diagnosis and treatment in healthcare settings. There was some lack of clarity in areas of reporting which impact on the ability to transfer results to other clinical settings, and also may be sources of bias. For example, there was lack of clarity around the selection criteria used, the time period between the localization studies and the surgery, and no study reported uninterpretable, indeterminate or intermediate results. Only one study (Lo et al. 2007) accounted for withdrawals from the study.

2.4 Study and subject characteristics

A summary of the subject and study characteristics of the articles is demonstrated in Table 4.

Six studies compared US and NM to surgical findings (Bhansali et al. 2006; Carlier et al. 2008, Lo et al. 2007; Prasannan et al. 2007; Shaheen et al. 2008; Sugg et al. 2004). Mihai et al (2006) differed by not directly comparing US to surgical findings, instead comparing it to NM only, then comparing NM to surgical findings.

Across the studies a total of 740 patients were examined, comprising 534 females (72 per cent) and 206 males (28 per cent), a distribution which closely reflects the epidemiology of PHPT (Ljunghall et al. 1991).The 740 patients had 798 pathologic parathyroid glands, comprising mostly of single adenomas (86 per cent), with a lower prevalence of double adenomas (3 per cent), hyperplasia (10 per cent), carcinoma (n=0.5 per cent) and one paraganglioma (n=0.5 per cent).

US was performed by experienced radiologists in two studies (Carlier et al. 200; Lo et al. 2007), experienced sonographers in two studies (Bhansali et al. 2006; Sugg et al. 2004), a parathyroid surgeon in one study (Prasannan et al. 2007) and the operator was not specified by Mihai et al. (2006) or Shaheen et al. (2008). Two studies (Lo et al. 2007; Shaheen et al. 2008) indicated that multiple operators were involved in performing the ultrasound examinations in their studies. US examinations were performed using linear array, small footprint or unspecified shaped transducers with frequencies of 5-12 MHz, all of which would be found to be used in current clinical practice.

		Bhansali et al. (2006)	**Carlier et al. (2008)**	**Lo et al. (2007)**	**Mihai et al. (2006)**	**Prasannan et al. (2007)**	**Shaheen et al. (2008)**	**Sugg et al. (2004)**
n		46 (33 female, 13 male)	51 (38 female, 13 male)	100 (70 female, 30 male)	155 (115 female, 40 male)	130 (97 female, 33 male)	25 (8 female, 17 male)	233 (173 female, 60 male)
Age	Mean	37.1	56	55.5 MEDIAN	62.1	59.1	18-25 RANGE	56

Table 4. Summary of patients

The most common NM tests were planar Tc^{99m} sestamibi, dual radionuclide subtraction (Tc^{99m}/Tl^{201}), and dual phase Tc^{99m} sestamibi. Patients underwent a range of NM techniques including conventional single photon emission computed tomography (C-SPECT) and pinhole SPECT (P-SPECT).

BNE was performed on 310 patients, and the remaining 430 underwent MIP. Two studies (Bhansali et al. 2006; Shaheen et al. 2008) performed BNE on all subjects. In the other studies the decision to perform MIP rather than BNE was made when the results of the US and NM localization examinations were concordant (Carlier et al. 2008), when suspected lesions were Tc^{99m} sestamibi positive (Lo et al. 2007), or on surgeon's preference (Carlier et al. 2008). It was common procedure in the studies to assess the success of the surgery in removing the parathyroid lesion(s) by performing a post-operative or intra-operative PTH assay, with or without corresponding serum calcium assays. A return of normal assay values was confirmatory for surgical success. Some studies reported that assays were undertaken intra-operatively (Lo et al. 2007; Shaheen et al. 2008; Sugg et al. 2004), and others reported the hormone assays to be taken postoperatively, with follow up which varied between 1 week and 3 years duration (Carlier et al. 2008; Bhansali et al. 2006; Mihai et al. 2006; Prasannan et al. 2007).

2.5 Results

Table 5 provides a summary of the results. Overall, US demonstrated lower sensitivities (51 to 86 per cent), to correctly localize parathyroid lesions compared to NM (64 to 98 per cent). Four studies reported the sensitivities of US to be comparable or slightly less than NM (Bhansali et al. 2006; Lo et al. 2007; Mihai et al. 2006; Shaheen et al. 2008). Two studies reported US to have higher detection rates than NM (Prasannan et al. 2007, Sugg et al. 2004). One study reported US to have significantly lower sensitivity (51 per cent) compared with planar Tc^{99m} sestamibi (75 per cent), conventional SPECT (82 per cent), and planar SPECT (87 per cent) (Carlier et al. 2008). Three studies analyzed data specifically for single gland disease (SGD) and multi-gland disease (MGD) and found US to have higher sensitivity (73-82 per cent) compared to NM (45 to 64 per cent) in identifying MGD (Bhansali et al. 2006; Shaheen et al. 2008; Sugg et al. 2004). There were no apparent trends to suggest that one NM imaging localization technique was better than any other.

2.6 Discussion

Our initial search revealed 892 articles, demonstrating a wide breadth of research into the pre-operative localization of parathyroid lesions. We restricted the review to include only prospective studies with consecutive or randomized sampling. Prospective studies are more easily controlled, and allow more rigorous methodologies including the use of blinding (Euser et al. 2009). The exclusion of retrospective studies significantly reduced the number of studies included in this review, as retrospective studies are more widely reported (Mihai, Simon & Hellman 2009) and prospective studies are less frequently reported due to long data collection periods when this study design is used. Articles prior to 2003 were excluded to capture the most advanced imaging technologies. Older studies using less sensitive equipment have demonstrated lower sensitivities for both US and NM (Ruda et al. 2005). However, the descriptions of US techniques were mostly limited to the operator and basic specifications of the transducer, rather than the make and model of the equipment, and it was not possible to assess if the differences in results were influenced by the capabilities of the technology used in each study.

Despite the limitations of our selection criteria, and resulting narrow range of studies included, we found wide variations in sensitivity rates for both US and NM localization examinations. Sensitivity rates for the detection of parathyroid lesions for preoperative US localization examinations ranged from 51 to 85.7 per cent and ranged from 64 to 98 per cent for NM localization examinations. In most cases successful localization was defined when the lesion(s) was correctly identified on the correct side of the neck. This is an important consideration for surgical planning. The sensitivities rates were similar to what was reported in a similar review (Mihai et al. 2009) which reported ultrasound sensitivity rates of 51 to 96 per cent, and NM sensitivity rates from 34 to 100 per cent. The wider variation reported by Mihai et al. (2009) is likely due to their inclusion of retrospective studies, short case series and older studies which were excluded from our review.

There are a number of factors that may impact on the performance of US in detecting parathyroid lesions including the expertise of the operator, the small size of some lesions, ectopic gland positions, multinodular thyroid goiter and parathyroid hyperplasia (Levy et al. 2011; Mihai et al. 2009; Ruda et al. 2005). Two studies in this review referred to the impact of lesion size on sensitivity rates; Prasannan et al. (2007) stated that US was more sensitive when detecting lesions over 1270 milligrams and Bhansali et al. (2006) stated that sensitivity reached 92.3 per cent sensitivity for glands weighing over five grams. While the sensitivity of US was shown to be lower in smaller glands (Bhansali et al. 2006; Prasannan et al. 2007), US still demonstrates the capability to detect lesions as small as 1.2 grams in weight (Bhansali et al. 2006). Colour Doppler US can be important in the differential diagnosis of a suspected lesion, demonstrating superior feeding vessels in parathyroid glands, as opposed to hilar flow in lymph nodes. However, the use of Doppler US in the differential diagnosis of parathyroid lesions was only reported in one study in this review (Prasannan et al. 2007).

The position of parathyroid lesions also influenced detection rates. The sensitivity of US to detect and localize ectopic parathyroid lesions was notably lower than the sensitivity when localizing those lesions in normal anatomical positions and appeared to be unrelated to the sizes of the ectopic lesions (Bhansali et al. 2006, Carlier et al. 2008). Across the seven studies, twenty ectopic glands were established at surgery. The overall detection rate of retro-sternal glands was low, regardless of their size. The study with the highest number of ectopic glands gave the lowest sensitivity (51 per cent) (Carlier 2008), and the highest sensitivity was recorded in studies with no or few ectopic glands in their series (Prasannan et al. 2007; Shaheen et al. 2008).

Bhansali et al. (2006) reported that US missed several ectopic glands which were located in retro-oesophageal and mediastinal positions. Both US and NM were more likely to identify ectopic lesions in the neck than those in retro-sternal positions (Carlier et al. 2008). For US, this is likely due to the difficulty in scanning through the narrow sternal notch, to avoid surrounding bony structures. NM is less affected by bone and gas than US, but despite this Bhansali et al. (2006) reported that NM missed the same retro-sternal lesions that were undetected using US.

It is not clear if the expertise of the US operator influences results. In studies which were clear in reporting the expertise of operators, radiologists appeared to be less successful in US localization compared to sonographers. Only one study (Prasannan et al. 2007) reported on surgeon performance of US localization, with good results (sensitivity 82%). Surgeons may have an advantage over other operators by receiving direct feedback on their performance when they perform surgery on the cases they examined with US.

Bhansali et al. (2006), Prasannan et al. (2007) and Sugg et al. (2004) assessed cases with single gland disease (SGD) separately to those with multi gland disease (MGD). US localization studies were better than NM in identifying MGD and also found that US was more effective in detection of MGD than SGD (Bhansali et al. 2006; Sugg et al. 2004), Caution should however be exercised when interpreting this finding due to the low prevalence of MGD compared to SGD.

The presence of thyroid nodules or multinodular goiter was also noted to reduce the sensitivity of US in the detection and localization of parathyroid lesions (Lo et al. 2007).

The variations in the reported performance of US and NM may also be influenced by other factors such as differences in selection criteria, and differences in cut off values of hormone assays both to diagnose PHPT in patients, and to confirm surgical success. These factors may have not had a large effect, but should not be discounted.

Differences in detection rates between US and NM may be due to the nature of the imaging in these techniques. Nuclear medicine scanning relies on a physiological process, and this is reflected in observations by Mihai et al. (2006) that there were lower detection rates for adenomas with predominantly chief cells, and higher detection rates for adenomas with oxyphil cells and mixed cells in NM scanning. Additionally, false positives may occur in NM scanning when non-parathyroid tissue uptakes Tc^{99m} sestamibi (Carlier et al. 2008). US instead relies on structural changes, and false negatives may result when sound reflective tissues such as bone and gas limits the identification of retro-sternal, retro-tracheal and retro-oesophageal lesions (Mihai et al. 2009). False positives may occur in US localization studies, when other structures such as lymph nodes are mistaken for parathyroid glands.

It has been suggested that both US and NM localization examinations should be performed for preoperative localization of parathyroid lesions (Mihai et al. 2009), to determine whether

		Bhansali et al. (2006)	Carlier et al. (2008)	Lo et al. (2007)	Mihai et al. (2006)	Prasannan et al. (2007)	Shaheen et al. (2008)	Sugg et al. (2004)
Surgery Type	BNE	46	28	34	63	28	25	86
	MIP	0	23	66	92	102	0	147
Ectopic glands		N=1 (retro-oesphageal)	N=11, (6 posterior, 3 thryothymic ligament, 1 mediastinal, 1 intra-thyroid)	N=1 (carotid sheath)	N=7 (retrosternal)	none	N=2 (mediastinum)	N=2 (mediastinum)
Conditions	US Operator	Experienced Sonographer	Experienced Radiologist	Radiologist	Single Experienced Operator	Surgeon	Not Stated	Experienced Sonographers
	US Transducer	Linear array 7.5-10 MHz	7-12 MHz	10 MHz	Linear Array Small Footprint 15 MHz	Linear Array 5-10 MHz	12 MHz	Linear Array 7-9 MHz
	NM Scan Type	Dual Phase Tc99m Sestamibi, Dual Radionuclide Subtraction Tc99m/Tl201, C-T SPECT	Dual Phase Subtraction Tc99mO4/Tc99m sestamibi, C-SPECT, P-SPECT	Tc99m sestamibi, C-SPECT	Tc99m sestamibi	Tc99m sestamibi	Tc99m sestamibi	Tc99m sestamibi
Reference Standard	Surgical Findings	√	√	√	√	√	√	√
	Histopathology	√	√	√	√	√		√
	Post/intra operative Assay	Post Ca and iPTH	Six Month	Quick PTH		Ca and iPTH	Intra PTH	Intra PTH
NM results known		no	no	no	Not stated	Not stated	no	no
Results	Total number of Lesions	53	55	100	155	130	28	278
	Lesions detected on US (n)	31/42 SGD 9/11 MGD	28/55	56/100	104/155	103/130	20/22 SGD, 4/6 MGD	150/204 SGD, 27/74 MGD
	US Sensitivity	73% (for correct side)	51%	57% (for correct side)	57% (for correct side)	82% (for correct side)	91% (for correct side)	73% (13 cases incorrect for side)
	Lesions Detected on NM (n)	41/42 SGD 5/11 MGD	Planar Scintigraphy 42/55, C-SPECT 45/55, P-SPECT 48/55	85/100	103/155	102/130	21/22 SGD, 5/6 MGD	130/204 SGD 15/74 MGD
	NM sensitivity	98%	76%, 82%, 87%	89%	93%	79%	95%	64%

Key: BNE = Bilateral Neck Exploration;Ca=serum calcium level; MIP = Minimally Invasive Parathyroidectomy; n.s. = Not Stated; % = per cent; MHz = megahertz; PTH = Parathyroid Hormone; iPTH = Intact Parathyroid Hormone; IOPTH = Intraoperative Parathyroid Hormone Assay; SGD = Single Gland Disease; MGD = Multi Gland Disease; C-SPECT = Conventional Single Photon Emission Computed Tomography; P-SPECT = Pinhole Single Photon Emission Computed Tomography; SPECT = Single Photon Emission Computed Tomography; Tc99m = Technetium 99m; Tl201 = Thallium 201; O4 = Oxygen 4

Table 5. Key findings

the patient is a viable candidate for MIP. The dependence of NM on physiologic changes, and the dependence of US on anatomic changes supports the argument to use the two techniques as complementary localization techniques. This approach was further supported in our review, with five studies demonstrating improvement in sensitivity when a combination of two localization examinations were employed (Bhansali et al. 2006; Lo et al. 2007; Prasannan et al. 2007; Shaheen et al. 2008; Sugg et al. 2004).

Most studies reported sensitivity (Bhansali et al. 2006, Carlier et al. 2008, Lo et al. 2007, Prasannan et al. 2007, Shaheen et al. 2008) as an outcome measure of the performance of the localization studies. Approximately half of the studies also reported positive predictive value (PPV) (Bhansali et al. 2006; Lo et al. 2007; Prasannan et al. 2007; Shaheen et al. 2008). PPV is influenced by the prevalence of the target condition, with high prevalence rates resulting in artificially elevated PPV rates. The sample populations in this review consisted of patients with recognized and confirmed parathyroid disease (i.e. 100 per cent prevalence), therefore limiting the relevance of the PPV. Other measurements of localization performance included detection rates (Mihai et al 2006; Shaheen et al. 2008; Sugg et al. 2004), accuracy (Lo et al. 2007) and specificity (Carlier et al. 2008). Specificity of US and NM in identifying and localizing parathyroid lesions is not widely reported. Patients are usually conclusively diagnosed using clinical examinations and blood tests prior to undergoing imaging, which is primarily for localization rather than diagnosis. In addition to this, most prospective studies using surgical findings as a reference standard only include patients that have at least one lesion as it is unethical to operate on an unaffected patient, and as such there should be no true-negative results from which to calculate specificity.

2.7 Conclusion

The aim of this review was to investigate the effectiveness of US as a localization technique for pre-operatively detecting and localizing parathyroid lesions. The rationale behind this was to establish benchmark sensitivity rates in order to set best practice goals for departmental audits. Audits are valuable not only as an assessment of performance, but also can be used to improve professional practice (Ridder et al. 2008). The results of the review determined that there was wide variability of US sensitivity in detecting parathyroid lesions, despite the studies being of similar quality and at the same level of evidence. Benchmarking is therefore difficult, without having a clear understanding of the reasons for the wide variability. Patient presentation, including the presence of pathologic ectopic parathyroid glands, are likely to have an impact on the sensitive rates for gland localization. Therefore benchmarking of detection rates will depend on the prevalence of ectopic glands in each setting. This review demonstrates that high detection rates using US can be achieved if there is low prevalence of pathologic ectopic glands.

3. References

Bhansali, A, Masoodi, S, Bhadada, S, Mittal, B, Behra, A & Singh, P (2006). Ultrasonography in detection of single and multiple abnormal parathyroid glands in primary hyperparathyroidism: Comparison with radionuclide scintigraphy and surgery. *Clinical Endocrinology*, vol. 65, no. 3, (September 2006), pp. 340-345, ISSN 1365-2265.

Byel, B, Brunken, R, DiFilippo, F, Neumnn, D, Wu, G, Cerqueira, M. (2008), SPECT /CT Imaging: Clinical Utility of an Emerging Technology, *Radiographics,* vo.28, no.4, (July-August 2008), pp.1097-1113, ISSN 0271-5333.

Carlier, T, Oudoux, A, Mirallie, E, Seret, A, Daumy, I, Leux, C, Bodet-Milin, C, Kraeber-Bodere, F & Ansquer, C (2008), 99mTc-MIBI pinhole SPECT in primary hyperparathyroidism: comparison with conventional SPECT, planar scintigraphy and ultrasonography, *European journal of nuclear medicine and molecular imaging,* vol. 35, no. 3, (March 2008), pp. 637-643, ISSN 1619-7070.

Clark O. (2003), How should patients with primary hyperparathyroidism be treated?[editorial], *Journal of Clinical Endocrinology and Metabolism,* vol.88, no. 7, (July 2003), pp. 3011–3014, ISSN 0021-972X.

Euser, AM, Zoccali, C, Jager, K & Dekker, F (2009), Cohort Studies: Prospective versus Retrospective, *Nephron Clinical Practice,* vol. 113, no. 3, (August 2009), pp. 214-217, ISSN 1660-8151.

Johnson, N, Tublin, M, Ogilvie, J. (2007), Review: Parathyroid Imaging: Technique and Role in the Preoperative Evaluation of Primary Hyperparathyroidism, *American Journal of Roentgenology,* vol. 188, no. 6, (June 2007), pp. 1706-1715, ISSN 1546-3141.

Kaplan, E, Yashiro, T, Salti, G. (1992), Primary hyperparathyroidism in the 1990s: choice of surgical procedures for this disease. *Annals of Surgery,* vol.215, no.215, no.4, (April 1992), pp. 300–316, 1528-1140.

Kobayashi, T, Man-I,M, Shin, E, Kikkawa, N, Kawahara, K, Kurata, A, Fukuda, H, Asakawa, H. (1999), Hyperfunctioning intrathyroid parathyroid adenoma: Report of two cases, *Surgery Today,* vol.29, no.8, (August 1999), pp.766-768, ISSN 0941-1291

Levy, J, Kandil, E, Yau, L, Cuda, J, Sheth, S & Tufano, R. (2011), Can ultrasound be used as the primary screening modality for the localization of parathyroid disease prior to surgery for primary hyperparathyroidism? A review of 440 cases, *Journal for oto-rhino-laryngology and its related specialties,* vol. 73, no. 2, (March 2011) pp. 116-120, ISSN 1423-0275.

Liou M, Huang H, Lin J, Huang BY, Hsueh C, Jeng L, Tzen KY. (1996), The accuracy of ultrasonography and 201Tl-99mTc subtraction scan in localization of parathyroid lesions, *Chang Gung Medical Journal,* vol. 19, no. 2, (June 1996) pp. 121-128.

Ljunghall S, Hellman P, Rastad J, Akerström G. (1991), Primary hyperparathyroidism: epidemiology, diagnosis and clinical picture, *World Journal Surgery,* vol. 15, no.6, (November-December 1991), pp.681-687, ISSN 0364-2313.

Lo, C, Lang, B, Chan, W, Kung, A & Lam, K. (2007), A prospective evaluation of preoperative localization by technetium-99m sestamibi scintigraphy and ultrasonography in primary hyperparathyroidism, *The American Journal of Surgery,* vol. 193, no. 2 February 2007), pp. 155-159, ISSN 0002-9610.

Mihai, R, Gleeson, F, Buley, I, Roskell, D & Sadler, G. (2006), Negative imaging studies for primary hyperparathyroidism are unavoidable: Correlation of sestamibi and high-resolution ultrasound scanning with histological analysis in 150 patients, *World Journal of Surgery,* vol. 30, no. 5, (May 2006) pp. 697-704, ISSN 0364-2313.

Mihai, R, Simon, D & Hellman, P. (2009), Imaging for primary hyperparathyroidism-an evidence-based analysis, *Langenbeck's Archives of Surgery,* vol. 394, no. 5, (September 2009) pp. 765-784, ISSN 1435-2443.

Mujtaba, B, Adenaike, M, Yaganti, V, Mujtaba, N & Jain, D. (2007), Anaphylactic reaction to Tc-99m sestamibi (Cardiolite) during pharmacologic myocardial perfusion imaging, *Journal of Nuclear Cardiology,* vol. 14, no. 2, (April 2007), pp. 256-258, ISSN 1071-3581.

Nguyen B. (1999), Parathyroid imaging with Tc-99m sestamibi, planar and SPECT scintigraphy, *Radiographics,* vol.19, no.3, (May-June 1999), pp. 601-614, ISSN 0271-5333.

Palazzo F. (2004), Minimally invasive parathyroidectomy [editorial], *British Medical Journal,* vol. 328, (April 2004), pp.849-850, ISSN 0959-8138.

Prasannan, S, Davies, G, Bochner, M, Kollias, J & Malycha, P. (2007), Minimally invasive parathyroidectomy using surgeon-performed ultrasound and sestamibi, *ANZ Journal of Surgery,* vol. 77, no. 9, (September 2007), pp. 774-777, ISSN 1445-1433.

Quiros, R, Alioto, J, Wilhelm, A, Prinz, R. (2004) An Algorithm to Maximize Use of Minimally Invasive Parathyroidectomy, *Archives of Surgery,* vol. 139, no. 5, (May 2004), pp. 506-507, ISSN 0272-5533

Reeder, S, Desser, T, Weigel, R, Jeffrey R. (2002), Sonography in Primary Hyperparathyroidism: Review With Emphasis on Scanning Technique, *Journal of Ultrasound in Medicine,* vol.21, no. 5, (May 2002), pp. 539-552, ISSN 0278-4297.

Ruda, J, Hollenbeak, C & Stack, B. (2005), A systematic review of the diagnosis and treatment of primary hyperparathyroidism from 1995 to 2003, *Otolaryngology - Head and Neck Surgery,* vol. 132, no. 3, (March 2005), pp. 359-372, ISSN 0194-5998.

Shaheen, F, Chowdry, N, Gojwari, T, Wani, A & Khan, S. (2008), Role of cervical ultrasonography in primary hyperparathyroidism, *Indian Journal of Radiology and Imaging,* vol. 18, no. 4, (November 2008), pp. 302-305, ISSN 0971-3026.

Sugg, S, Krzywda, E, Demeure, M & Wilson, S. (2004), Detection of multiple gland primary hyperparathyroidism in the era of minimally invasive parathyroidectomy, *Surgery,* vol. 136, no. 6, (December 2004), pp. 1303-1309, ISSN 0039-6060.

Udelsman R. (2002), Six hundred fifty-six consecutive explorations for primary hyperparathyroidism, *Annals of Surgery,* vol. 235, no. 5, (May 2002), pp.665-672, ISSN 0003-4932.

Udelsman, R, Donovan, P & Sokoll, L. (2000), One Hundred Consecutive Minimally Invasive Parathyroid Explorations, *Annals of Surgery,* vol. 232, no. 3, (September 2000), pp. 331-339, ISSN 0003-4932.

Van de Ridder, J, Stokking, K, mCGaghie, W, ten Cate, O. (2008), What is feedback in Medical Education?, Medical Education, vo. 42, no. 2, (February 2008), pp. 189-197, ISSN 0308-0110.

Whiting, P, Rutjes, A, Reitsma, J, Bossuyt, P & Kleijnen, J. (2003), The development of QUADAS: a tool for the quality assessment of studies of diagnostic accuracy included in systematic reviews, *BMC Medical Research Methodology,* vol. 3, no. 25, (November 2003), pp. 25-37, ISSN 1471-2288.

Yeh, M, Barraclough, B, Sidhu, S, Sywak, M, Barraclough, B & Delbridge, L. (2006), Two hundred consecutive parathyroid ultrasound studies by a single clinician: The impact of experience, *Endocrine Practice,* vol. 12, no. 3, (May-June 2006), pp. 257-263, ISSN 1530-891X.

6

Lung Sonography

Rahul Khosla
Pulmonary & Critical Care Medicine
Veterans Affairs Medical Center, Washington DC
USA

1. Introduction

Lung ultrasonography has come of age and is a well established technique that can be performed quickly at patient's bedside to evaluate for various pathological conditions. This is despite the fact that air is not a favorable medium for transmission of ultrasound waves, and lung being an air filled organ, it was considered not amneable to ultrasonographic evaluation. Dr. Daniel Lichtenstein is one of the pioneers who has developed the field of lung sonography over the last two decades. He has contributed immensely by publishing numerous landmark articles that built the basic concepts of lung sonography. Since then there have been many other groups around the world who have published their findings that have helped to expand this field even further. This chapter will review the utility of lung sonography to evaluate for the following conditions:

1. Pleural effusions
2. Pneumothorax
3. Alveolar interstitial syndromes
4. Acute respiratory distress
5. Peripheral lung masses

2. Basic principle and technique of lung sonography

Body is made up of different biologic media (bone, muscle, fat, air, blood etc). The speed of sound and the acoustic impedance (resistance of a tissue to the passage of ultrasound) varies for different biological media, but the average value is assumed to be 1,540 m/sec (constant) for most human soft tissues. The difference in acoustic impedances of the two tissues at the interface, determines the extent of reflection and partly the attenuation of ultrasound waves. Greater the difference, more the reflection and attenuation. The speed of sound through air is only 300 m/sec with very low acoustic impedance. Hence at the tissue-air interface (chest wall-lung) there is a large difference in the acoustic impedance leading to reflection of ultrasound waves. For this reason ultrasonography of lung appears as homogenous amorphic grayness rather than a discreet structural entity. Disease processes that reduce the amount of air in the lung, extend to the periphery, or result in collection of fluid in the pleural space make the ultrasonographic examination of the lung feasible. Because of the difference in acoustic impedance and velocity of ultrasound between tissues, certain artifacts (described in the chapter) arise at the air-tissue-fluid-bone interface. These artifacts were recognized and described by the pioneers in this field, and form the background of pleura-pulmonary ultrasonography.

3. Equipment

There are many ultrasound machines currently available in the market, and any one of those with 2 dimensional (2D) capability can be used for lung sonography (Photo 1a). Doppler ultrasound is not needed for lung sonography. The new generation machines may contain software and filters to optimize image quality, mainly for echocardiography. The fundamentals of lung sonography have been built on artifacts that were described by the original investigators using a simple 2D machine and probe, without these filters. Some machine may allow the user to override the filter settings. A sector or curved-array transducer with a frequency of 2-5 MHz is suitable for lung sonography. Higher frequency probes can be used to visualize the pleura (Photo 1b). One of the basic principle of sonography is, higher the frequency, lower the depth of penetration, with a higher resolution. The foot-print of the transducer should fit well between the rib spaces to avoid rib artifact. Probe should be in the cranio-caudal orientation with the probe marker towards the head. Radiologists while performing sonography keep the screen marker towards the left side of the screen and cardiologist keep it towards the right. Lung sonography is a new field being developed over the last two decades by intensivists and pulmonologist. It is important to maintain a standard probe orientation and screen marker position. In this chapter the screen marker will be seen on the right side of the screen, with the probe marker towards the head, in the cranio-caudal orientation. Prior to beginning an examination, gain and depth should be adjusted. One can start with a higher depth and then zoom in on nearer structures. Gain should be adjusted to optimize image quality. The gain function

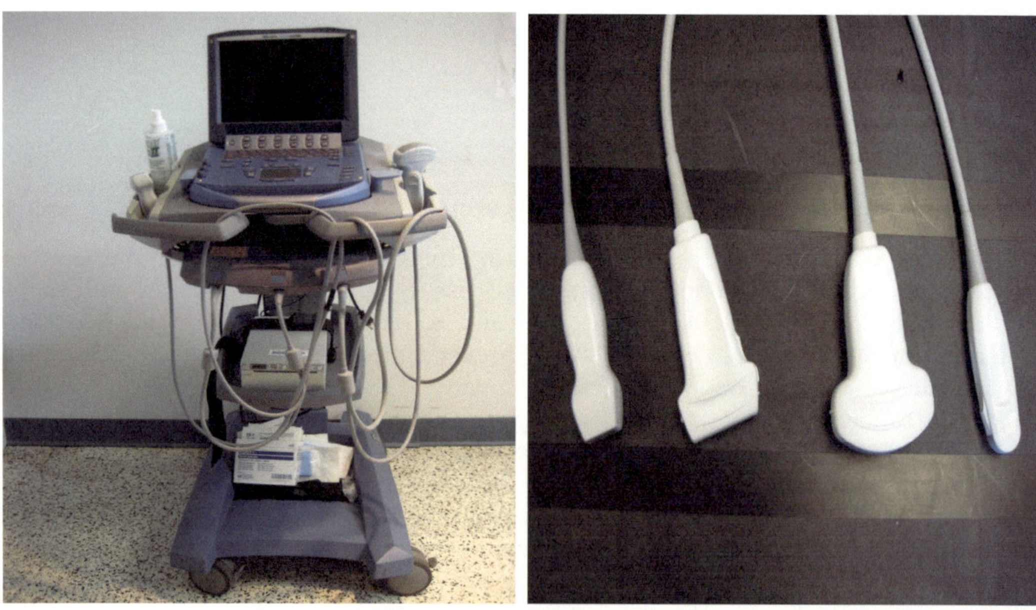

(a) (b)

Photo 1. (a) Portable ultrasound machine. (b) Various ultrasound probes compensates for attenuation (a reduction in sound amplitude) as sound travels deep into the body. The intensity of the returning signals can be amplified by the receiver upon arrival so that the displayed image is brighter and more visible on the screen. Gain can be adjusted for the near field, far field or the entire field (overall gain). If the gain is set too low, the image appears dark. Excessive increase in gain will add "noise" to the image, and make it appear too bright.

4. Ultrasound examination of lung

Depending upon patient's clinical condition and the reason for evaluation, the patient can be in supine, sitting, lateral decubitus, or semi-recumbent position. Critically ill patients in the intensive care unit are usually examined in supine, or partially rotated position. Transducer is in a cranio-caudal direction with the probe marker pointing cranially. The chest is divided into three zones, anterior (between sternum and anterior axillary line), lateral (between anterior and posterior axillary line), and posterior (between the posterior axillary line and spine) (Photo 2). The goal is to perform a complete lung examination by moving the probe along interspaces in a series of longitudinal scan lines. An organized approach is recommended with multiple points of examination in the anterior zone, followed by lateral zone, and if patients clinical condition permits, the posterior zone.

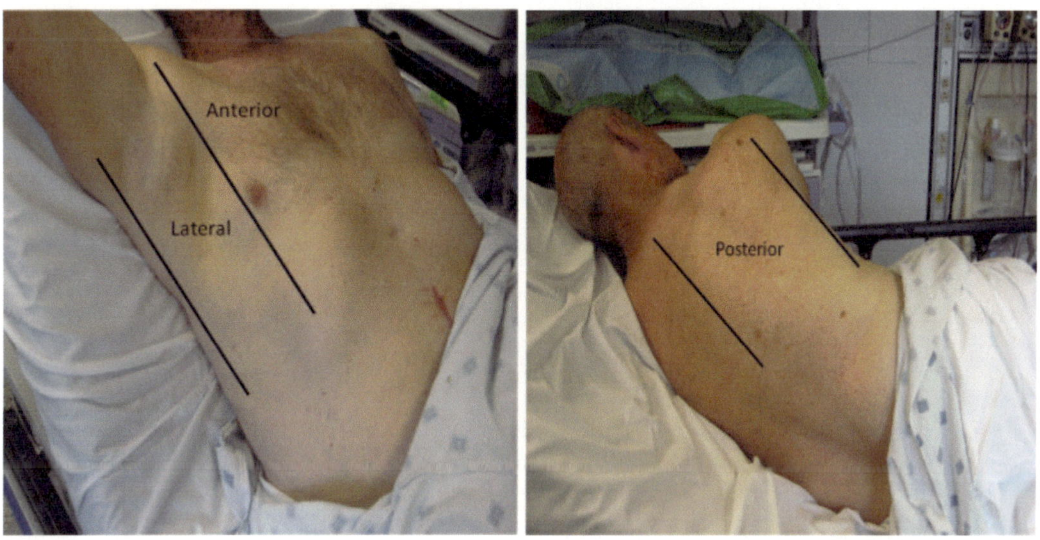

Photo 2. Anterior zone (between sternum and anterior axillary line). Lateral zone (between the anterior and posterior axillary line. Posterior zone (between posterior axillary line and the spine)

With the probe between two rib spaces, in the cranio-caudal direction, the normal ultrasound examination of the lung appears as shown in (Figure 7). Between the acoustic shadows of the two adjacent ribs, a hyperechoic horizontal pleural line is present, approximately 0.5 cm below the origin of the rib shadow. The pleural line is made up of the visceral and parietal pleural surfaces, and represents the interface between chest wall and aerated lung. With respiration pleural surfaces slide against each other, which on 2D mode appears as a shimmering white line moving in synchrony with respiration. This is called the lung sliding sign, a dynamic sign seen on 2D mode. There is a commonly seen artifact on 2D mode, called the A-line (Figure 13). Presence of A-line with lung sliding indicates the presence of a normally aerated lung. In the absence of lung sliding, their presence is non-specific. A-lines are horizontal artifacts, arising from reverberation of ultrasound waves between the skin and pleural surface. Repetition of this artifact occurs at a distance equal to the distance between the probe head on the skin surface, and the pleural line.

5. Pleural effusions

The utility of ultrasonography for the diagnosis of pleural effusion is well established. Ultrasound can detect pleural effusions as small as 3-5 milliliters (*Gryminski et al., 1976*). Physical examination is less accurate than ultrasonography in detecting a pleural effusion (*Diacon et al., 2003*). It can be difficult to distinguish between pleural thickening, atelectasis, pleural effusion, parenchymal infiltrates or a combination of these findings on a chest radiograph (*Overfors & Hedgecock, 1978;Yu et al., 1993*). Ultrasonography has been shown to be a better imaging modality than chest radiograph in distinguishing between these abnormalities (*Gryminski et al., 1976; Kelbel et al., 1991*). Ultrasonography was shown to have a diagnostic accuracy of 93% when compared with chest computerized tomography (CT) scan in detecting a pleural effusion (*Lichtenstein et al., 2004a*).

Free flowing fluid in the pleural space accumulates in the dependent portion of the thoracic cavity. Depending on patient's clinical condition and comfort, the patient can be in a sitting, supine, semi-recumbent or in a lateral decubitus position (Photo 4). The goal should be to examine as much of the hemithorax as possible to be able to detect even small or loculated pleural effusions.

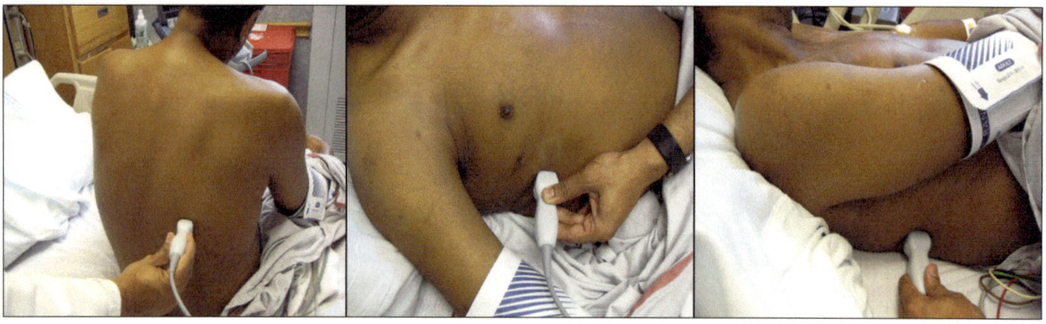

(a) (b) (c)

Photo 4. Patient in (a) sitting, (b) supine, and (c) slightly rotated position

There are three important findings that are useful in diagnosing a pleural effusion with the help of an ultrasound (Figure 1):

1. Anatomic boundaries of pleural effusions: the chest wall, the diaphragm, the lung and the subdiaphragmatic organs.
2. The presence of an anechoic space (black) between the visceral and parietal pleura.
3. Dynamic changes.

The probe should be in the cranio-caudal direction and the examiner needs to be aware of the position of the probe marker on the ultrasound screen for proper orientation. The first step is to identify the diaphragm as a curvilinear hyperechoic structure that moves with respiration. Pleural fluid in general is visualized as a hypoechoic or an anechoic collection above the diaphragm (Figure 1).

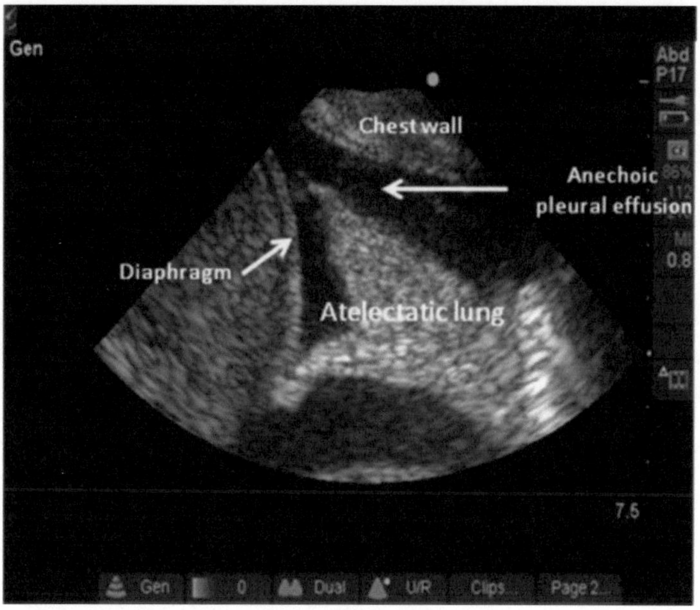

Fig. 1. Pleural effusion is present as an anechoic space with anatomic boundaries made up of chest wall, diaphragm and atelectatic lung

In the presence of moderate to large pleural effusions, the adjacent lung may become atelectatic and appears as tissue like structure flapping in the pleural effusion (flapping lung or the jellyfish sign). The compressed lung has an echogenicity similar to that of the liver, and this is termed as sonographic hepatization of the lung (Figure 1). Aerated lung may be seen moving over the pleural effusion with respiration. This is called the curtain sign. The movement of visceral pleural towards or away from the chest wall with inspiration and expiration creates a sinusoidal waveform pattern on M mode ultrasound (Figure 2). The sinusoid sign is a dynamic sign and is very specific for the diagnosis of pleural effusion, and can be helpful in distinguishing small pleural effusions from pleural thickening. Cellular or proteinaceous debris in the pleural fluid can be agitated by respiratory or cardiac motion creating a swirling pattern, which is called the plankton sign. Fibrin strands may be present and seen floating in the effusion or connected to each other in a lattice like pattern. Cellular debris in the effusion may settle down due to gravity, this creates an echogenic layering effect (hypocellular hypoechoic top layer with a cellular hyperechoic bottom layer) called the hematocrit sign.

Sonographic characteristics of the pleural fluid have been used to distinguish transudates from exudates. Effusions can have one of the following sonographic patterns, (1) anechoic: echo-free (black) space between the visceral and parietal pleura (2) complex non septated:

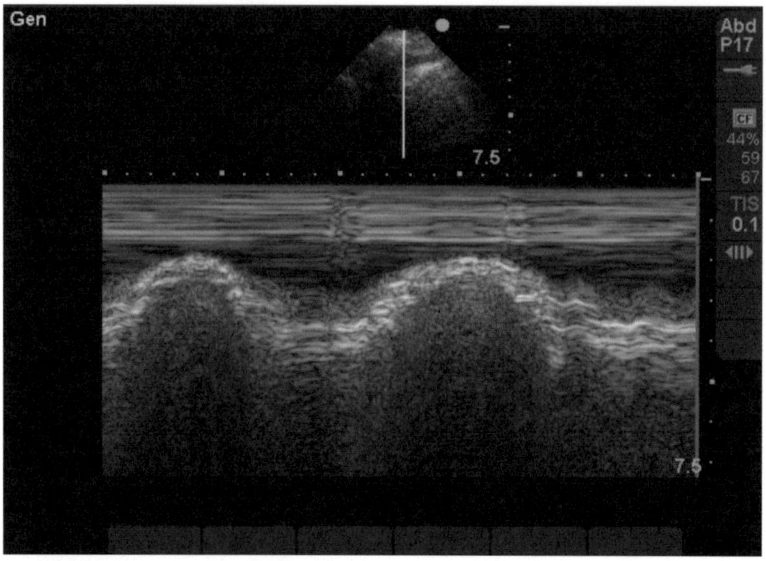

Fig. 2. Sinusoid sign on M mode (arrows)

echogenic material is present in a non homogenous pattern without septations (Figure 3). (3) complex septated: floating fibrin strands or septae in a lattice like pattern are present (Figure 4). This can be seen in parapneumonic effusions, empyemas, and malignant effusions. Ultrasonography has been shown to be superior to CT scan in detecting septations in pleural effusions (*McLoud & Flower, 1991*), and (4) homogenously echogenic: very cellular echogenic material is strewn homogenously in the effusion, as in an empyema or hemorrhagic effusions (Figure 5). Transudates are almost always anechoic (*Yang et al., 1992*). Exudates on the other hand can have any of the four patterns.

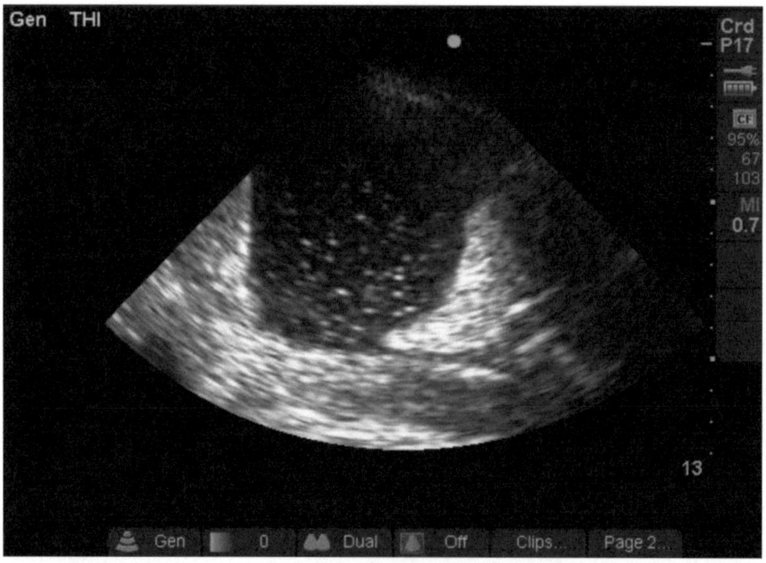

Fig. 3. Complex non septated pleural effusion

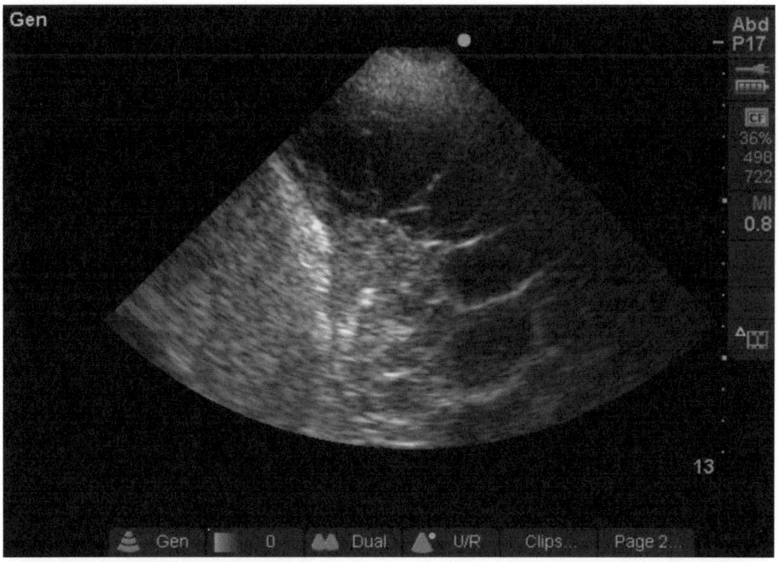

Fig. 4. Complex septated pleural effusion

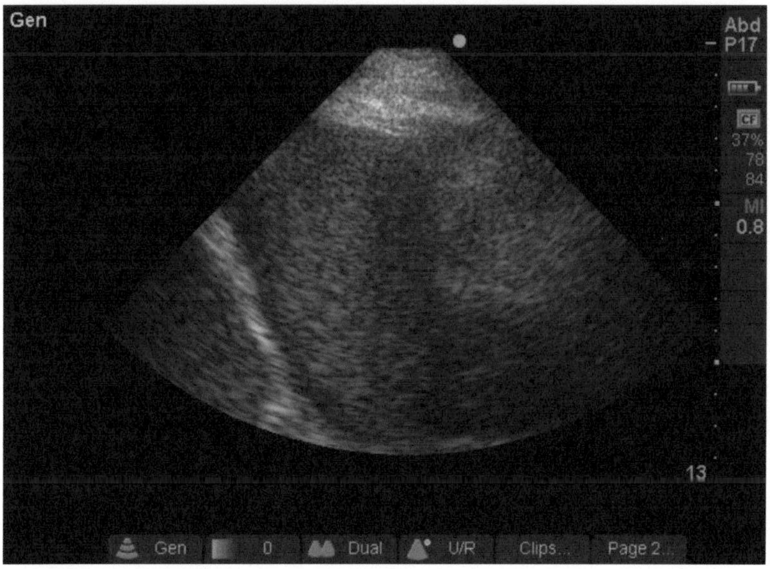

Fig. 5. Homogenously echogenic pleural effusion

Additional findings on sonography may be helpful to assess the etiology of pleural effusions. Echogenic swirling patterns or the presence of pleural nodules are suggestive of malignant effusions (*Chian et al., 2004*). The presence of adjacent consolidated lung with mobile hyperechoic air bronchograms indicates an effusion of infectious origin (Figure 6).

Loculated pleural effusions may be missed if the entire hemithorax is not examined, as they can be in non dependent areas. They do not change with body position, can be circular or elongated, with thick pleural linings.

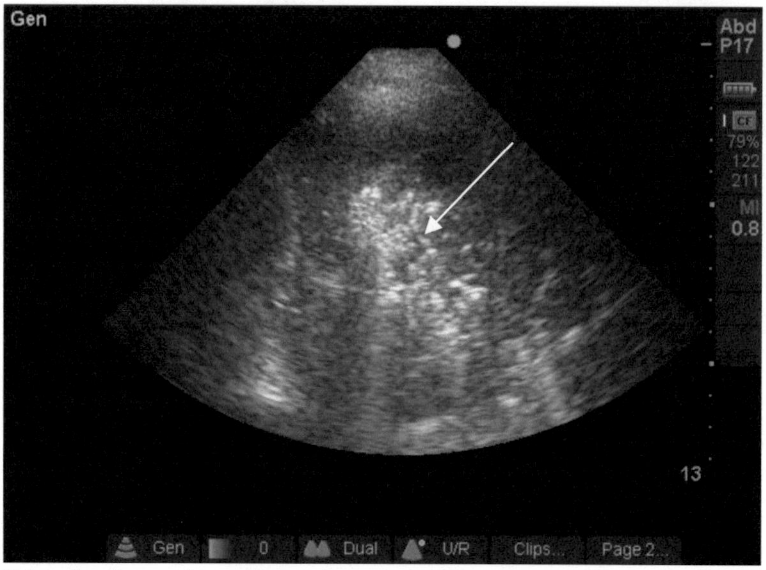

Fig. 6. Consolidated adjacent lung (arrow), suggesting a parapneumonic effusion

Many methods have been described to estimate the volume of pleural fluid (*Balik et al., 2006; Eibenberger et al., 1994*), and are reasonably accurate. It is best to classify the effusion as small: seen in one probe range, moderate: seen in two probe range and large: greater than two probe range.

Thoracentesis is a routinely performed procedure, although considered safe, the incidence of pneumothorax has been reported to be as high as 20 to 39% (*Grogan et al., 1990*). Several studies have shown that ultrasound guided thoracentesis has lower complication rates. In one study there was a significant reduction in pneumothorax rate when ultrasound was utilized for identification of needle placement (0% vs approximately 29%) (*Grogan et al., 1990*). A similar reduction in the rate of pneumothorax was reported in another study (18% vs 3%) (*Raptopoulos et al., 1991*). The procedure can be performed with real-time guidance for needle insertion with ultrasound, or the puncture site can be identified and marked. If the latter approach is used, it is important not to change patient's position, or delay the procedure, as this may displace freely flowing pleural fluid.

6. Pneumothorax

Early detection of pneumothorax is extremely important, especially in trauma patients and critically ill patients on mechanical ventilation. CT scan of chest is the gold standard test, but cannot be done immediately, may not be available in certain settings, and requires transport of patient to the radiology unit. Hence it is not an ideal test for a potentially life threatening situation such as pneumothorax. Chest radiographs are widely available, can be done relatively quickly and are routinely performed to evaluate a patient for pneumothorax. However, supine chest radiographs are not reliable, and have a high rate of misdiagnosis (*Chiles & Ravin, 1986, Tocino et al., 1985*). Ultrasonography can be performed quickly at patient's bedside, and has been shown to be very effective for rapidly ruling out pneumothorax (*Lichtenstein 1995, 1999, 2000, 2003, 2005*). Certain procedures, such as, thoracentesis, central line placements, lung biopsies etc carry a high risk of iatrogenic pneumothorax. Performing an ultrasound examination before and after the procedure can immediately rule out, or confirm a pneumothorax.

Lung sonography to detect pneumothorax should be performed with the transducer in cranio-caudal orientation. Free air in the pleural space collects in the non dependent anterior chest, making supine position ideal for evaluation for a pneumothorax (Photo 5). Between the acoustic shadows of the two adjacent ribs, a hyperechoic horizontal pleural line is present, approximately 0.5 cm below the origin of the rib shadow (Figure 7). The pleural line is made up of the visceral and parietal pleural surfaces, and represents the interface between chest wall and aerated lung. With respiration pleural surfaces slide against each other, which on 2D mode appears as a shimmering white line moving in synchrony with respiration. This is called the lung sliding sign, a dynamic sign seen on 2D mode. Air movement during respiration cause the lung to expand and contract, this sign indicates the presence of an expanded lung, with visceral pleural in contact, and sliding against parietal pleura. Detection of lung sliding at multiple sites of the chest virtually rules out a

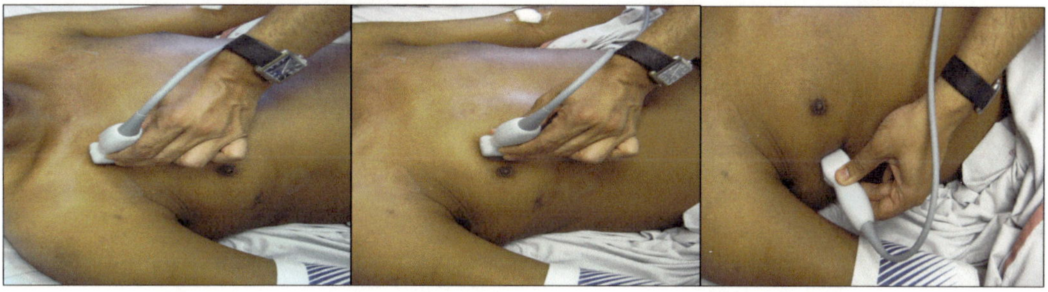

Photo 5. Supine position is ideal for the evaluation of pneumothorax. Multiple anterior and lateral points should be evaluated

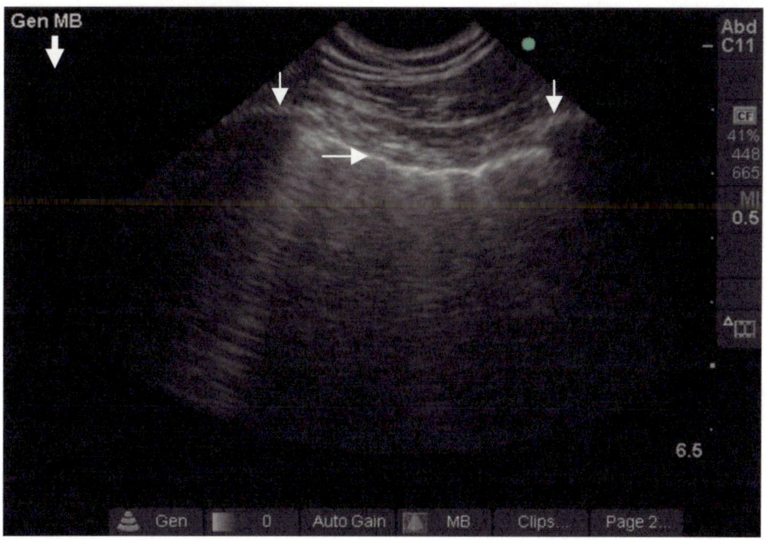

Fig. 7. Between the two ribs (vertical arrows), 0.5 cm below, shimmering white pleural line (horizontal arrow) is located

pneumothorax (*Lichtenstein & Menu, 1995*). Absence of lung sliding on the other hand can be seen in many other circumstances besides a pneumothorax. Conditions that prevent air movement into the lung (airway occlusion with mucous plug, tumor, foreign body), or inflation of the lung (ARDS, pneumonia, apnea) will abolish lung sliding. Pleural effusion from inflammatory or neoplastic processes will also abolish sliding. Therefore the absence of lung sliding is not very useful.

Lung sliding, a dynamic sign on 2D mode can be recorded as a static sign on M mode. In the presence of lung sliding, the characteristic pattern observed is the seashore sign (Figure 8). The pleural surface is the boundary, above it there is a wave like pattern (motion less chest wall), and below it is a granular or sandy beach like pattern (air filled lung). In the absence of lung sliding the pattern observed is called the stratosphere sign, also called the bar code sign (Figure 9). The granular or sandy beach pattern below the pleural line is replaced by horizontal lines.

There are two more dynamic findings, lung pulse (*Lichtenstein et al., 2003*) and comet-tail artifacts (B-lines) (*Lichtenstein et al., 1999*), seen on 2D mode, that rule out a pneumothorax. With lung pulse, the force of cardiac pulsation causes synchronous movement of the pleural line. Even in the absence of lung sliding in conditions that cause obstruction of air entry (mucous plug, airway tumor etc), lung pulse may be observed, indicating the presence of an expanded lung. B-lines, also called comet tail artifacts, are vertical artifacts that arise from the visceral pleura (Figure 10). They are well defined, do not fade, look like a laser beam, and move with lung sliding. Multiple B-lines indicate the presence of an interstitial syndrome. B-lines 7 mm apart, indicate thickened interlobular septa, an ultrasound equivalent of Kerly B-lines. B-lines 3 mm apart, correlate with ground glass opacities. Since B-lines originate from visceral pleura, their presence rules out pneumothorax.

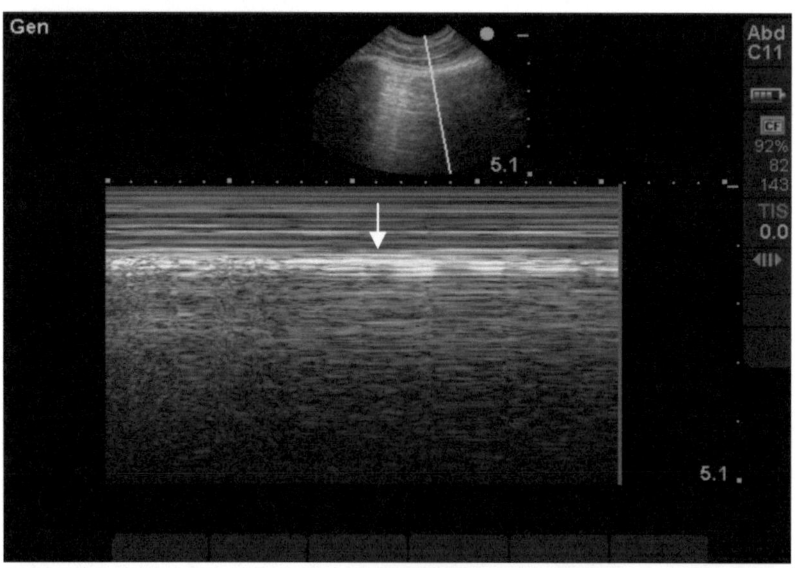

Fig. 8. Seashore sign on M mode, consistent with lung sliding. Above the pleural line (arrow), there is a wave like pattern created by the motionless chest wall. Below the pleural line is the granular, sandy beach like pattern, created by the air filled lung

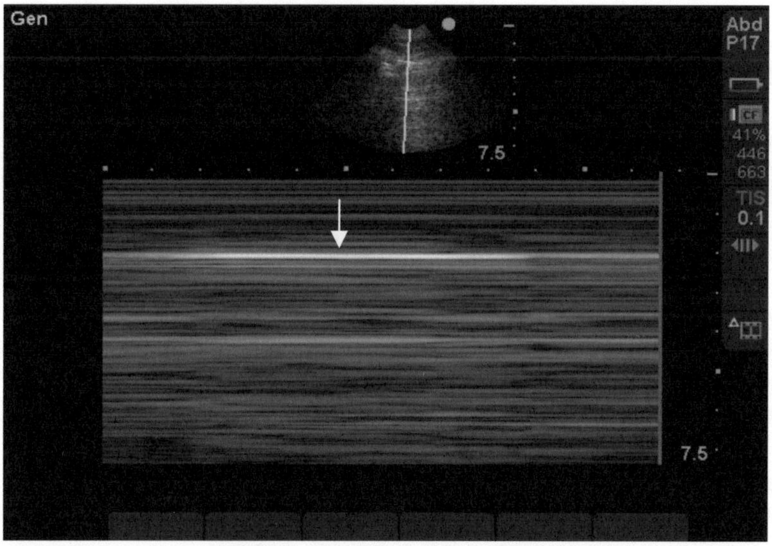

Fig. 9. Stratosphere sign on M mode, consistent with absent lung sliding. Horizontal lines above and below the pleural line (arrow), also called the barcode sign

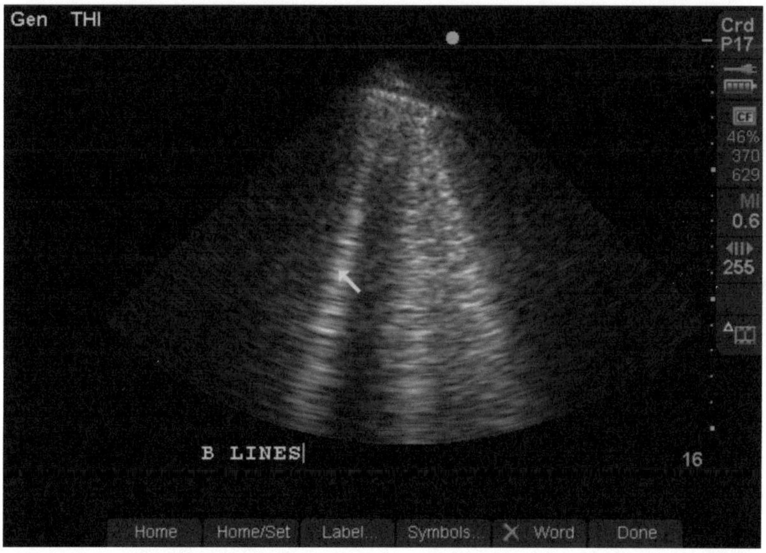

Fig. 10. B-lines (arrow). Vertical, laser like, hyperechoic, do not fade, arise from the visceral pleural, and move with lung sliding

There is one dynamic sign on 2D mode that confirms the presence of a pneumothorax, the lung point sign (*Lichtenstein et al., 2000*) (Figure 11). Partially collapsed lung is in contact with the chest wall at some point, where the visceral and parietal pleura are in contact, and slide against each other with respiration. A thorough examination may reveal this point where the pleura slides in with inspiration as the lung expands, but during expiration as the lung contracts, lung sliding disappears. This sign is 100% specific for pneumothorax, but has low sensitivity (*Lichtenstein & Menu, 1995*). Low sensitivity could be due to multiple reasons, operator skills, completely collapsed lung with no chest wall contact, incomplete examination, or the rib and sternum could be obscuring visualization. This sign can be recorded on M mode (Figure 12).

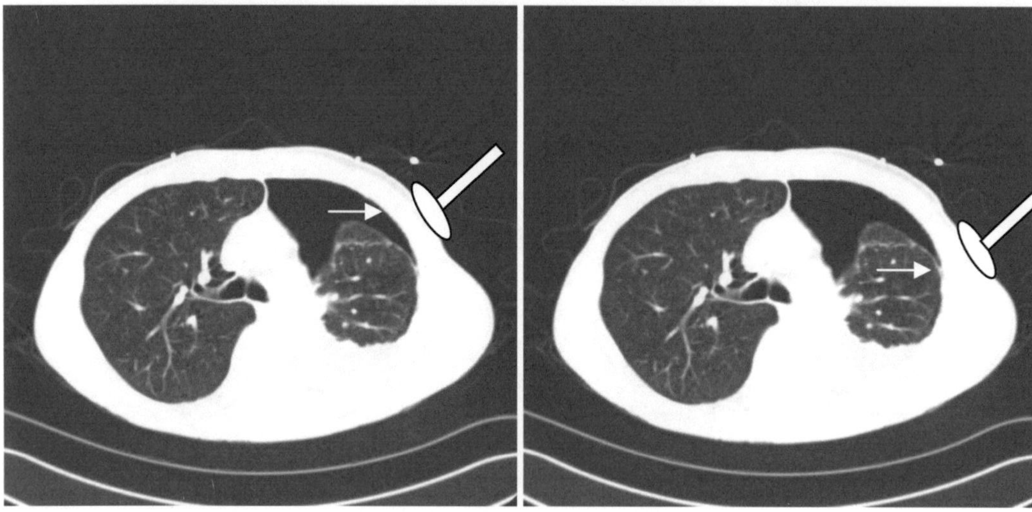

Fig. 11. Lung point sign. With the probe at this point, during expiration (1), the lung contracts, air comes between the pleural space (arrow). During inspiration (2), lung expands and slides in the ultrasound plane (arrow)

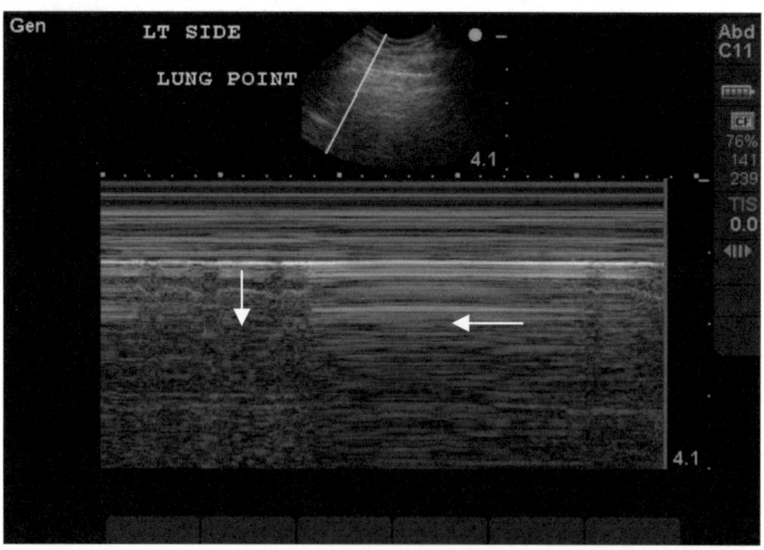

Fig. 12. Lung point sign on M mode. Alternating seashore sign (indicating lung sliding) (vertical arrow), with stratosphere sign (indicating absent lung sliding) (horizontal arrow)

There is another artifact commonly seen on 2D mode, called the A-line (Figure 13). The presence of A-line with lung sliding indicates the presence of a normally aerated lung. In the absence of lung sliding, their presence is non-specific, and can be seen with or without a pneumothorax. A-lines are horizontal artifacts, arising from reverberation of ultrasound waves between the skin and pleural surface. Repetition of this artifact occurs at a distance equal to the distance between the probe head on the skin surface, and the pleural line.

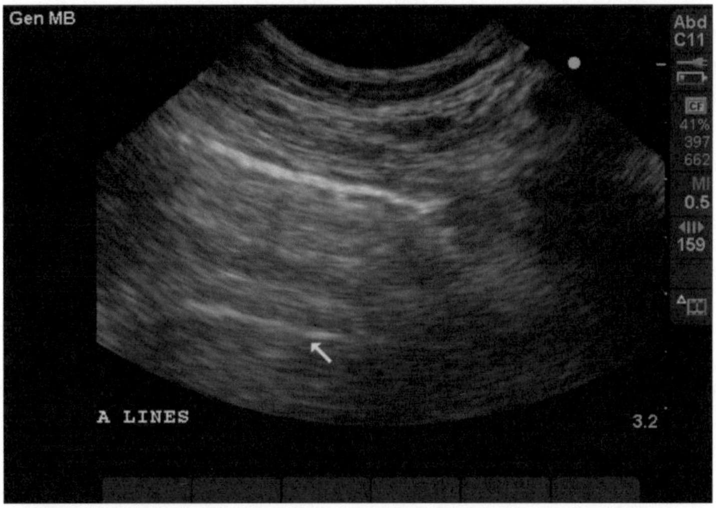

Fig. 13. Normal appearance of lung: A-line. Horizontal reverberation artifact, repetitive at a distance equal to the distance between the skin, and the pleural line

7. Alveolar consolidation

There are many causes of alveolar consolidation (pneumonia, ARDS, atelectasis etc), and its location can vary depending on the etiology. However 98.5% of cases of alveolar consolidation abut the pleura (*Lichtenstein et al., 2004b*), an important requisite for its detection by ultrasonography (Figure 14). Consolidated lung has a tissue like density on ultrasound with

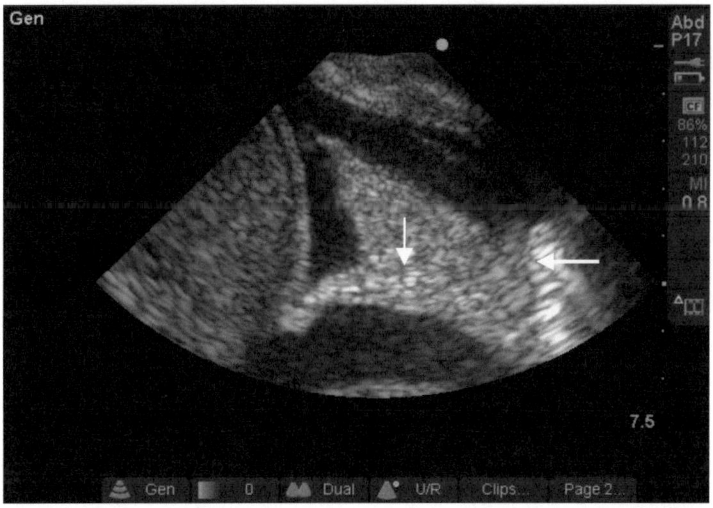

Fig. 14. Consolidated lung with tissue like density. The echogenicity is similar to that of the liver. Punctiform air bronchograms (vertical arrow) are present as hyperechoic artifacts, and the deep boundary is irregular, representing the shred sign (horizontal arrow)

an echogenicity similar to that of the liver, hence the term, sonographic hepatization of the lung. The deep interface between consolidated and aerated lung is irregular, called the shred sign. Air bronchograms when visualized, appear as punctiform or linear hyperechoic artifacts within the consolidated lung. When the centrifugal inspiratory movement of the air bronchogram is > 1mm, it is called a dynamic air bronchogram. The presence of dynamic air bronchogram indicates patent bronchi, with air bubbling within the bronchi with inspiration, and has a 94% specificity and a 97% positive predictive value for diagnosing pneumonia, and distinguishing it from resorptive atelectasis (*Lichtenstein et al., 2009*). Abscesses and necrotizing areas within the consolidated lung too can be detected with ultrasonography. Compared to CT scan, ultrasound has a sensitivity of 90% and a specificity of 98% for detecting alveolar consolidation (*Lichtenstein et al., 2004b*).

8. Alveolar-interstitial syndrome

The alveolar-interstitial syndrome (AIS) includes several heterogenous conditions, both chronic (pulmonary fibrosis) and acute (ARDS, cardiogenic pulmonary edema, interstitial pneumonia). Lung sonography is very useful in detecting AIS, and is an easy technique to learn. The patient should be examined in supine position with the probe in a cranio-caudal direction. Ideally the ultrasound examination should be performed by placing the probe in four discreet areas, two anterior and two lateral per hemithorax. Sonographic findings of AIS include multiple B-lines (comet tail artifact or lung rockets, described earlier) in a single view, disseminated diffusely over the antero-lateral thorax. Correlating with CT scan findings, B-lines 7 mm apart, indicate thickened interlobular septa, an ultrasound equivalent of Kerly B-lines. B-lines 3 mm apart, correlate with ground glass opacities. It is important to know that isolated B-lines, or confined to the last intercostals space above the diaphragm can be seen in healthy subjects and are of little clinical significance. It is critical to be able to distinguish B-line from two other vertical artifacts: the E-line and the Z-line. E-lines do not arise from the pleural line, and are seen in subcutaneous emphysema. The Z-lines arise from the pleural surface, are frequently seen artifacts without any clinical significance. They are ill-defined, fade away at a short distance, independent of lung sliding, and do not erase A-lines.

Finding of diffuse comet tail artifacts has a 93% sensitivity and 93% specificity for the diagnosis of diffuse interstitial syndrome, compared with radiography (*Lichtenstein et al., 1999*)· The finding of AIS by lung sonography is not very specific as many conditions can cause the sonographic pattern seen in AIS. *Prosen & Klemen, 2011* showed that in patients with acute dyspnea, the combination of comet tail artifacts and a elevated N-terminal pro-brain natriuretic peptide (NT-proBNP) level > 1000 pg/ml had a 100% sensitivity and specificity in differentiating acute heart failure from COPD and asthma. *Copetti et al., 2008* described pleuroparenchymal patterns seen on sonography that can differentiate ARDS/ALI from acute cardiogenic pulmonary edema. In their study on critically ill patients, the ultrasound finding of dyshomogeneous AIS with spared areas, pleural line modifications and lung consolidations were strongly predictive, in an early phase, of non-cardiogenic pulmonary edema. Lung sonography, looking at B line pattern of AIS has been shown to be of use in monitoring cardiogenic pulmonary edema (*Volpicelli et al., 2008*), effectiveness of hemodialysis in removing extravascular lung water (*Nobel et al., 2009*), and antibiotic failure in patients with ventilator associated pneumonia (*Bouhemad et al., 2010*).

9. Lung sonography in acute respiratory failure

Rapid evaluation for a diagnosis in patients presenting with acute respiratory failure is important, in order to institute proper management. Physical examination and chest radiography have limitations (*Lichtenstein et al., 2004a*). Chest CT scans involve time delays, risk of transport of unstable patients, and radiation exposure. *Lichtenstein & Meziere, 2008* showed in their study that lung ultrasound can immediately provide a diagnosis of acute respiratory failure in 90.5% of cases. They provide an algorithm, "Bedside Lung Ultrasound in Emergency- the BLUE protocol", to evaluate patients with acute respiratory distress (Figure 15). In their study, they assessed for (1) Lung sliding: present or absent (2) Artifacts: A or B-lines (Figure 16) (3) Alveolar consolidation and/or pleural effusion: absent or present, and (4) Deep venous thrombosis.

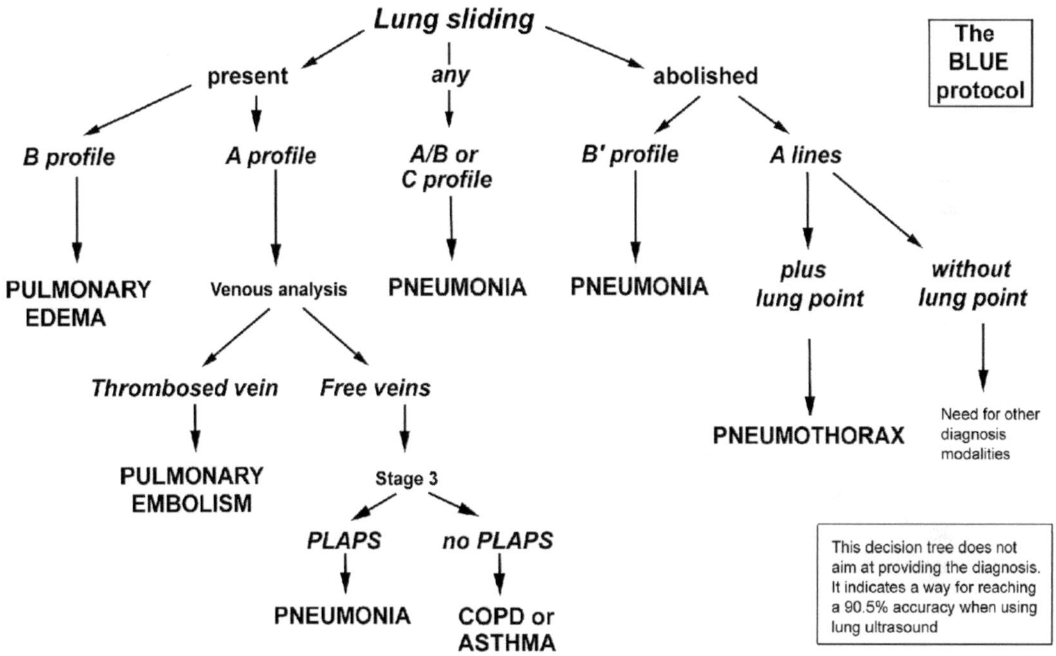

Fig. 15. A decision tree utilizing lung ultrasonography to guide diagnosis of severe dyspnea

Using this algorithm one can rapidly evaluate patients with acute dyspnea, in the emergency room, intensive care unit, or in rapid response team-events, at their bedside. Repeated examinations can be done, if needed, with a high diagnostic accuracy.

10. Peripheral lung masses

Peripheral intra-thoracic nodules and masses are (Figure 17) frequently encountered by pulmonary physicians and pose a diagnostic challenge, as the yield of bronchoscopy and sputum cytology is low for such lesions. Diagnostic options include percutaneous biopsy with image guidance (CT scan, fluoroscopy, and ultrasound), video-assisted thorascopy, or limited thoracotomy. Percutaneous image guided biopsy has a high diagnostic yield for malignant, compared with benign lesions. Ultrasound guided percutaneous biopsy of

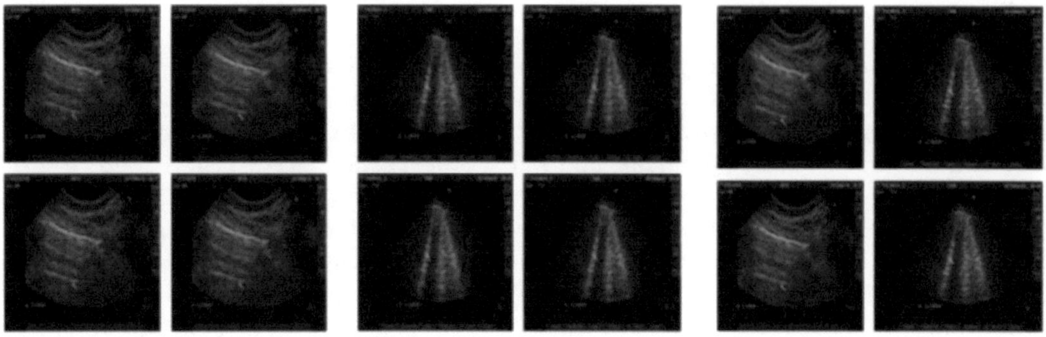

The A profile The B profile The AB profile

Fig. 16. Ultrasound profiles. Left panel: The A profile is defined as predominant A-lines plus lung sliding at the anterior surface in supine or half-sitting patients. This profile suggests COPD, embolism, and some posterior pneumonia. Pulmonary edema is nearly ruled out. Middle: The B profile is defined as predominant B +lines. This profile suggests cardiogenic pulmonary edema, and nearly rules out COPD, pulmonary embolism, and pneumothorax. Right panel: an A/B + profile, massive B-lines at the left lung, A-lines at the right lung. This profile is usually associated with pneumonia

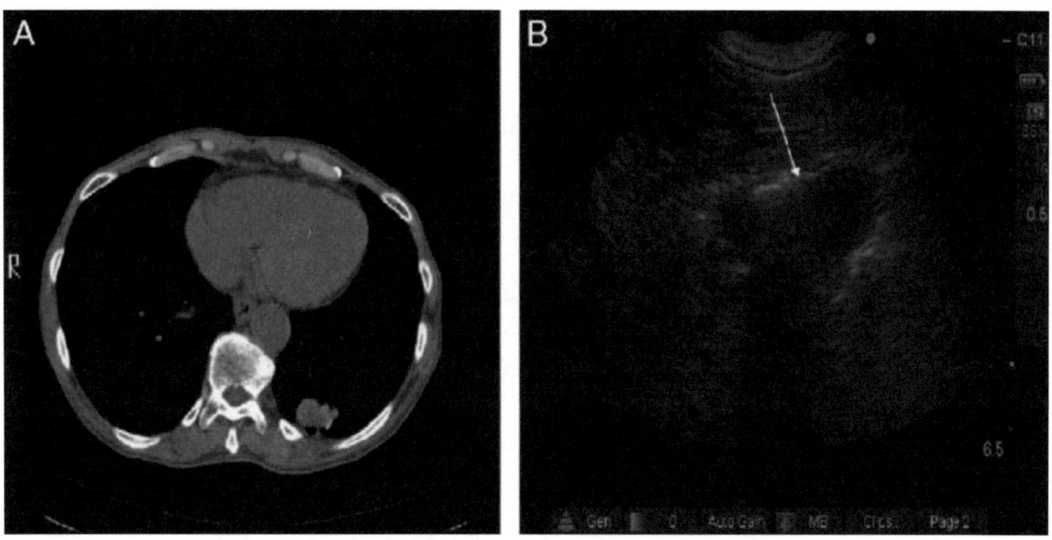

Fig. 17. (A) Transverse computed tomography scan of the chest in a 70-year-old male smoker with weight loss reveals 2.5 x 3 cm pleural-based left lower lobe mass. (B) Ultrasound examination of the mass shows a hypodense mass not invading the pleura (white arrow)

malignant peripheral pulmonary lesions has been shown to have a diagnostic accuracy (*Khosla et al., 2009*, higher than fluoroscopically guided biopsy and comparable to CT scan guided biopsy (*Liao et al., 2000*). Malignant lesions appear as hypoechoic or moderately echogenic, round or oval, inhomogeneous structures. They have well defined margins, which may be serrated with finger like projections into the lung tissue. Ultrasound guided biopsy of pleural-based intra-thoracic masses offers several advantages compared with CT guided procedure. There is no radiation exposure. Ultrasound is portable, allowing for performance of the procedure at bedside if needed. It is less expensive, less time consuming, and more readily available than CT scan. The procedure can be performed with the patient and physician in a comfortable position; and the physician does not have to wear a lead jacket which allows for greater freedom of movement. A significant advantage of ultrasound is real-time guidance that allows for dynamic evaluation of the target lesion, monitoring of the needle tip throughout the procedure, and fine adjustments that can be made quickly and precisely. Also, necrotic areas in the lesion and blood vessels can be avoided with real-time guidance. As small peripheral lesion may only be visible in one phase of the respiration, real-time guidance allows for the biopsy to be conducted in the respiratory phase, during which the lesion is most accessible with breath holding. Ultrasound examination allows for assessment of invasion of the chest wall by the tumor and has been reported to be superior to CT scan (*Bandi et al., 2008*). On ultrasound, reliable criteria for infiltration of the chest wall include: direct visualization of the infiltration on chest wall structure and rib destruction. Other indications include, interruption of the pleural line, and/or limited respiratory excursion of the mass.

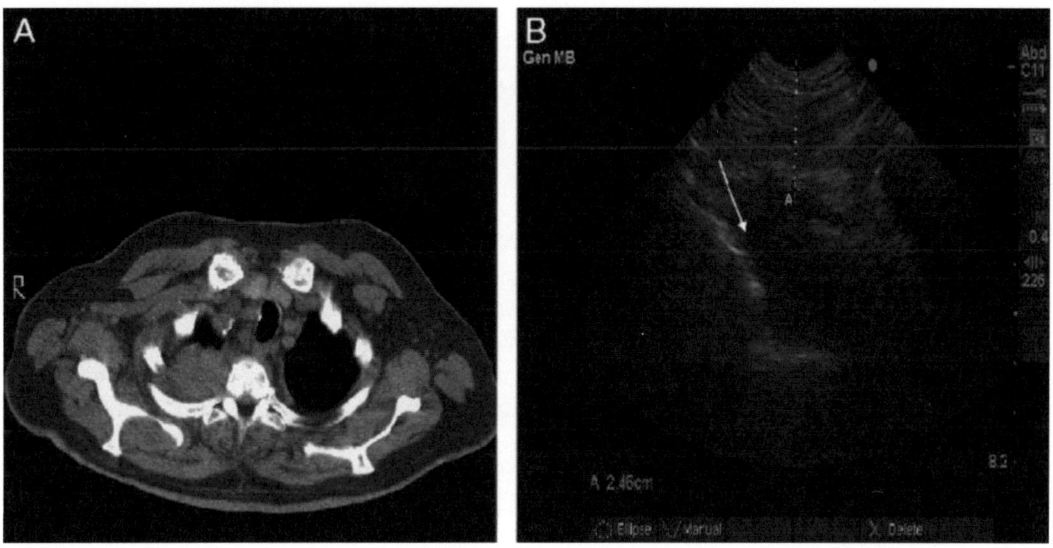

Fig. 18. (A) Transverse computed tomography scan of the chest in a 75 year old male smoker with right shoulder pain reveals a 4 x 5 cm pleural-based right upper lobe mass. (B) Ultrasound examination of the mass from the right supraclavicular fossa shows a hypodense mass. The mass is approximately 2.5 cm from the skin surface and is extending into the chest wall (white arrow)

11. Conclusion

Lung sonography has come of age and it is now a well established tool in the armamentarium of pulmonologists and intensivists. It has tremendous clinical utility, and provides rapid information at patient's bedside. It performs better than a chest radiograph in many clinical scenarios, and decreases the need for transporting critically ill patients for sophisticated, costly tests. The ultrasound probe is the stethoscope of the future (Photo 6).

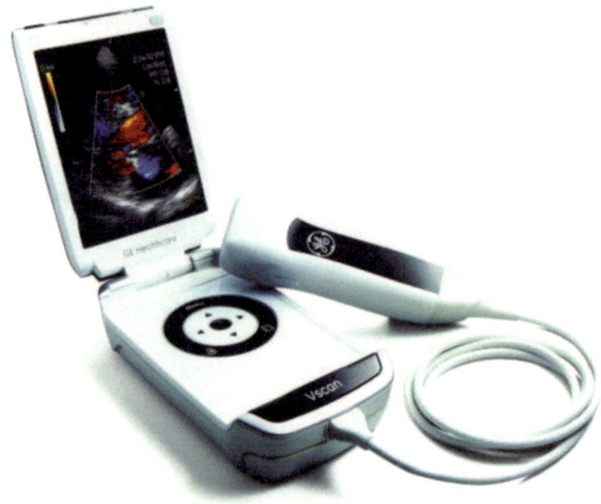

Photo 6. Pocket size ultrasound

12. Acknowledgment

The author acknowledges that photo 6 has been copied from the following website:
www.medgadget.com/archives/img/qr23nn.jpg

13. References

Balik M, Plasil P, Waldauf P, et al (2006). Ultrasound estimation of volume of pleural fluid in mechanically ventilated patients. *Intensive Care Med.* Vol 32(2):318–321.

Bandi V, Lunn W, Ernst A, et al (2008). Ultrasound vs. CT in detecting chest wall invasion by tumor: A prospective study. *Chest.* Vol 133(4):881–886.

Blaivas M, Lyon M, Duggal S. (2005). A prospective comparison of supine chest radiography and bedside ultrasound for the diagnosis of traumatic pneumothorax. *Acad Emerg Med.* Vol 12(9):844–849.

Bouhemad B, Liu Z, Aerbelot C, et al (2010). Ultrasound assessment of antibiotic-induced pulmonary reareation in ventilator-associated pneumonia. *Crit Care Med.* Vol 38(1):84-92.

Chian CF, Su WL, Soh LH, et al (2004). Echogenic swirling pattern as a predictor of malignant pleural effusions in patients with malignancies. *Chest.* Vol 126 91):129–134.

Chiles C, Ravin CE. (1986).Radiographic recognition of pneumothorax in the intensive care unit. *Crit Care Med.* Vol 14(8):677-80.

Copetti R, Soldati G, Copetti P. (2008). Chest sonography: a useful tool to differentiate acute cardiogenic pulmonary edema from acute respiratory distress syndrome. *Cardiovascular Ultrasound.* Vol. 6(16):1-10.

Diacon AH, Brutsche MH, Soler M. (2003). Accuracy of pleural puncture sites: a prospective comparison of clinical examination with ultrasound. *Chest.* Vol 123(2): 436-41.

Eibenberger KL, Dock WI, Ammann ME, et al (1994). Quantification of pleural effusions: sonography versus radiography. *Radiology.* Vol 191(3):681–684.

Grogan DR, Irwin RS, Channick R, et al. (1990). Complications associated with thoracentesis: a prospective, randomized study comparing three different methods. *Arch Intern Med.* Vol 150(4):873–877.

Gryminski J, Krakowka P, Lypacewicz G. (1976). The diagnosis of pleural effusion by ultrasonic and radiologic techniques. *Chest.* Vol 709(1):33-7.

Kelbel C, Borner N, Schadmand S, et al. (1991). Diagnosis of pleural effusions and atelectasis: sonography and radiology compared. *Rofo.* Vol. 154(2): 159-63.

Khosla R, Rohatgi PK, Seam N. (2009). Ultrasound-guided Fine Needle Aspiration Biopsy of Pleural-based Intrathoracic Lesions. *J Bronchol Intervent Pulmonol.* Vol 16(2):87–90.

Liao WY, Chen MZ, Chang YL, et al (2000). US-guided transthoracic cutting biopsy for peripheral thoracic lesions less than 3 cm in diameter. *Radiology.* Vol 217(3): 685–691.

Lichtenstein DA, Menu Y. (1995). A bedside ultrasound sign ruling out pneumothorax in the critically ill. Lung sliding. *Chest.* Vol 108(5):1345–1348.

Lichtenstein D, Meziere G, Biderman P, Gepner A. (1999). The comet-tail artifact: an ultrasound sign ruling out pneumothorax. *Intensive Care Med.* Vol 25(4):383–388.

Lichtenstein D, Mezière G, Biderman P, Gepner A. (2000). The "lung point": an ultrasound sign specific to pneumothorax. *Intensive Care Med.* Vol 26(10):1434-40.

Lichtenstein DA, Lascols N, Prin S, Mezière G. (2003). The "lung pulse": an early ultrasound sign of complete atelectasis. *Intensive Care Med.* Vol 29(12):2187-2192.

Lichtenstein D, Goldstein I, Mourgeon E, et al. (2004). Comparative diagnostic performances of auscultation, chest radiography, and lung ultrasonography in acute respiratory distress syndrome. *Anesthesiology.* Vol 100(1):9–15.

Lichtenstein D, Lascols N, Meziere G, et al. (2004). Ultrasound diagnosis of alveolar consolidation in the critically ill. *Intensive Care Med.* Vol 30(2):276–281.

Lichtenstein DA, Meziere G, Lascols N, et al. (2005). Ultrasound diagnosis of occult pneumothorax. *Crit Care Med.* Vol 33(6):1231–1238.

Lichtenstein DA, Meziere GA. (2208). Relevance of lung ultrasound in the diagnosis of acute respiratory failure: The BLUE protocol. *Chest.* Vol 134(1):117–125.

Lichtenstein D, Mezière G, Seitz J. (2009). The dynamic air bronchogram. A lung ultrasound sign of alveolar consolidation ruling out atelectasis. *Chest.* Vol 135(6):1421-5.

McLoud TC, Flower CD. (1991). Imaging the pleura: sonography,CT, and MR imaging. *Am J Roentgenol.* Vol 156(6):1145–1153.

Nobel EV, Murray AF, Capp R, et al. (2009). Ultrasound Assessment for Extravascular Lung Water in Patients Undergoing Hemodialysis. Time Course for Resolution. *Chest.* Vol 135(6):1433-1439.

Overfors C, HedgecockMW. (1978). Intensive care unit radiology: problems of interpretation. *Radiol Clin North Am.* Vol 16(3):407–409.

Prosen G, Klemen P, Strnad M, et al. (2011). Combination of lung ultrasound (a comet-tail sign) and N-terminal pro-brain natriuretic peptide in differentiating acute heart failure from chronic obstructive pulmonary disease and asthma as cause of acute dyspnea in prehospital emergency setting. *Critical Care.* Vol 5(2):R114.

Raptopoulos V, Davis LM, Lee G, et al. (1991). Factors affecting the development of pneumothorax associated with thoracentesis. *AJR Am J Roentgenol.* Vol 156(5):917–920.

Tocino IM, Miller MH, Fairfax WR. (1985). Distribution of pneumothorax in the supine and semirecumbent critically ill adult. *AJR*. Vol 144(5):901-905.

Volpicelli G, Caramello V, Cardinale L, et al. (2008). Bedside ultrasound of the lung for the monitoring of acute decompensated heart failure. *American Journal of Emergency Medicine*. Vol 26(5):585–591.

Yang PC, Luh KT, Chang DB, et al. (1992). Value of sonography in determining the nature of pleural effusion: analysis of 320 cases. *AJR Am J Roentgenol*. Vol 159(1):29–33.

Yu CJ, Yang PC, Wu HD, et al. (1993). Ultrasound study in unilateral hemithorax opacification: image comparison with computed tomography. *Am Rev Respir Dis*. Vol 147(2):430–434.

7

The Use of Ultrasonography in Conservative Management of Cervical Pregnancy

Bing Xu[1], Jo Kitawaki[2], Yuying Duan[1] and Jilian Ding[3]
[1]Department of Obstetrics and Gynecology, The Affiliated Hospital of Medical College, Qingdao University,
[2]Department of Obstetrics and Gynecology, Kyoto Prefectural University of Medicine,
[3]Department of Obstetrics and Gynecology, Shanghai East Hospital Affiliated Tongji University,
[2]Japan
[1,3]P.R.China

1. Introduction

Cervical pregnancy is defined as an implantation of a fertilized ovum in the cervical canal. It is a very rare and dangerous form of ectopic pregnancy. The incidence ranges from 1/2500 to 1/12,000 pregnancies, which accounts for approximately 0.15% of all ectopic pregnancies. Rapid crossing of the fertilized ovum through the endometrial cavity and the travel speed of the ovum could be the cause of cervical implantation. An unfertilized ovum may reach the cervical canal and implantation occurs. Although the etiology of cervical pregnancy is unclear, previous uterine procedures such as dilation and curettage (D & C) and cesarean section, pelvic inflammatory disease, use of an intrauterine device (IUD), and in vitro fertilization (IVF) are likely causative or contributing factors. Particularly, with the use of assisted reproductive technology in recent years, the incidence of cervical pregnancy is expected to rise.

Cervical pregnancy is characterized by profuse, even life-threatening hemorrhage, which may lead to an emergency hysterectomy. In cervical pregnancy, the trophoblastic tissue directly invades into the cervix which is predominantly composed of fibrous connective tissue, with only 15% of smooth muscle. Such a cervical environment cannot satisfy the needs of the growing ovum. Pregnancy may eventually terminate when invasion, erosion, or rupture of large vessels results in bleeding. Clinically, the patients present a history of amenorrhea followed by uterine bleeding without cramping pain.

Before the routine use of ultrasound in gynecologic care, cervical pregnancy is rarely diagnosed at early gestational age. Prior to late 1980s, clinical diagnosis of cervical pregnancy was usually made when curettage for misdiagnosed incomplete spontaneous abortion resulted in uncontrollable hemorrhage. Such a condition often presented with life-threatening hemorrhage that frequently required an emergent hysterectomy and even resulted in maternal death. To avoid heavy bleeding and preserve uterus it is crucial to obtain an early and accurate diagnosis. In recent years, the widespread use of high resolution ultrasound, particularly of the transvaginal sonography, has enabled the early diagnosis of cervical pregnancy, thereby allowing the application of conservative measures for women who desire to preserve fertility and/or obviate hysterectomy. Treatments tend to be more conservative and minimally invasive. In various conservative measures for cervical pregnancy, ultrasonography has progressively become an indispensable tool in diagnosis, interventional guidance, follow-up monitoring and clinical outcomes assessment.

2. Diagnosis of cervical pregnancy

Transvaginal or transabdominal ultrasound has become a standard and indispensible tool in the diagnosis of cervical pregnancy. An ultrasound examination will reveal a gestational sac in a widened cervical canal, with the absence of a gestational sac in the uterus (Figures 1, 2 and 3). The diagnosis is commonly established according to the following criteria described by Hofmann and Timor-Tritsch:

1. Presence of gestational sac or placental texture dominantly within the cervix;
2. No evidence of intrauterine pregnancy;
3. Visualization of an endometrial stripe;
4. Hourglass uterine shape with ballooned cervical canal;
5. Sac with active cardiac motion below the internal os for viable pregnancy.

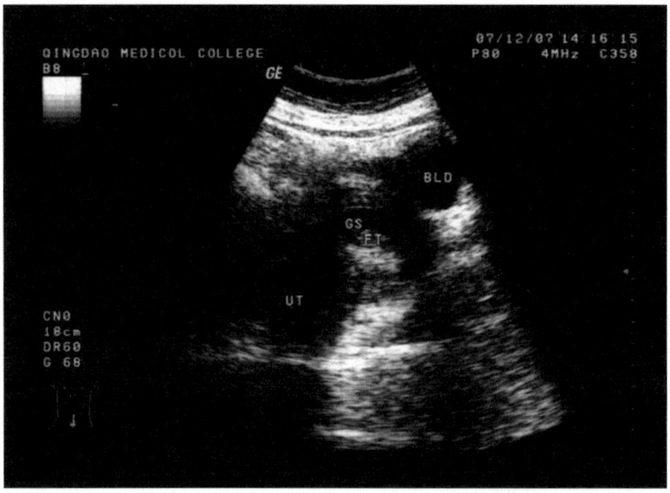

Fig. 1. Transabdominal ultrasound image of the cervical pregnancy. A 45-year-old woman, gravida 3, para 1 was admitted at 7 weeks and 5 days' gestation, presenting with a small amount of bloody vaginal discharge. Transabdominal sonography revealed normal-sized uterus with empty cavity. The gestational sac with a viable fetus is evident under the closed internal os. The β-hCG level was 59,313 mIU/L. UT: uterus; BLD: bladder; GS: gestational sac; FT: fetus

Ultrasound is used to localize and measure the gestational mass. Color Doppler imaging is applied to detect the blood flow of the gestational mass and surrounding tissues (Figure 4A and 4B). For the cases with acute bleeding or the cases that have been treated improperly with misdiagnosis, the combination use of transvaginal and transabdominal ultrasound will supply more accurate information. Besides, serum β-hCG value is important for the diagnosis and assessment of treatment effect. A cautious vaginal speculum examination should be performed when the patient's physical condition permits.

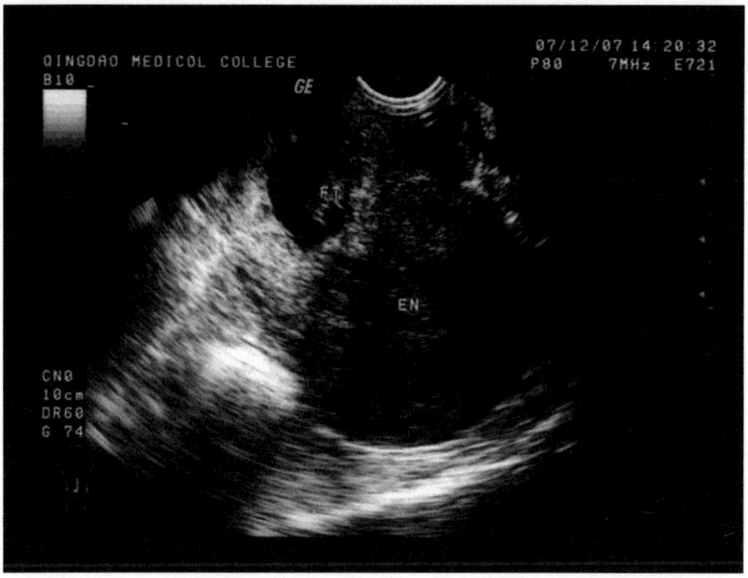

Fig. 2. Tranvaginal ultrasound image of the cervical pregnancy. The same case as described in Figure 1. An empty cavity of uterus with a 35 mm gestational sac containing fetal cardiac activity is evident under the closed internal os. EN: endometrium; FT: fetus

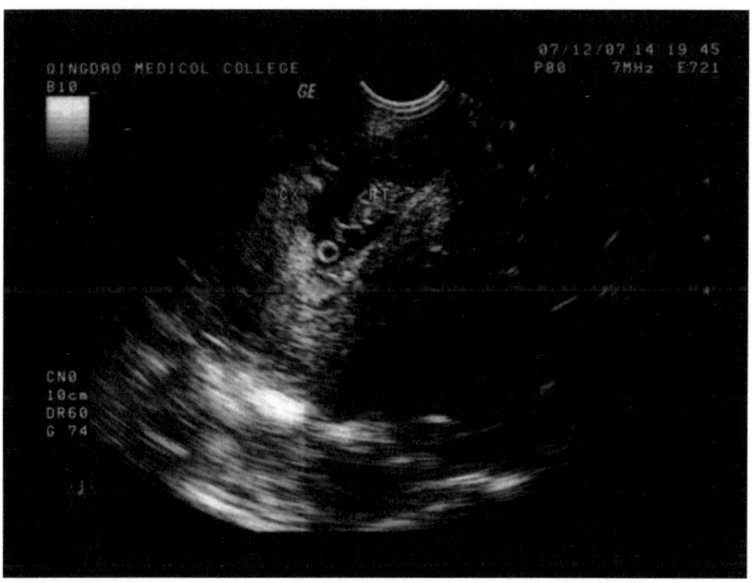

Fig. 3. Tranvaginal ultrasound image of the cervical pregnancy. The same case as described in Figure 1. An enlarged cervix with a viable fetus in a gestational sac is evident under the closed internal os. CX: cervix; FT: fetus

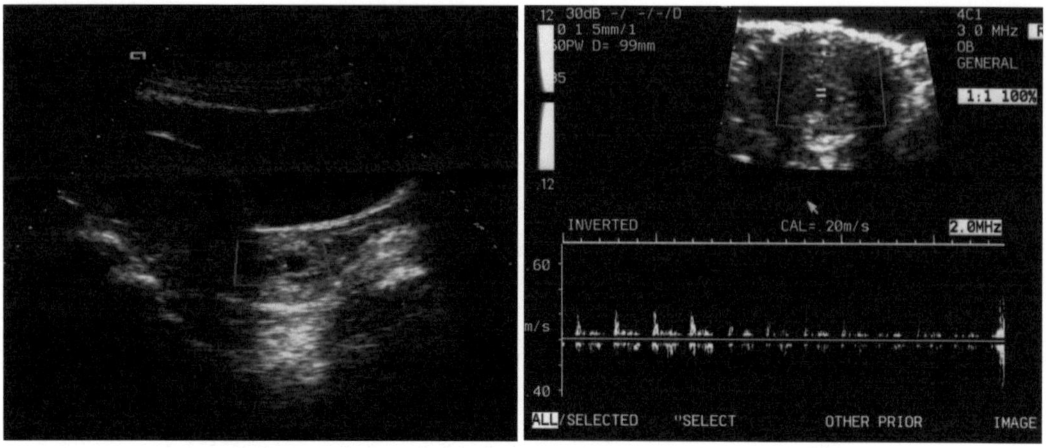

(a) (b)

Fig. 4. (a) Ultrasonographic scan of a case of cervical pregnancy. The gestational sac is evident under the closed internal os. (b) Doppler flow velocimetry depicting fetal cardiac activity. (Xu, et al. J Obstet Gynaecol Res. 2007;33:190-4)

2.1 Differential diagnosis of cervical pregnancy

The differential diagnosis of a cervical pregnancy includes other possible abnormal implantations, such as cesarean scar, low uterine corpus and abortion in progression pregnancies.

Caesarean scar pregnancy

A cesarean scar pregnancy is a gestation separated from the endometrial cavity and completely surrounded by the myometrium and the fibrous tissue of the scar. It is also a very rare form of ectopic pregnancy. However, with the caesarean deliveries increased all over the world, the incidence is rising in recent years. The most possible mechanism of cesarean scar pregnancy is because the invasion of the myometrium through a microscopic tract. The microscopic tract is believed to develop from trauma from previous uterine surgeries like caesarean section, myomectomy, and dilatation and curettage. Early diagnosis can promptly offer treatment options to decrease the likelihood of uterine rupture and heavy bleeding. Therefore, it is important to suspect the possibility of scar pregnancy when the gestational sac is found at the level of the uterine isthmus in a patient with a previous caesarean section. Transvaginal ultrasonography combined with Doppler is a reliable tool for diagnosis. Ultrasound imaging presents a gestational sac located in the anterior uterine wall at the isthmus (Figure 5).

Spontaneous abortion in progress

Differentiation from a spontaneous abortion of an early pregnancy can be accomplished by the shape of the uterus, which is generally globular in an intrauterine pregnancy, as well as by the absence of a "sliding sign," where an aborted gestational sac slides against the endocervical canal in response to gentle pressure by the sonographer. On transvaginal scan the gestational sac should be seen in the cervical canal and the sac should appear avascular, reflecting the fact that the sac has been detached from its implantation site.

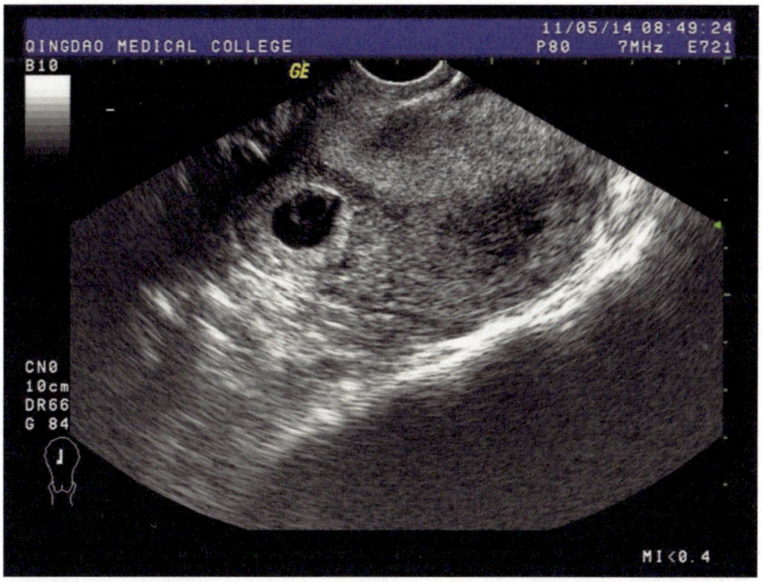

Fig. 5. Transvaginal ultrasound image of a cesarean scar pregnancy. Transvaginal scan revealed a 26 mm gestational sac with fetal pole outside the lower uterine cavity at the level of the isthmus in the anterior uterine wall

Low uterine corpus pregnancy

Low uterine corpus pregnancy should be differentiated from cervical pregnancy. The implantation usually takes place in the lower part of the cavity of the uterus. The gestational sac is located above the internal os of the cervix (Figure 6).

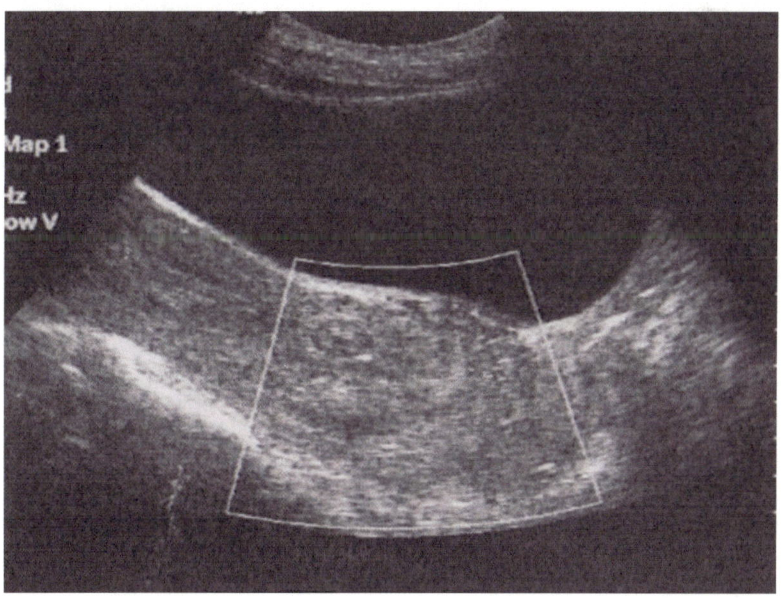

Fig. 6. Transabdominal ultrasound image of pregnancy in low uterine corpus

3. Conservative treatments of cervical pregnancy

The treatment options for cervical pregnancy largely depend on the severity of vaginal bleeding, gestational age, initial serum hCG levels, absence or presence of fetal heartbeat, and the woman`s desire to preserve fertility and/or to obviate hysterectomy. Treatments tend to be more conservative and minimally invasive in recent years. Hysterectomy is performed only as a radical treatment in cases of intractable hemorrhage.

Various conservative treatments have been reported previously, such as local or systemic administration of methotrexate (MTX), Foley catheter tamponade, curettage and local prostaglandin injection, cervical cerclage and intra-cervical injections of vasoconstricting agents, laparoscopy-assisted uterine artery ligation combined with hysteroscopic endocervical resection, angiographic uterine artery embolization (UAE). These procedures are used either alone or in combination. However, there is no consensus to date about the best approach mainly due to a lack of evidence derived from large series of clinical cases. Moreover, a risk of hemorrhage accompanies all options available.

UAE has been widely used as a highly effective technique for treating cervical pregnancy. However, recent studies indicate that rebleeding or delayed bleeding can occur after UAE. It is speculated that after complete occlusion of the uterine arteries by UAE, the extensive collateral circulation to the cervix will be established within hours. If the cervical pregnancy is not evacuated soon after UAE, some gestational tissues may remain alive and result in bleeding once again. We recently reported a promising conservative modality treatment--UAE followed by immediate curettage. We recommend this method for the cases with fetal cardiac activity, high serum hCG levels and late gestational age when fertility capacity is desired. The procedure is performed as the following: the UAE procedure is performed using digital subtraction angiography. After the bilateral arteries embolization is confirmed, an experienced gynecologist performed vacuum evacuation and curettage of the cervical canal under ultrasound guidance. After the procedure, vaginal bleeding is closely monitored for at least 48 hours. Outpatient follow-up, including sonographic examinations and β-hCG measurements are performed routinely twice in the first week after the procedure, and then once a week until decreased to normal range. After follow-up, the UAE and curettage technique, complications, vaginal bleeding, the changes of serum hCG level, regression of the uterine cervical mass, recovery of menses, pregnancy and pregnancy outcome are evaluated for the assessment of clinical outcomes. Of the patients treated by this method, quick regression of serum hCG level and cervical mass, fertility preservation, and a short hospital stay are observed.

4. Ultrasound guidance during medical and surgical intervention

During the medical or surgical intervention, ultrasound is used to accurately locate the gestational mass and guide medical injection. Direct injection of potassium chloride (KCl) or MTX into the gestational sac or fetal heart under ultrasound guidance is often used to kill embryo and destruct trophoblast tissues in cervix. It has been proved effective in clinical practice. Combined medical treatment with UAE has been proved to reduce the risk of bleeding. Local injection of prostaglandin and vasoconstricting agents are reported to effectively reduce bleeding. In the recently reported new treatment modality--UAE followed by immediate curettage, under ultrasound guidance an experienced gynecologist performs vacuum evacuation and curettage of the cervical canal immediately after the bleeding is controlled by the bilateral arteries embolization. With a special emphasis on the clinical outcome, an advantage of this procedure is to complete bleeding control and evacuate gestational tissue in one step, which can lead to a quick recovery.

5. Ultrasound examination in follow-up and clinical outcomes assessment

After the medical or surgical treatment, the vaginal bleeding, the changes of serum hCG level and regression of the uterine cervical mass should be closely monitored. The clinical outcome assessment should be made. Thus, serial sonographic examinations and β-hCG measurements are required in follow-up routinely until cervical contour is recovered to a normal shape on sonogram and gynecological examination, serum β-hCG is reduced to undetectable, and normal menstrual cycle returns. In our previous report, a case of cervical pregnancy treated with UAE only presented intermittent vaginal bleeding again although serious bleeding was successfully controlled by UAE. The ultrasound images consistently revealed a heterogeneous mass in the cervix (Figure 7).

By contrast, in the patients treated by UAE followed by immediate curettage, a quick regression of cervical mass and serum hCG level, fertility preservation and a short hospital stay are observed (Figure 8).

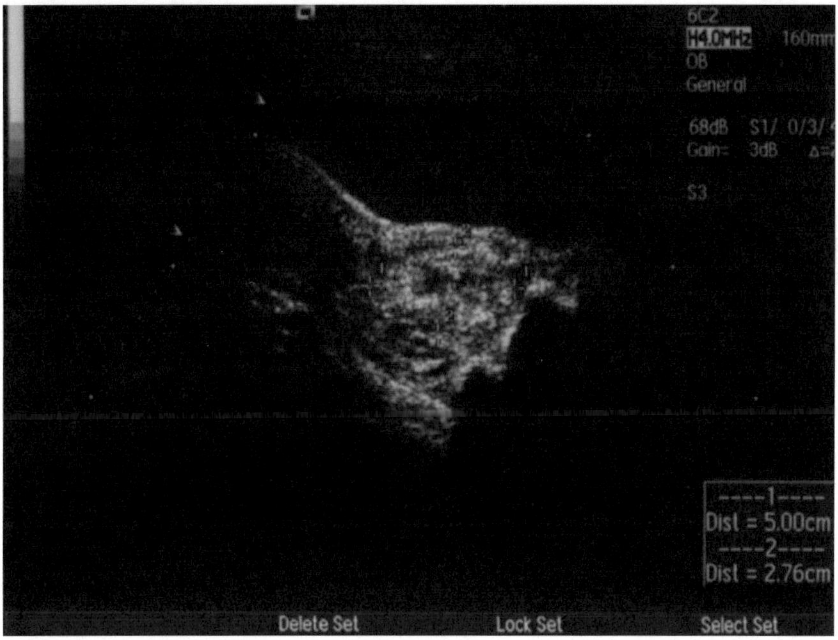

Fig. 7. A failure case of cervical pregnancy treated by UAE only. The sonography consistently revealed a heterogeneous mass in the cervix although serious bleeding was successfully controlled by UAE. The patient presented intermittent vaginal bleeding again. The patient underwent second UAE followed by immediate curettage and obtained complete solution. (Xu, et al. J Obstet Gynaecol Res. 2007;33:190-4)

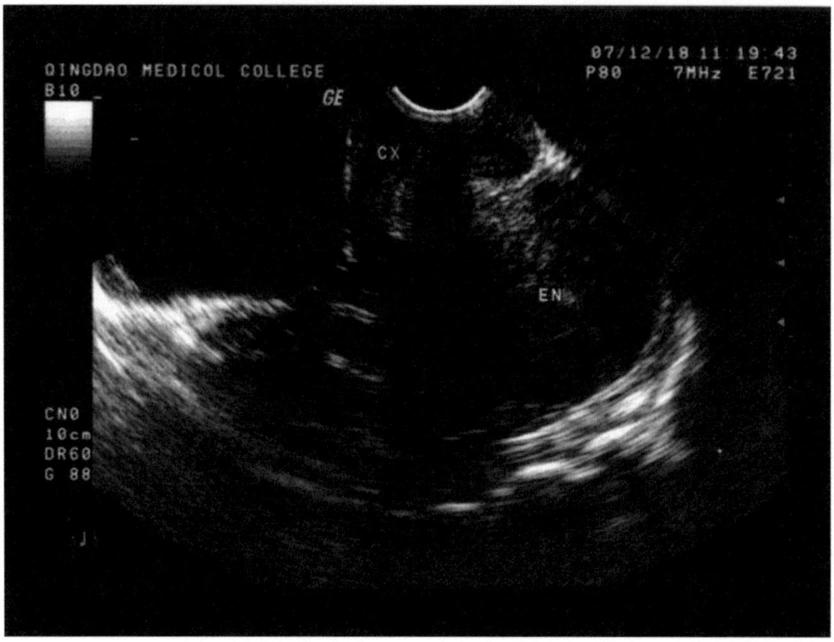

Fig. 8. Tranvaginal ultrasound image of the cervical pregnancy after treatment. The same case as described in Figure 1. Eight days after treatment by UAE followed by curettage, the cervix recovered to normal in contour

6. Conclusion

Cervical pregnancy is a very rare and dangerous form of ectopic pregnancy. It is characterized by profuse, even life-threatening hemorrhage, which may lead to an emergency hysterectomy. Recent widespread use of high-resolution ultrasound has enabled the early and accurate diagnosis of cervical pregnancy, thereby allowing the application of conservative measures for women who desire to preserve fertility. In various conservative measures for cervical pregnancy, ultrasonography has progressively become an indispensable tool in diagnosis, interventional guidance, follow-up monitoring and clinical outcomes assessment.

7. References

[1] Ushakov, FB, Elchalal U, Aceman PJ, Schenker JG. Cervival pregnancy: past and future. Obstet Gynecol Surv 1997;52:45-59.

[2] Frates MC, Benson CB, Doubilet PM et al. Cervical ectopic pregnancy: results of conservative treatment. Radiology 1994; 191: 773-5.

[3] Sherer DM, Dalloul M, Santoso P et al. Complete abortion of a nonviable cervical pregnancy following methotrexate treatment. Am J Perinatol 2004; 21: 223-6.

[4] Hofmann HM, Urdl W, Höfler H, Hönigl W, Tamussino K. Cervical pregnancy: case reports and current concepts in diagnosis and treatment. Arch Gynecol Obstet. 1987;241:63-9.

[5] Timor-Tritsch IE, Monteagudo A, Mandeville EO et al. Successful management of viable cervical pregnancy by local injection of methotrexate guided by transvaginal untrasonography. Am J Obstet Gynecol 1994; 170: 737-9.
[6] Gun M, Mavrogiorgis M. Cervical ectopic pregnancy: a case report and literature review. Ultrasound Obstet Gynecol 2002;19:297–301.
[7] Jurkovic D, Hacket E, Campbell S. Diagnosis and treatment of early cervical ectopic pregnancy: a review and report of two cases treatedconservatively. Ultrasound Obstet Gynecol 1996;8:373– 80.
[8] Sherer DM, Lysikiewicz A, Abulafia O. Viable cervical pregnancy managed with systemic Methotrexate, uterine artery embolization, and local tamponade with inflated Foley catheter balloon. Am J Perinatol 2003; 20: 263-7.
[9] Spitzer D, Steiner H, Graf A et al. Conservative treatment of cervical pregnancy by curettage and local prostaglandin injection. Hum Reprod 1997;12:860-6.
[10] Davis LB, Lathi RB, Milki AA, Dahan MH. Transvaginal ligation of the cervical branches of the uterine artery and injection of vasopressin in a cervical pregnancy as an initial step to controlling hemorrhage: a case report. J Reprod Med. 2008;53:365-8.
[11] Kung FT, Lin H, Hsu TY, Chang CY, Huang HW, Huang LY, Chou YJ, Huang KH. Differential diagnosis of suspected cervical pregnancy and conservative treatment with the combination of laparoscopy-assisted uterine artery ligation and hysteroscopic endocervical resection. Fertil Steril. 2004;81:1642-9.
[12] Trambert JJ, Einstein MH, Banks E, Frost A, Goldberg GL. Uterine artery embolization in the management of vaginal bleeding from cervical pregnancy: a case series. J Reprod Med. 2005 ;11:844-50.
[13] Cosin JA, Bean M, Grow D et al. The use of methotrexate and arterial embolization to avoid surgery in a case of cervical pregnancy. Fertil Steril 1997;67:1169-71.
[14] Vedantham S, Goodwin CS, Mclucas B et al. Uterine artery embolization: an underused method of controlling pelvic hemorrhage. Am J Obstet Gynecol 1997; 176: 938-48.
[15] Xu B, Wang YK, Zhang YH, Wang S, Yang L, Dai SZ. Angiographic uterine artery embolization followed by immediate curettage: an efficient treatment for controlling heavy bleeding and avoiding recurrent bleeding in cervical pregnancy. J Obstet Gynaecol Res. 2007;33:190-4.
[16] Wang Y, Xu B, Dai S, Zhang Y, Duan Y, Sun C. An efficient conservative treatment modality for cervical pregnancy: angiographic uterine artery embolization followed by immediate curettage. Am J Obstet Gynecol. 2011 Jan;204(1):31.e1-7.
[17] Nakao Y, Yokoyama M, Iwasaka T. Uterine artery embolization followed by dilation and curettage for cervical pregnancy. Obstet Gynecol. 2008;111:505-7.
[18] Yu B, Douglas NC, Guarnaccia MM, Sauer MV. Uterine artery embolization as an adjunctive measure to decrease blood loss prior to evacuating a cervical pregnancy. Arch Gynecol Obstet. 2009;279:721-4.
[19] Hajenius PJ, Roos D, Ankum WM, Van der Veen F. Are serum human chorionic gonadotropin clearance curves of use in monitoring methotrexate treatment in cervical pregnancy? Fertil Steril.1998;70:362-5.
[20] Akutagawa N, Nishikawa A, Saito T, Sagae S, Kudo R. Conservative vaginal surgery for cervical pregnancy. BJOG. 2001;108:888-9.

[21] Ash S, Farrell SA. Hysteroscopic resection of a cervical ectopic pregnancy. Fertil Steril. 1996;66:842-4.

[22] Suzumori N, Katano K, Sato T et al. Conservative treatment by angiographic artery embolization of an 11-week cervical pregnancy after a period of heavy bleeding. Fertil Steril 2003; 80:617-619.

[23] Nappi C, D'Elia A, Di Carlo C et al. Conservative treatment by angiographic uterine artery embolization of a 12 week cervical ectopic pregnancy. Hum Reprod. 1999; 14: 1118-21.

[24] Takano M, Hasegawa Y, Matsuda H et al. Successful management of cervical pregnancy by selective uterine artery embolization: a case report. J Reprod Med 2004; 49: 986-8.

[25] Hirakawa M, Tajima T, Yoshimitsu K, Irie H, Ishigami K, Yahata H, Wake N, Honda H. Uterine artery embolization along with the administration of methotrexate for cervical ectopic pregnancy: technical and clinical outcomes. AJR Am J Roentgenol. 2009;192;6:1601-7.

[26] Einarsson JI, Michel S, Young AE. Delayed spontaneous expulsion of a cervical ectopic pregnancy: a case report. J Minim Invasive Gynecol 2005; 12: 165-7.

[27] Hidalgo LA, Peñafiel J, Chedraui PA. Management of cervical pregnancy: risk factors for failed systemic methotrexate. J Perinat Med. 2004;32:184-6.

[28] Hung TH, Shau WY, Hsieh TT, Hsu JJ, Soong YK, Jeng CJ. Prognostic factors for an unsatisfactory primary methotrexate treatment of cervical pregnancy: a quantitative review. Hum Reprod. 1998;13:2636-42. Review.

[29] Song MJ, Moon MH, Kim JA, Kim TJ. Serial transvaginal sonographic findings of cervical ectopic pregnancy treated with high-dose methotrexate. J Ultrasound Med. 2009;1:55-61.

[30] Jeng CJ, Ko ML, Shen J. Transvaginal ultrasound-guided treatment of cervical pregnancy. Obstet Gynecol. 2007;5:1076-82.

[31] Leeman L, Wendland C. Cervical ectopic pregnancy: diagnosis with endovaginal ultrasound examination and successful treatment with methotrexate. Arch Fam Med 2000;9:72–7.

[32] Sherer DM, Lysikiewicz A, Abulafia O. Viable cervical pregnancy managed with systemic Methotrexate, uterine artery embolization, and local tamponade with inflated Foley catheter balloon. Am J Perinatol 2003; 20: 263-7.

8

Clinical Utility of Ultrasonographic Detection of Pleural Effusion for Evaluation of Heart Failure Patients

H. Kataoka
Nishida Hospital
Japan

1. Introduction

Because heart failure is a clinical syndrome that is caused by abnormal cardiac function, the major goals in the evaluation of patients with heart failure are: 1) to identify the nature and severity of the cardiac abnormality; 2) to characterize the nature and severity of the patient's functional limitation; and 3) to assess the presence and severity of body fluid retention (Packer & Cohn, 1999). An accurate objective measurement of the presence of body fluid retention is necessary in order to evaluate whether or not heart failure status deteriorates. The difficulty in clinically defining such patients, however, stems from the fact that no simpler or more objective sign of body fluid accumulation is currently available because there is no clear cut-off sign of fluid accumulation that can be used reliably to identify subjects with worsening or decompensated heart failure (Gheorghiade et al., 2010). In the recent years, technologies available for the assessment of body fluid status in heart failure patients are increasing in number, variety, and availability (Abraham et al., 2011; Blair et al., 2009; Kataoka, 2009a, 2009b; McDonald, 2010; Tang & Tong, 2009). Chest ultrasound to evaluate pleural effusion or changes in lung status is an evolving imaging technique with novel uses in critically ill patients, including those with heart failure (Bouhemad et al., 2007; Evans & Gleeson, 2004; Havelock et al., 2010; Stefanidis et al., 2011). In uncontrolled heart failure, fluid accumulates throughout the body, including in the thorax. The accumulation and retention of body fluid in the pleural (Kataoka & Takada, 2000; Kataoka, 2007, 2010) and/or pericardial (Kataoka, 2000; Movahed et al., 2006) cavities could be suitable targets for clinical evaluation by chest ultrasound in heart failure patients. This review article describes the application of this technique for the evaluation of pleural effusion in heart failure patients.

2. Pathophysiology of heart failure-associated pleural effusion

The pleural cavity contains a relatively small amount of fluid – approximately 10 ml on each side (Sahn, 1988). Pleural fluid volume is maintained by a balance between fluid production and removal, and changes in the rates of either can potentially result in the presence of excess fluid, traditionally known as pleural effusion (Miserocchi, 1997; Natanzon & Kronzon, 2009). Pathologic pleural effusion can be caused by a wide variety of intrathoracic and systemic diseases (Sahn, 1988). Pleural effusions are classified as either exudates, which indicate a structural pleural abnormality, or transudates, which indicate an imbalance of the hydrostatic and oncotic pressures across the normal pleura (Agostoni et al., 1957; Paddock, 1940). The main causes of structural pleural abnormalities include pulmonary infection, malignancy, pulmonary embolism, or collagen disease. Imbalanced pressure across the normal pleura, on the other hand, is due to heart failure, pulmonary atelectasis, hypoalbuminemia, hepatic hydrothorax, or nephritic syndrome (Azoulay, 2003; Golshan et al., 2002; Light et al., 1972; Mattison et al., 1997; Sahn, 1988). Decompensated heart failure with transudative pleural effusion is the most common cause of pleural effusion in many parts of the world.

The syndrome of heart failure is the response of the body to the heart's inability to maintain an adequate blood supply at a rate commensurate with the requirements of the metabolizing tissues. Arterial underfilling due to worsening of heart failure, either by diminished cardiac output or arterial vasodilatation, triggers activation of neurohormonal systems and derangement of renal function, that in turn incite heart failure-related body fluid retention (Ronco & Maisel, 2010; Schrier & Abraham, 1999; Sica, 2006), including pleural cavity. In decompensated heart failure, the accumulation of pleural effusion is more closely associated with left atrial pressure than right atrial pressure, suggesting that high-pressure pulmonary edema due to left-sided heart failure, accumulating fluid in the lung passes through the visceral pleura and enters the pleural space (Wiener-Kronish et al., 1985, 1987). In this condition, an elevated right atrial pressure might help to sustain or worsen pleural effusion by interfering with lymphatic drainage from the lung (Szabo & Magyar, 1967). The volume of pleural effusion, however, is not known to be associated with pericardial effusion in decompensated heart failure patients (Kataoka, 2000).

Early studies reported a right-sided predominance of heart-failure associated pleural effusion (Bedford & Lovibond, 1941; McPeak & Levine, 1946; White et al., 1947), but subsequent studies report mixed results regarding the lateralization of pleural effusion in heart failure, presumably due to differences in the assessment methods (Kataoka, 2000). A recent review article (Wong et al., 2009) systematically examined a large number of heart failure-associated pleural effusion studies and concluded: (1) most of the studies reported bilateral effusion, and (2) when asymmetry occurred, effusion was predominantly right-sided (either unilateral or one side larger than the other) with summary prevalence for unilateral or larger right-sided effusion at 47% compared with left-sided prevalence of 19%. The findings of a previous study, in which heart failure-associated pleural effusion was quantitatively assessed using computed tomography, support the observations summarized above (Kataoka, 2000). In that study, as many as 52 (87%) of 60 acutely decompensated heart failure patients had pleural effusion. Of 52 heart failure patients with pleural effusion, 45 (87%) had bilateral effusion, 5 (10%) had right-sided effusion only, and 2 (3%) had left-sided effusion only. Among the 45 patients with bilateral pleural effusion, 20 (44%) patients had predominantly right-sided effusion (interhemithoracic difference of the pleural volume > 100 ml), 23 (51%) patients had equally bilateral effusion, and only 2 (5%) had predominantly left-sided effusion.

Multiple explanations for the asymmetry in heart failure-associated pleural effusion have been proposed based on the results of several studies. Among these studies of the right-side preponderance of pleural effusion in heart failure patients, one study presented impressive evidence that the anatomic and hydrostatic factors relating to blood flow from the pulmonary venous bed to the left ventricle strongly favored the predominance of pleural effusion in the right hemithorax (Dock, 1935). In addition, these factors are augmented by the generally preferred right lateral decubitus position of heart failure patients as revealed by studies on trepopnea (Wood, et al., 1937; de Araujo et al., 2011). An older study attributed the right side predominance of pleural effusion to the greater extent of lung and pleural surfaces on the right side relative to the left side (White et al., 1947). To date, however, none of the theories regarding the right-sided polarity of pleural effusion in patients with heart failure has been universally accepted (Natanzon & Kronzon, 2009).

3. Sonographic evaluation of pleural effusion in heart failure

The classical symptoms of heart failure are dyspnea, palpitation, and fatigue. Dyspnea on exertion is common in the general population, particularly in patients with respiratory disease or in the obese, and, therefore, it cannot be used as the selection criterion for the diagnosis of heart failure. Orthopnea and paroxysmal nocturnal dyspnea are less common in the general population than dyspnea alone, but less sensitive, for the diagnosis of heart failure (Ahmed et al., 2004; Fonseca et al., 2004; Mueller et al., 2005).

Body fluid retention in worsening heart failure is reflected in physical signs of congestion, such as fluid body weight gain, leg edema, jugular venous distension and pulmonary crackles. As for pleural effusion, some studies suggest the possibility of physical examination maneuver to detect pleural effusion as little as 50 ml (Bernstein & White, 1952; Guarino & Guarino, 1994). However, none of these physical signs of fluid retention is particularly sensitive, though specificity varies among studies (Fonseca et al., 2004; Mueller et al., 2005; Rohde et al, 2004; Stevenson & Perloff, 1989; Tresch, 1997). These limited roles of heart failure-associated physical findings and poor prediction of symptoms for identifying worsening heart failure status emphasize the need for additional diagnostic tools. Chest ultrasound might be one of these diagnostic tools, but this modality is not yet in widespread use. Evaluation of the clinical utility of this method for assessing heart failure patients is therefore important.

3.1 Chest ultrasound technique

The patient is placed in a sitting position on a bed or chair, and chest ultrasound is performed on each hemithorax using a transducer through the intercostal space, and scanning is performed along the paravertebral, scapular, and posterior axillary lines (Kataoka & Takada, 2000; Kataoka, 2007; Piccoli et al., 2005; Waggoner et al., 1995). Using a high resolution (3.5-5.0 MHz) transducer applied to the chest wall, the parietal pleura lining the bony thorax and the visceral pleura covering the lung are seen just beneath the chest wall as two thin and bright echogenic lines. Normally, the two pleural lines are smooth and less than 2 mm thick (Mathis, 1997). These higher frequency transducers, while providing superior spatial resolution, may be limited by insufficient penetration (Warakaulle & Traill, 2004) and thus inadequate for obese patient. The pleural space can be identified by observing the normal motion of the lung during breathing. The liver and spleen, and occasionally the kidney, are used as guides to chest ultrasound searching for the pleural effusion. The air-filled lung surface totally reflects the ultrasound beam and produces a bright, echogenic line of sound reflection (Figure 1A). This characteristic pattern of bright echoes produced by a reverberation artifact is recognized as normal for the air-filled lung and indicates the absence of a pleural effusion, but there is an observation that pointed out an appearance of 2-mm-thick pleural fluid layer in healthy individuals (Kocijančič et al., 2005). The presence of a pleural effusion is diagnosed by the appearance of an anechoic space between the parietal pleura and the highly reflective visceral pleura-lung interface. The amount of pleural effusion visualized on an ultrasonogram can be assessed quantitatively (Remérand et al., 2010; Vignon et al., 2005) or semi-quantitatively (Kataoka, 2007; Tsai et al., 2008). The following categories are one example of the semi-quantification of pleural effusion (Kataoka, 2007): small if the echo-free space is within the costophrenic angle, moderate if the echo-free space extends over the costophrenic angle and causes near separation of basal lung from the diaphragm, and large if the space is bigger and separates the basal lung from the diaphragm (Figures 1- B, C, D).

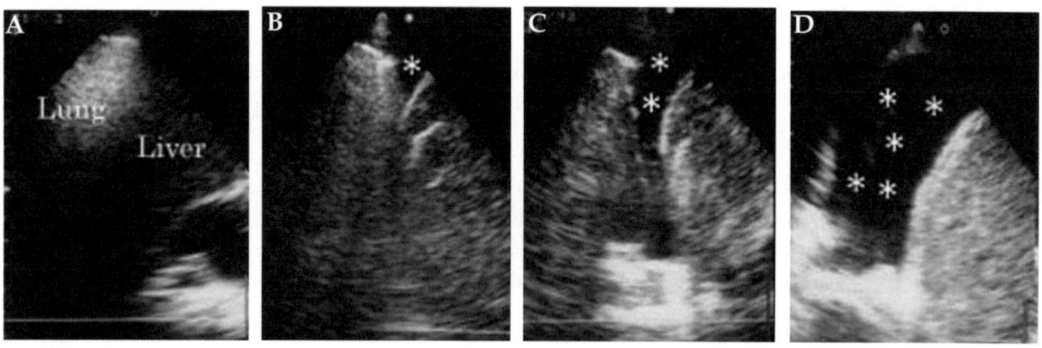

Fig. 1. Examples of pleural effusion. (A) absent, (B) small, (C) moderate, (D) large collection of fluid. Asterisks indicate pleural effusion. Adapted from Kataoka (2007). (Adapted and reproduced with permission from Wiley Periodicals, Inc.)

3.2 Accuracy of sonographic detection of pleural effusion

Radiographic identification of pleural effusion is reported to be insensitive and detects only moderate to large accumulation of pleural fluid. Pleural effusion becomes visible on the upright lateral radiograph at a volume of approximately 50 ml as a meniscus in the posterior costophrenic sulcus. The meniscus becomes visible on the postero-anterior projection at a volume about 175 to 525 ml (Woodring, 1984) or 200 ml (Blackmore et al., 1996). To determine the accuracy of chest ultrasound for detecting pleural effusion in acutely decompensated heart failure patients, previous study evaluated the usefulness of chest ultrasound in comparison with physical signs, erect postero-anterior chest x-ray, and thoracic x-ray computed tomography (Kataoka & Takada, 2000). The incidence of pleural effusion detected by chest ultrasound was high when compared to plain chest radiograph (Table 1): postero-anterior projection of chest x-ray could not identify a very small amount (less than 100 ml) of pleural effusion, but chest ultrasound detected most of the pleural effusion. Many other studies have also confirmed the superiority of chest ultrasound for detection of small pleural effusion compared to simple chest radiographic technique (Gryminski et al., 1976; Kohan et al., 1986; Lipscomb et al., 1981; Yu et al., 1992; Zanobetti et al., 2011). Thus, the diagnosis of pleural effusions in critically ill patients has been revolutionized with the advent of chest ultrasound allowing easy bedside quantification of pleural fluid and making thoracentesis a safe procedure (Pneumatikos & Bouros, 2008).

	Right Hemithorax			Left Hemithorax		
Pleural Effusion by CT	**n**	**X-ray**	**Ultrasound**	**n**	**X-ray**	**Ultrasound**
Normal controls (n = 22)						
Absent	22	0	0	22	0	1 (5%)
Patient group (n = 60)						
Absent	10	0	1 (10%)	14	0	2 (14%)
Present (ml)						
Very small (≤100)	15	2 (13%)	13 (87%)	15	0	12 (80%)
Small (≤400)	20	9 (45%)	18 (90%)	23	6 (26%)	23 (100%)
Moderate (≤700)	8	6 (75%)	8 (100%)	6	4 (67%)	6 (100%)
Large	7	7 (100%)	7 (100%)	2	2 (100%)	2 (100%)
Total	50	24 (48%)	46 (92%)	46	12 (26%)	43 (93%)

Table 1. Comparison of the presence of signs of pleural effusion between plain chest x-ray and chest ultrasound in normal controls and patients with decompensated chronic heart failure. Adapted from Kataoka & Takada (2000). (Adapted and reproduced with permission from the American College of Cardiology)

3.3 Clinical significance of ultrasound pleural effusion in heart failure patients

In acutely worsening heart failure patients, the reported incidence of pleural effusion on chest ultrasound is high when compared to other heart failure-associated examinations (Kataoka & Takada, 2000). Namely, an observation of 60 acutely decompensated heart failure patients indicated that the incidence of pulmonary rales or wheezing was modest (56%) but that of other physical signs of jugular venous distension (38%) and peripheral edema (33%) was low. On erect postero-anterior plain chest radiograph, combined frequency of radiographic heart failure signs, consisting of the pulmonary edema (45%) and/or pleural effusion (41%), was low (61%), but the presence of ultrasound pleural effusion was high (90%). As such, diagnostic utility of chest ultrasound searching for pleural effusion in heart failure patients seems to be high in emergent situation.

Recent studies have reported that ultrasound signs of pleural effusion were a common presenting heart failure-related sign for established heart failure patients during follow-up (Kataoka, 2007; Kataoka, 2011), and were strongly associated with the appearance of other heart failure-related symptoms and signs (Kataoka, 2010). The results also demonstrated that the ultrasound signs of pleural effusion had high diagnostic value for identifying heart failure status worsening, confirming that this sign was a useful marker in such patients during follow-up (Kataoka, 2010). Importantly, ultrasound-detected pleural effusion signs were often present in asymptomatic heart failure worsening with the minimal appearance of other heart failure-related signs, which was supported by recent observation (Kataoka, 2011). Other than in the severity of leg edema, there were no differences in heart failure-related signs between symptomatic (n = 45) and asymptomatic clinic visits (n = 38) with a positive ultrasound pleural effusion sign (Table 2). Unsuspected and not clinically apparent pleural effusion is easily detected by a simple chest ultrasound examination and may have an important bearing on therapeutic decisions and outcome. Detection of the ultrasound pleural effusion can potentially become one of the leading signs of deterioration in heart failure during follow-up of established heart failure patients. Thus, chest ultrasound should appropriately be performed in established heart failure patients, with or without symptomatic change, in order to obtain objective evidence of worsening heart failure status.

Variables	Symptomatic Events (n = 45)	Asymptomatic Events (n = 38)	*P* Value
Amount of ultrasound pleural effusion			
Small degree	20 (44%)	24 (63%)	0.0257
Moderate degree	18 (40%)	14 (37%)	0.0257
Large degree	7 (16%)	0	0.0257
Heart failure-related signs			
Leg edema			
Mild	12 (27%)	17 (45%)	<0.0001
Moderate to severe	19 (42%)	0	<0.0001
Total	31 (69%)	17 (45%)	0.044
Audible third heart sound	11 (24%)	3 (8%)	0.075
Pulmonary rales	12 (27%)	8 (21%)	0.613
Fluid body weight gain	35 (78%)	23 (61%)	0.099

Table 2. Comparison of heart failure-related signs between positive ultrasound pleural effusion events with (n = 45) and without (n = 38) symptomatic change. Values are presented as numbers (percentages)

In established heart failure patients during follow-up, effects of the volume of pleural effusion on heart failure-associated symptoms, signs, and the requirement of hospitalization are still unknown. Based on my clinical records of heart-failure monitoring in 83 established heart failure patients, I evaluated the pleural fluid volume dependency of symptoms and signs, and/or the requirement of hospitalization. The results of this analysis have shown that heart failure-related symptoms were not different, and only several signs were different between worsening heart failure events in patients with moderate to large pleural fluid retention and those in patients with small pleural effusion (Table 3). However, worsening heart failure events with moderate to large pleural fluid retention required more hospitalization than those with small pleural effusion. Thus, determining the volume of pleural effusion is clinically important because the amount of pleural effusion can affect the clinical course of individual heart failure patients.

3.4 Differentiation of heart failure-associated pleural effusion from other causes

Pleural effusion can be caused by a variety of intrathoracic and systemic diseases (Golshan et al., 2002; Mattison et al., 1997) which may necessitate thoracentesis to determine the cause of the effusion as described below in this section. In established heart failure patients, pleural effusion usually appears in relation to worsening heart failure during follow-up. Treatment with additional diuretics could resolve the pleural effusion in such cases, confirming the cause of effusion with high probability due to worsening heart failure. Persistent or increased amounts of pleural effusion despite added diuretic therapy during follow-up of established heart failure patients should first be considered a reflection of refractory heart failure and/or worsening of renal function, and requires concomitant consideration of other causes of pleural effusion. A review of my clinical records for heart-failure monitoring of 83 established heart failure patients (follow-up period of 652 ± 456 days) revealed unresolved pleural effusion due to refractory heart failure and/or renal failure in 12 study patients, but thoracentesis was required to reveal the cause in two other patients, one due to lung cancer and the other due to bacterial pneumonia (unpublished data).

Chest ultrasound provides information regarding the nature of pleural effusion, e.g., transudates are echo-free, whereas echoic effusions are likely to be exudates (Yang et al., 1992; Yu et al., 1992), but might be of limited value for identifying the cause of the pleural effusion. Thus, a persistent or increased amount of effusion on ultrasound despite the augmented treatment for decompensated heart failure status should be an indication for thoracentesis to evaluate the possible cause of effusions other than heart failure through analysis of the pleural fluid (Bartter et al., 1994; Light et al., 1972; Pneumatikos & Bouros, 2008; Porcel et al., 2009; Porcel, 2011). In general, the traditional criteria of Light et al. (1972) (i.e., pleural fluid/serum total protein ratio > 0.5, pleural fluid/serum LDH ratio > 0.6, and pleural fluid LDH > 200 for identifying exudative pleural effusions) can be used to differentiate exudates from transudates with a negative predictive value of 96% and a sensitivity of 98%. A high incidence of misclassifications by Light's criteria has been reported, however, in heart failure patients on diuretic therapy (Eid et al., 2002; Porcel et al., 2009; Romero-Candeira et al., 2001; Roth et al., 1990). In such heart failure patients, differences in the amount of albumin in the serum and pleural fluid (discriminating level; around 1.2 g/dl) are useful for differentiating exudates from transudates (Eid et al., 2002; Romero-Candeira et al., 2001; Roth et al., 1990).

	Volume of Pleural Effusion by Ultrasound		
Heart Failure-related Variable	**Small (n = 44)**	**Moderate to Large (n = 39)**	***P* Value**
Heart failure-related symptoms	20 (45%)	25 (64%)	0.123
Heart failure-related signs			
Leg edema			
Mild	15 (34%)	27 (69%)	0.0001
Moderate to severe	9 (20%)	10 (26%)	
Total	24 (55%)	37 (95%)	P<0.0001
Audible third heart sound	4 (9%)	10 (26%)	0.045
Pulmonary rales	10 (23%)	10 (26%)	0.757
Fluid body weight gain	27 (61%)	31 (79%)	0.073
Required hospitarization	12 (27%)	20 (51%)	0.025

Table 3. Pleural effusion volume dependency of symptoms and signs of heart failure. Values are presented as numbers (percentages)

Recently, the pleural fluid level of natriuretic peptide, either B-type natriuretic peptide (BNP) or the amono-terminal fragment N-terminal pro-BNP (NT-pro-BNP), has been suggested as a useful adjunct for the diagnosis of heart failure-associated pleural effusion, including cardiac effusion misclassified as exudates by the criteria of Light (Kolditz et al., 2006; Liao, et al., 2008; Long et al., 2010; Porcel et al., 2004, 2009; Tomcsányi et al., 2004). Some studies have shown a strong correlation of natriuretic peptide concentrations in serum and pleural fluid and equal diagnostic accuracies for serum and pleural fluid natriuretic peptide measurements for the discrimination of pleural effusions attributable to heart failure (Kolditz et al., 2006; Tomcsányi et al., 2004). Therefore, it could be claimed that it may not be necessary to perform diagnostic thoracentesis in patients with serum natriuretic concentrations exceeding a cut-off value with a high positive predictive value, making the diagnosis of heart failure as the underlying cause of the pleural effusion very likely in these patients. However, in all other patients with serum natriuretic concentrations below such a cut-off value, early diagnostic thoracentesis may be necessary to determine whether the effusion is exudates or transudates in nature (Mueller & Haltmayer, 2006).

3.5 Advantages and limitations of thoracic sonography for evaluating heart failure

This technique has several advantages for evaluating heart failure patients: 1) high diagnostic accuracy for diagnosing worsening heart failure through identifying ultrasound pleural effusion, e.g., bedside chest radiography is routinely performance under emergent conditions, but this technique offers limited diagnostic performance and efficacy for identifying pleural effusion (see sections "3.2" and "4"); 2) portability and performance ease at outpatient clinic or bedside with a hand-held device (Piccoli et al., 2005; Roelandt, 2003), e.g., though x-ray computed tomography has high diagnostic performance for identifying pleural effusion, this modality is not available or is not available quickly enough because it requires transportation of the patient to the radiology department; 3) short examination time, e.g., acquisition time to assess both hemithorax searching for pleural effusion is approximately 2 minutes (Tayal et at., 2006); 4) safety of the procedure due to the non-ionizing nature of the examination; and 4) lower cost. Additionally, several studies have demonstrated that chest ultrasound can detect pulmonary edema (Agricola et al., 2005; Copetti et al., 2008; Jambrik et al., 2004; Lichtenstein et al., 1997, 2004; Zanobetti et al., 2011) and help to discriminate among the most important causes of acute dyspnea like pulmonary or cardiovascular diseases. The presence of diffuse "comet-tails" or B-line artifacts on chest ultrasound indicates diffuse alveolar-interstitial syndrome, which is often a sign of acute pulmonary edema. This condition rules out exacerbation of chronic obstructive pulmonary disease as the main cause of acute dyspnea (Lichtenstein & Mezière, 1998; Volpicelli et al., 2008). These advantages make chest ultrasound a useful diagnostic tool with great potential for assisting decision-making and management of patients with heart failure. Several disadvantages include: 1) technical difficulty in obtaining a high quality of image in obese patients; 2) restricted field of view; and 3) somewhat operator-dependent findings.

4. Reappraisal of chest x-ray for evaluation of heart failure patients

Because chest radiography is still a standard method for evaluating fluid status in heart failure patients (Evans & Gleeson, 2004; Logue et al., 1963; McHugh et al., 1972; Meszaros, 1973; Milne et al., 1985; Wiener et al., 1991), it is appropriate to briefly summarize the limitation of this modality for assessing heart failure status for comparison with the clinical role of chest ultrasound. Two important specific markers of fluid accumulation on plain chest radiograph are pleural effusion and interstitial edema (hilar haziness, peribronchial cuffing, Kerley's B lines, or septal lines) or alveolar pulmonary edema. An erect postero-anterior chest x-ray should be performed wherever possible, including a lateral decubitus film, when necessary, for detecting small pleural effusions (Moskowitz et al., 1973). Though chest x-ray signs of interstitial/alveolar pulmonary edema and pleural effusion are important markers of fluid retention, the diagnostic accuracy of these x-ray signs of pulmonary congestion in chronic heart failure is not very high (Chakko et al., 1991; Collins et al., 2006; Gadsbøll et al., 1989; Mahdyoon et al., 1989), presumably due to increased lymphatic drainage clearing of the flooded interstitium/alveoli (Szidon et al., 1972). Also, as described above (see section "3.2"), chest x-ray identification of pleural effusion is not sensitive and only detects moderate to large amounts of accumulation. Thus, clinicians cannot rule out body fluid retention in heart failure patients without radiographic signs of pulmonary congestion, particularly in those without chest x-ray signs of pleural effusion. Chest ultrasound allows accurate evaluation of fluid accumulation in the thorax, including pleural effusion, and pulmonary congestion due to worsening heart failure (Agricola et al., 2005; Jambrik et al., 2004; Lichtenstein, et al., 1997, 2004; Zanobetti et al., 2011).

5. Case presentation

5.1 Patient no.1

A 75-year-old female patient visited the hospital emergently with a complaint of New York Heart Association functional class III dyspnea and night cough. Physical examination disclosed an audible third heart sound and mild ankle edema. Electrocardiographic findings included sinus tachycardia of 105 beats/minute and non-specific ST-T changes. Echocardiography revealed dilated, generalized hypokinesis of the left ventricle with an ejection fraction of 23% and a diastolic volume of 200 ml. An erect postero-anterior chest x-ray film showed moderate cardiomegaly with mild hypervascularity in the upper lung field, but no apparent pleural effusion (Figure 2). Chest ultrasound revealed the collection of a large pleural effusion in both hemithoraces. Computed tomography confirmed the chest ultrasound findings. Worsening of heart failure status due to dilated cardiomyopathy was confirmed by the marked elevation of serum B-type natriuretic peptide level of 1865 pg/ml. The selected therapeutic option using extra-diuretics improved her clinical status; she lost 2.6 kg body weight and chest ultrasound confirmed complete resolution of the pleural effusion.

5.2 Patient no.2

During follow-up of a 78-year-old male patient with a history of decompensated heart failure due to hypertension, he experienced New York Heart Association functional class III dyspnea at a regular clinic visit, and underwent a scheduled examination. Physical examination revealed mild leg edema and diffuse basal rales on auscultation. The electrocardiogram showed a regular sinus rhythm of 72 beats/minute and left ventricular hypertrophy. On echocardiogram, left ventricular size and function were normal based on a left ventricular diastolic volume of 68 ml, ejection fraction of 65%, and Doppler index of the ratio of mitral E wave to the A wave of 0.8. Plain erect postero-anterior chest x-ray was

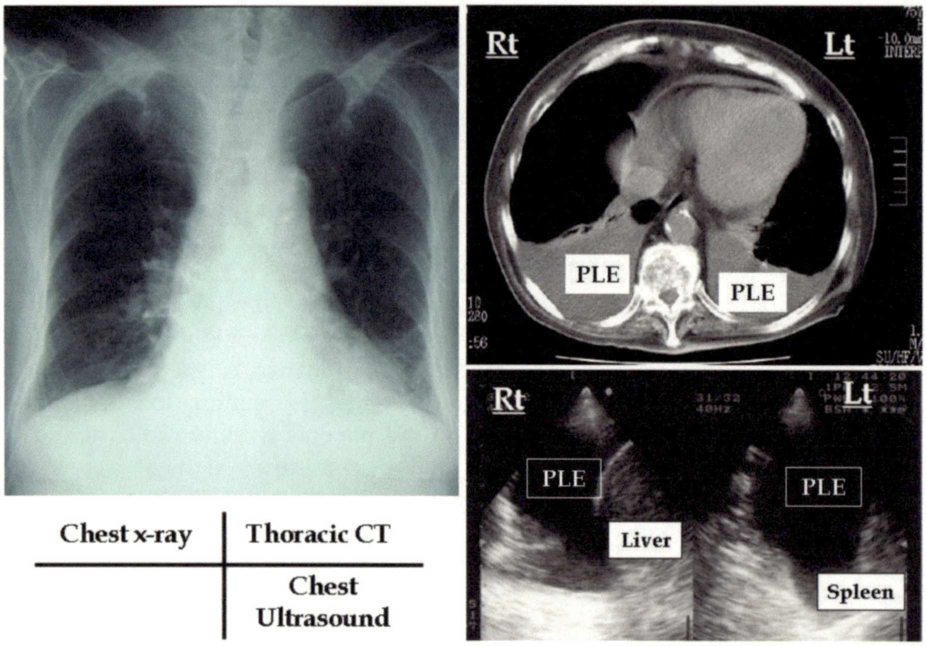

Fig. 2. Chest x-ray film, x-ray computed tomogram, and chest ultrasound obtained from a 75-year-old female with worsening heart failure due to idiopathic dilated cardiomyopathy. Lt = left; PLE = pleural effusion; Rt = right

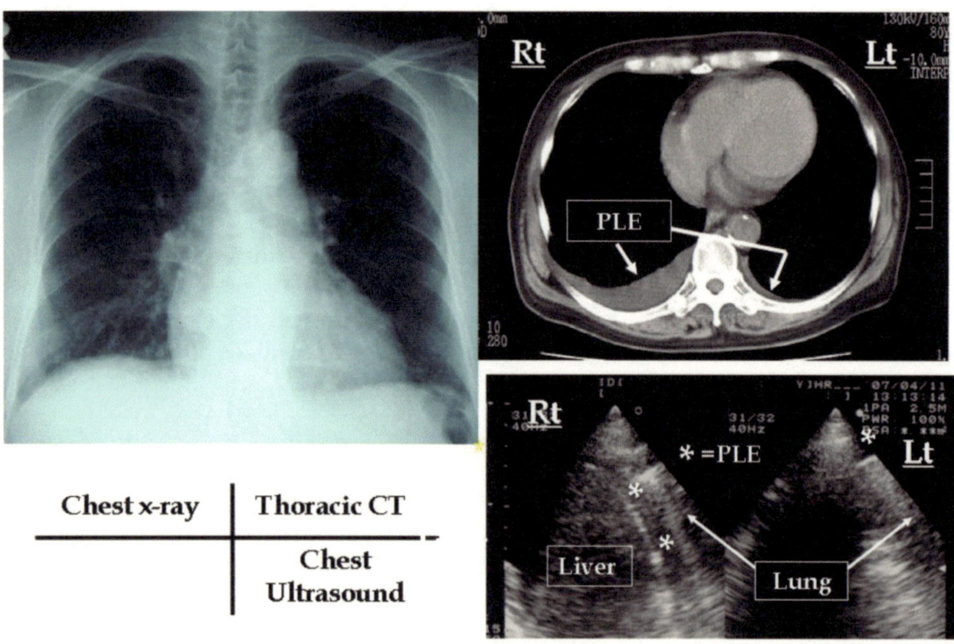

Fig. 3. Chest x-ray film, x-ray computed tomogram, and chest ultrasound obtained from a 78-year-old male with worsening heart failure due to hypertensive heart disease. Lt = left; PLE = pleural effusion; Rt = right

normal except moderate cardiomegaly (Figure 3). There was no evidence of pleural effusion on postero-anterior chest x-ray. Chest ultrasound disclosed a moderate amount of pleural effusion in the right hemithorax and a small collection in the left. Computed tomography confirmed the chest ultrasound findings. Serum B-type natriuretic peptide was increased to 381 pg/ml from 65 pg/ml measured at a recent clinic visit for clinical stability. Use of extra-diuretics improved his clinical status with improvement of symptoms and lost of body weight of 3.1 kg, and the pleural effusion disappeared on chest ultrasound.

6. Conclusion

Heart failure is a leading cause of hospitalization, particularly in the elderly population, and the frequency of heart failure-related hospital re-admission in heart failure patients within the first 3 to 6 months is high (Vinson et al., 1990; Krumholz et al., 1997; Fonarow et al., 2008). Heart failure-related hospitalizations are not benign events, with an increased (and independent) risk of mortality following the initial and each subsequent hospitalization for heart failure (Setoguchi et al., 2007; Solomon et al., 2007). Body fluid retention or congestion is the main characteristic feature for worsening heart failure, leading to hospitalization (Gheorghiade et al., 2006; Pang & Levy, 2010). Thus, early detection of excess body fluid accumulation is crucial for identifying worsening heart failure events in patients with heart failure. As described in this chapter, the use of chest ultrasound to determine pleural effusion allows for sensitive detection of worsening heart failure and will improve diagnosis and facilitate decision-making in heart failure patients. Widespread use of ultrasound, a method that is not technically difficult to perform or analyze, to evaluate pleural effusion in patients with heart failure is therefore warranted, irrespective of the accompanying symptoms, and will lead to a more accurate diagnosis. Of course, it should be kept in mind that, a lot of patients without pleural effusion on chest ultrasound have deterioration of heart failure status. Fortunately, physicians rarely use single observation in clinical decision-making. Proper diagnosis of worsening heart failure requires clinicians to integrate elements of patient history, physical examination, and diagnostic test results together with knowledge of multiple pharmacologic and non-pharmacologic treatments.

7. Future research

Up to date, there is a paucity of data on the feasibility of using ultrasound pleural effusion as part of the diagnostic approach in patients with heart failure. Thus, additional study is necessary to answer the question of whether chest ultrasound pleural effusion may emerge as clinically useful in identifying worsening heart failure status.

8. References

[1] Abraham, WT., Adamson, PB., Bourge, RC., Aaron, MF., Costanzo, MR., Stevenson, LW., Strickland, W., Neelagaru, S., Raval, N., Krueger, S., Weiner, S., Shavelle, D., Jeffries, B. & Yadav, JS., for the CHAMPION Trial Study Group. (2011). Wireless Pulmonary Artery Haemodynamic Monitoring in Chronic Heart Failure: A Randomised Controlled Trial. *Lancet*, Vol.377, No.9766, pp.658-666

[2] Agostoni, E., Taglietti, A. & Setnikar, I. (1957). Absorption Force of the Capillaries of the Visceral Pleura in Determination of the Intrapleural Pressure. *American Journal of Physiology*, Vol.191, No.2, pp. 277-282

[3] Agricola, E., Bove, T., Oppizzi, M., Marino, G., Zangrillo, A., Margonato, A. & Picano, E. (2005). "Ultrasound Comet-Tail Images": A Marker of Pulmonary Edema – A Comparative Study with Wedge Pressure and Extravascular Lung Water. *Chest*, Vol.127, No.5, pp. 1690-1695

[4] Ahmed, A., Allman, RM., Aronow, WS. & DeLong, JF. (2004). Diagnosis of Heart Failure in Older Adults: Predictive Value of Dyspnea at Rest. *Archives of Gerontology and Geriatrics*, Vol.38, No.3, pp. 297-307

[5] Azoulay, E. (2003). Pleural Effusions in the Intensive Care Unit. *Current Opinion in Pulmonary Medicine*, Vol.9, No.4, pp. 291-297

[6] Bartter, T., Santarelli, R., Akers, SM. & Pratter, MR. (1994). The Evaluation of Pleural Effusion. *Chest*, Vol.106, No.4, pp. 1209-1214

[7] Bedford, DE. & Lovibond, JL. (1941). Hydrothorax in Heart Failure. *British Heart Journal*, Vol.3, No.2, pp. 93-111

[8] Bernstein, A. & White, FZ. (1952). Unusual Physical Findings in Pleural Effusion: Intrathoracic Manometric Studies. *Annals of Internal Medicine*, Vol.37, Vol.4, pp. 733-738

[9] Blackmore, CC., Black, WC., Dallas, RV. & Crow, HC. (1996). Pleural Fluid Volume Estimation: A Chest Radiograph Prediction Rule. *Academic Radiology*, Vol.3, No.2, pp. 103-109

[10] Blair, JE., Brennan, M., Goonewardena, SN., Shah, D., Vasaiwala, S. & Spencer, KT. (2009). Usefulness of Hand-Carried Ultrasound to Predict Elevated Left Ventricular Filling Pressure. *American Journal of Cardiology*, Vol.103, No.2, pp. 246-247

[11] Bouhemad, B., Zhang, M., Lu, Q. & Rouby, JJ. (2007). Clinical Review: Bedside Lung Ultrasound in Critical Care Practice. *Critical Care*, Vol.11, 205 (doi:10.1186/cc5668)

[12] Chakko, S., Woska, D., Martinez, H., de Marchena, E., Futterman, L., Kessler, KM. & Myerburg, RJ. (1991). Clinical, Radiographic, and Hemodynamic Correlations in Chronic Congestive Heart Failure: Conflicting Results May Lead to Inappropriate Care. *American Journal of Medicine*, Vol.90, No.3, pp. 353-359

[13] Collins, SP., Lindsell, CJ., Storrow, AB., Abraham, WT., on behalf of the ADHERE Scientific Advisory Committee, Investigators and Study Group. (2006). Prevalence of Negative Chest Radiography Results in the Emergency Department Patient with Decompensated Heart Failure. *Annals of Emergency Medicine*, Vol.47, No.1, pp. 13-18

[14] Copetti, R., Soldati, G. & Copetti, P. (2008). Chest Sonography: A Useful Tool to Differentiate Acute Cardiogenic Pulmonary Edema from Acute Respiratory Distress Syndrome. *Cardiovascular Ultrasound*, Vol.6: 16 (doi:10.1186/1476-7120-6-16)

[15] de Araujo, BS., Reichert, R., Eifer, DA., Soder, SA., dos Santos, MBS., Clausell, N. & Beck-da-Silva, L. (2011). Trepopnea May Explain Right-Sided Pleural Effusion in Patients with Decompensated Heart Failure. *American Journal of Emergency Medicine*, doi:10.1016/j.ajem.2011.04.013

[16] Dock, W. (1935). The Anatomical and Hydrostatic Basis of Orthopnea and of Right Hydrothorax in Cardiac Failure. *American Heart Journal*, Vol.10, No.8, pp. 1047-1055

[17] Eid, AA., Keddissi, JI., Samaha, M., Tawk, MM., Kimmell, K. & Kinasewitz, GT. (2002). Exudative Effusions in Congestive Heart Failure. *Chest*, Vol.122, No.5, pp. 1518-1523

[18] Evans, AL. & Gleeson, FV. (2004). Radiology in Pleural Disease: State of the Art. *Respirology*, Vol.9, No.3, pp. 300-312

[19] Fonarow, GC., Abraham, WT., Albert, NM., Stough, WG., Gheorghiade, M., Greenberg, BH., O'Connor, CM., Pieper, K., Sun, JL., Yancy, CW. & Young, JB., for the OPTIMIZE-HF Investigators and Hospitals. (2008). Factors Identified as Precipitating Hospital Admissions for Heart Failure and Clinical Outcomes: Findings from OPTIMIZE-HF. *Archives of Internal Medicine*, Vol.168, No.8, 847-854

[20] Fonseca, C., Morais, H., Mota, T., Matias, F., Costa, C., Gouveia-Oliveira, A. & Ceia, F., on behalf of the EPICA Investigators. (2004). The Diagnosis of Heart Failure in Primary Care: Value of Symptoms and Signs. *European Journal of Heart Failure*, Vol.6, No.6, pp. 795-800

[21] Gadsbøll, N., Høilund-Carlsen, PF., Nielsen, GG., Berning, J., Brunn, NE., Stage, P., Hein, E., Marving, J., Løngborg-Jensn, H. & Jensen, BH. (1989). Symptoms and Signs of Heart Failure in Patients with Myocardial Infarction: Reproducibility and Relationship to Chest X-ray, Radionuclide Ventriculography and Right Heart Catheterization. *European Heart Journal*, Vol.10, No.11, pp. 1017-1028

[22] Gheorghiade, M., Filippatos, G., De Luca, L. & Burnett, J. (2006). Congestion in Acute Heart Failure Syndromes: An Essential Target of Evaluation and Treatment. *American Journal of Medicine*, Vol.119, No.12 (Supplement 1), pp. S3-S10

[23] Gheorghiade, M., Follath, F., Ponikowski, P., Barsuk, JH., Blair, JEA., Cleland, JG., Dickstein, K., Drazner, MH., Fonarow, GC., Jaarsma, T., Jondeau, G., Lopez Sendon, J., Mebazaa, A., Metra, M., Nieminen, M., Pang, PS., Seferovic, P., Stevenson, LW., van Veldhuisen, DJ., Zannad, F., Anker, SD., Rhodes, A., McMurray, JJV. & Filippatos, G. (2010). Assessing and Grading Congestion in Acute Heart Failure: A Scientific Statement from the Acute Heart Failure Committee of the Heart Failure Association of the European Society of Cardiology and Endorsed by the European Society of Intensive Care Medicine. *European Journal of Heart Failure*, Vol.12, No.5, pp. 423-433

[24] Golshan, M., Faghihi, M., Ghanbarian, K. & Ghanei, M. (2002). Common Causes of Pleural Effusion in Referral Hospital in Isfahan, Iran 1997-1998. *Asian Cardiovascular & Thoracic Annals*, Vol.10, No.1, pp. 43-46

[25] Gryminski, J., Krakówka, P. & Lypacewicz, G. (1976). The Diagnosis of Pleural Effusion by Ultrasonic and Radiographic Techniques. *Chest*, Vol.70, No.1, pp. 33-37

[26] Guarino, JR. & Guarino, JC. (1994). Auscultatory Percussion: A Simple Method to Detect Pleural Effusion. *Journal of General Internal Medicine*, Vol.9, No.2, pp. 71-74

[27] Havelock, T., Teoh, R., Laws, D., Gleeson, F., on behalf of the BTS Pleural Disease Guideline Group. (2010). Pleural Procedures and Thoracic Ultrasound: British Thoracic Society Pleural Disease Guideline 2010. *Thorax*, Vol.65, Supplement 2, pp. ii61-ii76

[28] Jambrik, Z., Monti, S., Coppola, V., Agricola, E., Mottola, G., Miniati, M. & Picano, E. (2004). Usefulness of Ultrasound Lung Comets as a Nonradiologic Sign of Extravascular Lung Water. *American Journal of Cardiology*, Vol.93, No.10, pp. 1265-1270

[29] Kataoka, H. & Takada, S. (2000). The Role of Thoracic Ultrasonography for Evaluation of Patients with Decompensated Chronic Heart Failure. *Journal of American College of Cardiology*, Vol.35, No.6, pp. 1638-1646

[30] Kataoka, H. (2000). Pericardial and Pleural Effusions in Decompensated Chronic Heart Failure. *American Heart Journal*, Vol.139, No.5, pp. 918-923.

[31] Kataoka, H. (2007). Utility of Thoracic Sonography for Follow-Up Examination of Chronic Heart Failure Patients with Previous Decompensation. *Clinical Cardiology*, Vol. 30, No.7, pp. 336-341

[32] Kataoka, H. (2009a). A New Monitoring Method for the Estimation of Body Fluid Status by Digital Weight Scale Incorporating Bioelectrical Impedance Analyzer in Definite Heart Failure Patients. *Journal of Cardiac Failure*, Vol.15, No.5, pp. 410-418

[33] Kataoka, H. (2009b). Novel Monitoring Method for the Management of Heart Failure: Combined Measurement of Body Weight and Bioimpedance Index of Body Fat Percentage. *Future Cardiology*, Vol.5, No.6, pp. 541-546

[34] Kataoka, H. (2010). UltraSound Pleural Effusion (US-PE) Sign as a Useful Marker for Identifying Worsening of Established Heart Failure Patients during Follow-Up. *European Heart Journal*, Vol.31, Supplement 1, pp. 278

[35] Kataoka, H. (2011). Detection of Preclinical Body Fluid Retention in Established Heart Failure Patients during Follow-Up by a Digital Weight Scale Incorporating a Bioelectrical Impedance Analyzer. *Congestive Heart Failure*, doi: 10.1111/j.1751-7133.2011.00230.x

[36] Kocijančič, K., Kocijančič, I. & Vidmar, G. (2005). Sonography of Pleural Space in Healthy Individuals. *Journal of Clinical Ultrasound*, Vol.33, No.8, pp. 386-389

[37] Kohan, JM., Poe, RH., Israel, RH., Kennedy, JD., Benazzi, RB., Kallay, MC. & Greenblatt, DW. (1986). Value of Chest Ultrasonography versus Decubitus Roentgenography for Thoracentesis. *American Review of Respiratory Disease*, Vol.133, No.6, pp. 1124-1126

[38] Kolditz, M., Halank, M., Schiemanck, CS., Schmeisser, A. & Höffken, G. (2006). High Diagnostic Accuracy of NT-proBNP for Cardiac Origin of Pleural Effusions. *European Respiratory Journal*, Vol.28, No.1, pp. 144-150

[39] Krumholz, HM., Parent, EM., Tu, N., Vaccarino, V., Wang, Y., Radford, MJ. & Hennen, J. (1997). Readmission after Hospitalization for Congestive Heart Failure among Medicare Beneficiaries. *Archives of Internal Medicine*, Vol.157, No.1, pp. 99-104

[40] Liao, H., NA, MJ., Dikensoy, O., Lane, KB., Randal, B. & Light, RW. (2008). Diagnostic Value of Pleural Fluid N-Terminal Pro-Brain Natriuretic Peptide Levels in Patients with Cardiovascular Diseases. *Respirology*, Vol.13, No.1, pp. 53-57

[41] Lichtenstein D., Mézière, G., Biderman, P., Gepner, A. & Barré, O. (1997). The Comet-Tail Artifact: An Ultrasound Sign of Alveolar-Interstitial Syndrome. *American Journal of Respiratory and Critical Care Medicine*, Vol.156, No.5, pp. 1640-1646

[42] Lichtenstein, D. & Mezière, G. (1998). A Lung Ultrasound Sign Allowing Bedside Distinction between Pulmonary Edema and COPD: The Comet-Tail Artifact. *Intensive Care Medicine*, Vol.24, No.12, pp. 1331-1334

[43] Lichtenstein, D., Goldstein, I., Mourgeon, E., Cluzel, P., Grenier, P. & Rouby, JJ. (2004). Comparative Diagnostic Performances of Auscultation, Chest Radiography, and Lung Ultrasonography in Acute Respiratory Distress Syndrome. *Anesthesiology*, Vol.100, No.1, pp. 9-15

[44] Light, RW., MacGregor, I., Luchsinger, PC. & Ball, WC. Jr. (1972). Pleural Effusions: The Diagnostic Separation of Transudates and Exudates. *Annals of Internal Medicine*, Vol.77, No.4, pp. 507-513

[45] Lipscomb, DJ., Flower, CDR. & Hadfield, JW. (1981). Ultrasound of the Pleura: An Assessment of its Clinical Value. *Clinical Radiology*, Vol.32, No.3, pp. 289-290

[46] Logue, RB., Rogers, JV. Jr. & Gay, BB. Jr. (1963). Subtle Roentgenographic Signs of Left Heart Failure. *American Heart Journal*, Vol.65, No.4, pp. 464-473

[47] Long, AC., O'Neal, HR. Jr., Peng, S., Lane, KB. & Light, RW. (2010). Comparison of Pleural Fluid N-Terminal Pro-Brain Natriuretic Peptide and Brain Natriuretic-32 Peptide Levels. *Cheat*, Vol.137, No.6, pp. 1369-1374

[48] Mahdyoon, H., Klein, R., Eyler, W., Lakier, JB., Chakko, SC. & Gheorghiade, M. (1989). Radiographic Pulmonary Congestion in End-Stage Congestive Heart Failure. *American Journal of Cardiology*, Vol.63, No.9, pp. 625-627

[49] Mathis, G. (1997). Thoraxsonography - Part I: Chest Wall and Pleura. *Ultrasound in Medicine & Biology*, Vol.23, No.8, pp. 1131-1139

[50] Mattison, LE., Coppage, L., Alderman, DF., Herlong, JO. & Sahn, SA. (1997). Pleural Effusions in the Medical ICU: Prevalence, Causes, and Clinical Implications. *Chest*, Vol.111, No.4, pp. 1018-1023

[51] McDonald, K. (2010). Monitoring Fluid Status at the Outpatient Level: The Need for More Precision. *Congestive Heart Failure*, Vol.16, Supplement 1, pp. S52-S55

[52] McHugh, TJ., Forrester, JS., Adler, L., Zion, D. & Swan, HJC. (1972). Pulmonary Vascular Congestion in Acute Myocardial Infarction: Hemodynamic and Radiologic Correlations. *Annals of Internal Medicine*, Vol.76, No.1, pp. 29-33

[53] McPeak, EM. & Levine, SA. (1946). The Preponderance of Right Hydrothorax in Congestive Heart Failure. *Annals of Internal Medicine*, Vol.25, No.6, pp. 916-927

[54] Meszaros, WT. (1973). Lung Changes in Left Heart Failure. *Circulation*, Vol.47, No.4, pp. 859-871

[55] Milne, ENC., Pistolesi, M., Miniati, M. & Giuntini, C. (1985). The Radiologic Distinction of Cardiogenic and Noncardiogenic Edema. *American Journal of Roentgenology*, Vol.144, No.5, pp. 879-894

[56] Miserocchi, G. (1997). Physiology and Pathophysiology of Pleural Fluid Turnover. *European Respiratory Journal*, Vol.10, No.1, pp. 219-225

[57] Moskowitz, H., Platt, RT., Schachar, R. & Mellins, H. (1973). Roentgen Visualization of Minute Pleural Effusion: An Experimental Study to Determine the Minimal Amount of Pleural Fluid Visible on a Radiograph. *Radiology*, Vol.109, No.1, pp. 33-35

[58] Movahed, MR., Saito, Y., Ahmadi-Kashani, M. & Kasravi, B. (2006). Relation of Pericardial Effusion to Degree of Fractional Shortening. *American Journal of Cardiology*, Vol.97, No.6, pp. 910-911

[59] Mueller, C., Frana, B., Rodriguez, D., Laule-Kilian, K. & Perruchoud, AP. (2005). Emergency Diagnosis of Congestive Heart Failure: Impact of Signs and Symptoms. *Canadian Journal of Cardiology*, Vol.21, No.11, pp. 921-924

[60] Mueller, T. & Haltmayer, M. (2006). Natriuretic Peptide Measurements as Part of the Diagnostic Work-Up in Pleural Effusions: An Emerging Concept? *European Respiratory Journal*, Vol.28, No.1, pp. 7-9

[61] Natanzon, A. & Kronzon, I. (2009). Pericardial and Pleural Effusions in Congestive Heart Failure—Anatomical, Pathophysiologic, and Clinical Considerations. *American Journal of Medical Sciences*, Vol. 338, No.3, pp. 211-216

[62] Packer, MP. & Cohn, JN. (1999). Consensus Recommendations for the Management of Chronic Heart Failure: Part I. Evaluation of Heart Failure. *American Journal of Cardiology*, Vol.83, No.2 (Supplement 1), pp. 2A-8A

[63] Paddock, FK. (1940). The Diagnostic Significance of Serous Fluids in Disease. *New England Journal of Medicine*, Vol.223, No.25, pp. 1010-1015

[64] Pang, PS. & Levy, P. (2010). Pathophysiology of Volume Overload in Acute Heart Failure Syndromes. *Congestive Heart Failure*, Vol.16, Supplement 1, pp. S1-S6

[65] Piccoli, M., Trambaiolo, P., Salustri,A., Cerquetani, E., Posteraro, A., Pastena, G., Amici, E., Papetti, F., Marincola, E., La Carruba, S. & Gambelli, G. (2005). Bedside Diagnosis and Follow-Up of Patients with Pleural Effusion by a Hand-Carried Ultrasound Device Early after Cardiac Surgery. *Chest*, Vol.128, No.5, pp. 3413-3420

[66] Pneumatikos, I. & Bouros, D. (2008). Pleural Effusions in Critically Ill Patients. *Respiration*, Vol.76, No.3, pp. 241-248

[67] Porcel, JM., Vives, M., Cao,G., Esquerda, A, Rubio, M. & Rivas, C. (2004). Measurement of Pro-Brain Natriuretic Peptide in Pleural Fluid for the Diagnosis of Pleural Effusions due to Heart Failure. *American Journal of Medicine*, Vol.116, No.6, pp. 417-420

[68] Porcel, JM., Martínez-Alonso, M., Cao, G., Bielsa, S., Sopena, A. & Esquerda, A. (2009). Biomarkers of Heart Failure in Pleural Fluid. *Chest*, Vol.136, No.3, pp. 671-677

[69] Porcel, JM. (2011) Pearls and Myths in Pleural Fluid Analysis. *Respirology*, Vol.16, No.1, pp. 44-52

[70] Remérand, F., Dellamonica, J., Mao, Z., Ferrari, F., Bouhemad, B., Jianxin, Y., Arbelot, C., Lu, Q., Ichaï, C. & Rouby, JJ. (2010). Multiplane Ultrasound Approach to Quantify Pleural Effusion at the Bedside. *Intensive Care Medicine*, Vol.36, No.4, pp. 656-664

[71] Roelandt, JRTC. (2003). Ultrasound Stethoscopy: A Renaissance of the Physical Examination? *Heart*, Vol.89, No.9, pp. 971-974

[72] Rohde, LE., Beck-da-Silva, L., Goldraich, L., Grazziotin, TC., Palombini, DV., Polanczyk, CA. & Clausell, N. (2004). Reliability and Prognostic Value of Traditional Signs and Symptoms in Outpatients with Congestive Heart Failure. *Canadian Journal of Cardiology*, Vol.20, No.7, pp. 697-702

[73] Romero-Candeira, S., Fernández, C., Martín, C., Sánchez-Paya, J. & Hernández, L. (2001). Influence of Diuretics on the Concentration of Proteins and other Components of Pleural Transudates in Patients with Heart Failure. *American Journal of Medicine*, Vol.110, No.9, pp. 681-686

[74] Ronco, C. & Maisel, A. (2010). Volume Overload and Cardiorenal Syndromes. *Congestive Heart Failure*, Vol.16, Supplement 1, pp. S1-S4

[75] Roth, BJ., O'Meara, TF. & Cragun, WH. (1990). The Serum-Effusion Albumin Gradient in the Evaluation of Pleural Effusions. *Chest*, Vol.98, No.3, pp. 546-549

[76] Sahn, SA. (1988). State of the Art: The Pleura. *American Review of Respiratory Disease*, Vol.138, No.1, pp. 184-234

[77] Schrier, RW. & Abraham, WT. (1999). Hormones and Hemodynamics in Heart Failure. *New England Journal of Medicine*, Vol.341, No.8, pp. 577-585

[78] Setoguchi, S., Stevenson, LW. & Schneeweiss, S. (2007). Repeated Hospitalizations Predict Mortality in the Community Population with Heart Failure. *American Heart Journal*, Vol.154, No.2, pp 260-266

[79] Sica, DA. (2006). Sodium and Water Retention in Heart Failure and Diuretic Therapy: Basic Mechanisms. *Cleveland Clinic Journal of Medicine*, Vol.73, Supplement 2, pp. S2-S7

[80] Solomon, SD., Dobson, J., Pocock, S., Skali, H., McMurray, JJV., Granger, CB., Yusuf, S., Swedberg, K., Young, JB., Michelson, EL. & Pfeffer, MA., for the Candesartan in Heart Failure: Assessment of Reduction in Mortality and morbidity (CHARM) Investigators. (2007). Influence of Nonfatal Hospitalization for Heart Failure on Subsequent Mortality in Patients with Chronic Heart Failure. *Circulation*, Vol.116, No.13, pp. 1482-1487

[81] Stefanidis, K., Dimopoulos, S. & Nanas, S. (2011). Basic Principles and Current Applications of Lung Ultrasonography in the Intensive Care Unit. *Respirology*, Vol.16, No.2, pp. 249-256

[82] Stevenson, LW. & Perloff, JK. (1989). The Limited Reliability of Physical Signs for Estimating Hemodynamics in Chronic Heart Failure. *Journal of American Medical Association*, Vol.261, No.6, pp. 884-888

[83] Szabo, G. & Magyar, Z. (1967). Effect of Increased Systemic Venous Pressure on Lymph Pressure and Flow. *American Journal of Physiology*, Vol.212, No.6, pp. 1469-1474

[84] Szidon, JP., Pietra, GG. & Fishman, AP. (1972). The Alveolar-Capillary Membrane and Pulmonary Edema. *New England Journal of Medicine*, Vol.286, No.22, pp. 1200-1204

[85] Tang, WHW. & Tong, W. (2009). Measuring Impedance in Congestive Heart Failure: Current Options and Clinical Applications. *American Heart Journal*, Vol.157, No.3, pp. 402-411

[86] Tayal, VS., Nicks, BA. & Norton, HJ. (2006). Emergency Ultrasound Evaluation of Symptomatic Nontraumatic Pleural Effusions. *American Journal of Emergency Medicine*, Vol.24, No.7, pp. 782-786

[87] Tomcsányi, J., Nagy, E., Somlói, M., Moldvay, J., Bezzegh, A., Bózsik, B. & Strausz, J. (2004). NT-Brain Natriuretic Peptide Levels in Pleural Fluid Distinguish between Pleural Transudates and Exudates. *European Journal of Heart Failure*, Vol.6, No.6, pp. 753-756

[88] Tresch, DD. (1997). The Clinical Diagnosis of Heart Failure in Older Patients. *Journal of American Geriatric Society*, Vol.45, No.9, pp. 1128-1133

[89] Tsai, T-H., Jerng, J-S. & Yang, P-C. (2008). Clinical Applications of Transthoracic Ultrasound in Chest Medicine. *Journal of Medical Ultrasound*, Vol.16, No.1, pp. 7-25

[90] Vignon, P., Chastagner, C., Berkane, V., Chardac, E., François, B., Normand, S., Bonnivard, M., Clavel, M., Pichon, N., Preux, PM., Maubon, A. & Gastinne, H. (2005). Quantitative Assessment of Pleural Effusion in Critically Ill Patients by Means of Ultrasonography. *Critical Care Medicine*, Vol.33, No.8, pp. 1757-1763

[91] Vinson, JM., Rich, MW., Sperry, JC., Shah, AS. & McNamara, T. (1990). Early Readmission of Elderly Patients with Congestive Heart Failure. *Journal of American Geriatrics Society*, Vol.38, No.12, pp. 1290-1295

[92] Volpicelli, G., Cardinale, L., Garofalo, G. & Veltri, A. (2008). Usefulness of Lung Ultrasound in the Bedside Distinction between Pulmonary Edema and Exacerbation of COPD. *Emergency Radiology*, Vol.15, No.3, pp. 145-151

[93] Waggoner, AD., Baumann, CM. & Stark, PA. (1995). "Views from the Back" by Subscapular Retrocardiac Imaging: Technique and Clinical Application. *Journal of American Society of Echocardiography*, Vol.8, No.3, pp. 257-262

[94] Warakaulle, DR. & Traill, ZC. (2004). Imaging of Pleural Disease. *Imaging*, Vol.16, No.1, pp. 10-21

[95] White, PD., August, S. & Michie, CR. (1947). Hydrothorax in Congestive Heart Failure. *American Journal of Medical Sciences*, Vol.214, No.3, pp. 243-247

[96] Wiener-Kronish, JP., Matthay, MA., Callen, PW., Filly, RA., Gamsu, G. & Staub, NC. (1985). Relationship of Pleural Effusions to Pulmonary Hemodynamics in Patients with Congestive Heart Failure. *American Review of Respiratory Disease*, Vol.132, No.6, pp. 1253-1256

[97] Wiener-Kronish, JP., Goldstein, R., Matthay, RA., Biondi, JW., Broaddus, VC., Chatterjee, K. & Matthay, MA. (1987). Lack of Association of Pleural Effusion with Chronic Pulmonary Arterial and Right Atrial Hypertension. *Chest*, Vol.92, No.6, pp. 967-970

[98] Wiener, MD., Garay, SM., Leitman, BS., Wiener, DN. & Ravin, CE. (1991). Imaging of the Intensive Care Unit Patient. *Clinics in Chest Medicine*, Vol.12, No.1, pp. 169-198

[99] Wong, CL., Holroyd-Leduc, J. & Straus, SE. (2009). Does this Patient have a Pleural Effusion? *Journal of American Medical Association*, Vol.301, No.3, pp. 309-317

[100] Wood, FC. Jr., Wolferth, CC. & Terrell, AW. (1937). Trepopnea as an Etiological Factor in Paroxysmal Nocturnal Dyspnea. *American Heart Journal*, Vol.14, No.3, pp. 255-267

[101] Woodring, JH. (1984). Recognition of Pleural Effusion on Supine Radiographs: How Much Fluid is Required? *American Journal of Roentgenology*, Vol.142, No.1, pp. 59-64

[102] Yang, P-C., Luh, K-T., Chang, D-B., Wu, H-D., Yu, C-J. & Kuo, S-H. (1992). Value of Sonography in Determining the Nature of Pleural Effusion: Analysis of 320 Cases. *American Journal of Roentgenology*, Vol.159, No.1, pp. 29-33

[103] Yu, C-J., Yang, P-C., Chang, D-B. & Luh, K-T. (1992). Diagnostic and Therapeutic Use of Chest Sonography: Value in Critically Ill Patients. *American Journal of Roentgenology*, Vol.159, No.4, pp. 695-701

[104] Zanobetti, M., Poggioni, C. & Pini, R. (2011). Can Chest Ultrasonography Replace Standard Chest Radiography for Evaluation of Acute Dyspnea in the ED? *Chest*, Vol.139, No.5, pp. 1140-1147

9

Ultrasound Guided Vascular Access

Hamid Shokoohi, Ali Pourmand and Keith Boniface
George Washington University Medical Center, Washington DC, USA

1. Introduction

Vascular access is an important procedure for clinicians to master. Chronic medical conditions, intravenous drug use, and obesity can all make placements of vascular catheters in central and peripheral veins challenging and time-consuming. External landmarks have traditionally guided the placement of the needle for the performance of central venous catheterization. The proximity of such structures as the large arteries of the chest and neck as well as the apex of the lung results in a 6.2-11.3% rate of immediate mechanical complications when performing subclavian or internal jugular catheterization.[1] In recent years there have been significant improvements in portable ultrasound technology including the development of relatively inexpensive ultrasound machines with sufficient resolution to guide needle placement through tissues. These machines are now found throughout the house of medicine by the bedside of patients. Multiple studies have been performed demonstrating the benefits of ultrasound guidance of central venous catheter placement by multiple specialties, and the same technique has been extended to the placement of peripheral intravenous catheters.[2,3,4,5,6] In this chapter, we describe the use of ultrasound for guidance of vascular access.

2. Use of ultrasound for vascular access

2.1 Transducer selection

Transducer characteristics, such as frequency and shape, determine ultrasound image quality. For the purpose of vascular access, it is ideal to use high frequency and small footprint transducers. The high-frequency linear array transducer provides higher resolution of the superficial areas of soft tissue including artery and veins. The flat and small footprint shape of the linear array transducer is less prone to slip off of the vessel of interest. Modern transducers are designed to generate a range of frequencies. For example, linear 5-12 MHz transducer can be used to adequately scan deeper targets if it used in lower range of frequencies. In general, transducers in the range of 5-12 MHz are preferred as the depths of target vessels for accesses are often limited to 2-4 cm below the skin surface.[7]

2.2 Modes

B-Mode and color Doppler are the main ultrasound modes used for the purpose of venous access. B-mode ultrasound produces recognizable two dimensional (2D) gray scale images.

Color Doppler is an application to characterize blood flow. The doppler effect occurs when blood flow of red blood cells move toward or away the ultrasound transducer. If the flow in a vessel is moving towards the transducer, the color displayed in the vessel is RED and when the flow is moving away from the transducer, the perceived frequency display is BLUE (BART - Blue Away and Red Toward). (Figure 1A, B) To clearly display the presence of a flow in an artery or vein, it is necessary to create an angle between the transducer and the direction of the flow. The color Doppler detection of flow is optimal when the transducer is parallel (0 degrees) to the flow and it is worst when the transducer is perpendicular (90 degrees) to the vessel, so in clinical practice, some angulations of the transducer are necessary to optimize color Doppler signal.

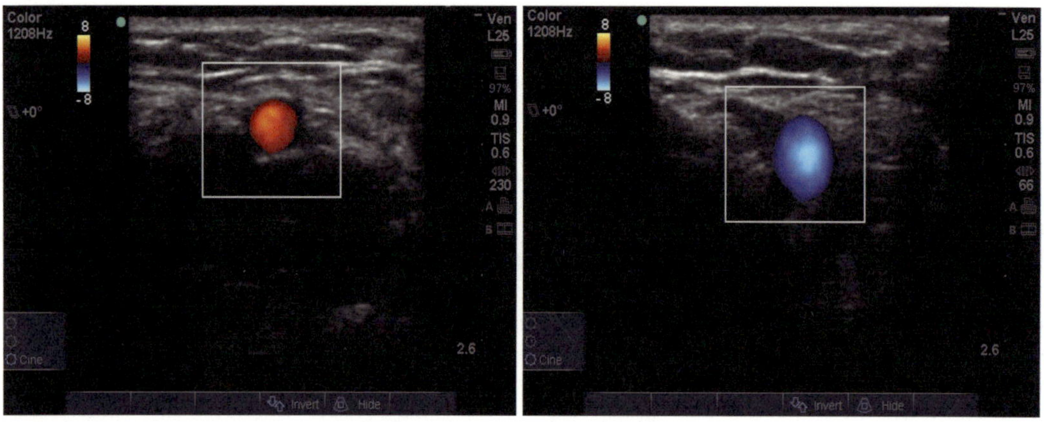

Fig. 1. (A) Transverse view, the brachial artery without compression with color flow TOWARD the transducer, (B) Transverse view, the brachial artery without compression with color flow AWAY from the transducer

2.3 Optimizing image quality

Best visualization of target vessels with ultrasound requires an optimal machine setting. In general, proper transducer selection and the selection of pre-programmed vascular ultrasound settings provide acceptable quality images. Additional controls that can further improve the image quality include gain, depth, focus and frequency.

Depth: Proper depth adjustment provides better target vessel imaging and facilitates tracking the needle through the tissues. By increasing the depth setting, the target vessel gets smaller and smaller. With too shallow a depth setting, important structures in the vicinity of the target vessel (such as a neighboring artery) may be lost off the far edge of the screen. It is therefore important to select the appropriate depth setting according to the target vessel location.

Gain: The brightness of the image on the screen is controlled by the gain setting of the ultrasound machine, and the quality of images displayed on monitor also depends on the selected gain. Increasing the gain makes the image brighter, while decreasing the gain makes the image darker. In addition to the overall gain, selected regions of the screen can be adjusted by selecting gain controls for the near field or far field. Inappropriately increased gain will add "noise" artifact to the image that adversely impact the quality of images.

Focus: The highest resolution of the displayed image is at the focal zone. Some machines automatically adjust the focal zone to the center of the screen, however, in systems with a manually adjustable focus, it is important to place the 'focus' at the level of the target vessel of interest.

3. Image orientation

Proper transducer orientation is an important step to accomplish a successful procedure. Most transducers have an indicator of some sort on one side of the probe that corresponds to a mark displayed on one side of the displayed image on the screen. (Figure 2A and 2B)

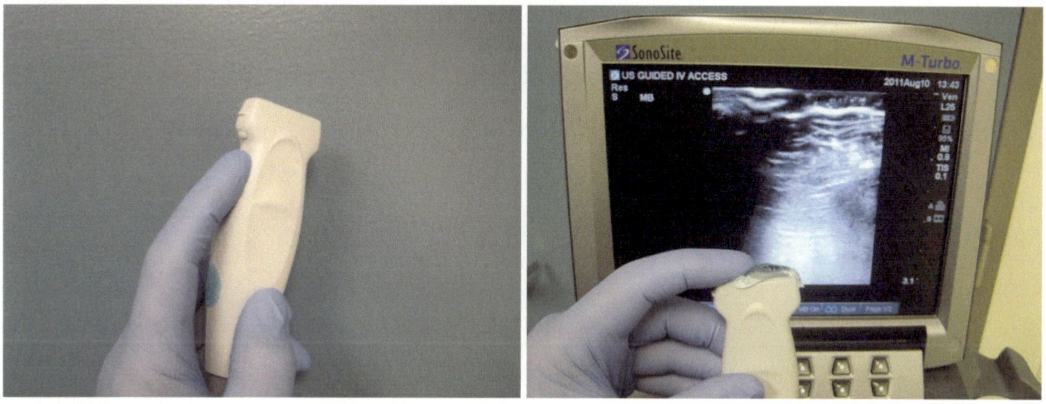

Fig. 2. (A) A high frequency linear transducer for vascular procedure, with orientation indicator (B) Localization and matching orientation indicator with ultrasound indicator on screen (green dot)

The aim is to keep the indicator on the side of the probe oriented in the same direction as the orientation mark side of the monitor. By default, the orientation mark is usually displayed at the left side of the image and keeping the indicator toward the left side of provider will largely prevent further confusion about the orientation. If there is any confusion about the orientation of the probe, a finger can be rubbed on one side of the transducer surface after gel application to produce an image on the screen and confirm the orientation.

3.1 Preparing a sterile transducer

Central venous access is a sterile procedure. In order to use ultrasound, the probe needs to become part of the sterile field. When preparing for the procedure a sterile ultrasound sheath should be placed on the sterile field. Ask your assistant to apply ample sterile or non-sterile gel into the sterile sheath. Place the ultrasound transducer inside the sterile sheath and ensure that gel is applied generously between the transducer and inside of the sheath covering. Smooth the sheath covering over the transducer surface to avoid any wrinkles or trapped air that could impede full contact. Wrap the sterile rubber band supplied with most commercially available probe covers around the transducer to avoid transducer movement inside the sheath during ultrasound scanning.[8,9]

Alternatively, if a sterile probe cover is not available, a sterile glove can be used to cover the transducer surface, although this does not cover the cable of the ultrasound probe and care must be taken during the procedure to prevent contamination of the sterile field by the cable. Applying generous amount of gel into the sterile glove and sliding the transducer into the glove's thumb may prevent air trapping or wrinkle on the contact surface. (Figure 3)

1.	Sterilize the skin surface thoroughly with an antiseptic solution
2.	Surround the CVC placement location with full body sterile fenestrated drape
3.	Using sterile technique, open the probe cover packet onto the sterile work field
4.	The gowned and gloved provider places ½ of the contents of the sterile gel inside the sheath
5.	Place the transducer inside the sheath, taking care to displace any air bubbles between the probe face and the probe cover
6.	Extend the sterile sheath to cover the cord completely
7.	Hold the sheath in place with a rubber band around the transducer head
8.	Place the transducer on the sterile field
9.	Use a package of sterile acoustic gel
10.	Apply sufficient amount of sterile gel over the site of scanning
11.	Place the transducer over the procedure site, identify target vessel, and proceed with cannulation

Table 1. Preparing the ultrasound transducer for central venous catheterization

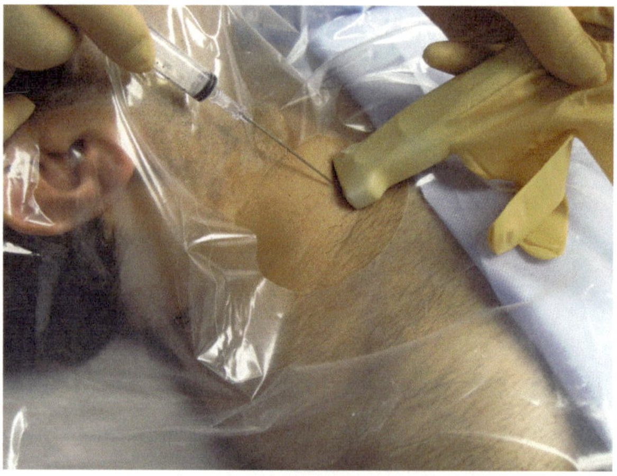

Fig. 3. Probe position and needle insertion to approach internal jugular Central line access by using a sterile glove as an alternative to sterile probe cover

4. Planes and views

Transverse and longitudinal views are two main planes used for the purpose of vascular access. In transverse view, the transducer plane is in cross section of the target vessel and the vessel is displayed on the screen as a circle. In longitudinal view, transducer plane and vessel plane are parallel and the vessel is displayed on the screen as a long tube running across the screen. A longitudinal view allows visualization of entire vessel of interest, but it requires that transducer beam, needle and target vessel be held parallel, which can be challenging for the novice user.[10,11]

In general, we recommend starting with transverse view as it allows visualizing adjacent structures including artery and nerve in the area and is easier to visualize the tip of needle and its insertion. The provider can switch between the two views during the procedure as needed to track the progress of the needle moving toward the target vessel.

4.1 Differentiating artery and vein

Differentiating between artery and vein is essential to safely perform ultrasound guided vascular access. Compressibility of veins is the simplest way to distinguish artery from vein. Veins typically compress with minimal pressure applied from the probe, while arteries retain much of their original shape and appearance. When performing internal jugular vein placement one may visualize the influence of respiratory variation on the vein diameter. Valsalva maneuvers and trendelenberg positioning make the vein larger but have minimal affect on the carotid artery. The application of color Doppler is also very useful in differentiating artery from vein. Arteries have pulsatile flow visualized on color Doppler, while the vein has minimal flow. (Figure 4A and 4B)

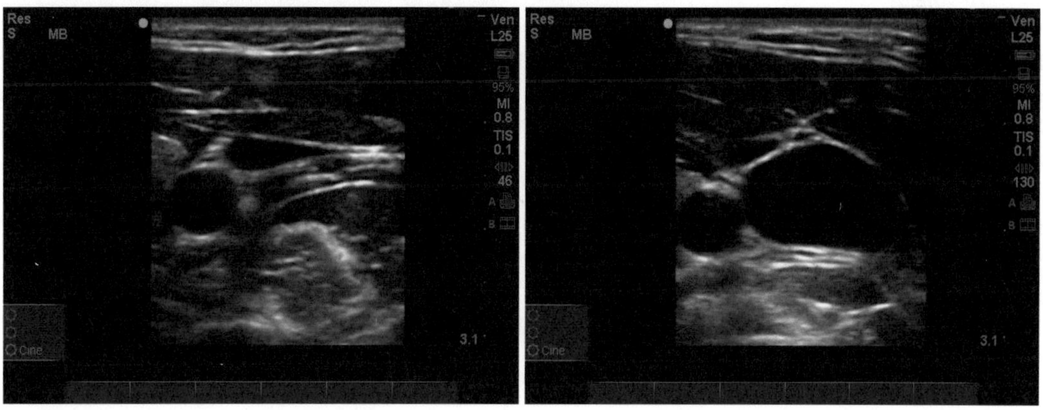

Fig. 4. (A) Transverse view of right internal jugular vein (with mild compression) and adjacent carotid artery (B) Transverse view of a distended right internal jugular vein during Valsalva maneuver and adjacent carotid artery

4.2 Scanning techniques

Static vs. Dynamic: The guidance of vascular access using ultrasound can be categorized as static or dynamic. In the static use of ultrasound, the provider would apply ultrasound to localize the vein and mark the site of needle insertion on the skin; after that the procedure will be performed much like a traditional landmark-based approach.

In dynamic guidance, the provider uses the ultrasound in "real time," with continuous visualization of the needle insertion throughout the procedure. The authors highly recommend the dynamic approach on performing central venous access considering the possibility of changes due to patient movement in the time interval between marking and needle insertion in the static approach. The success rates for dynamic guidance as compared with the static technique is significantly higher. Direct ultrasound guidance gives the opportunity of visualizing the needle in real time to puncture the vein and avoid puncturing adjacent artery and nerves but it is more technically demanding because it requires significant eye–hand coordination and it requires a sterile probe cover throughout the procedure.

One-provider vs. Two-provider: The dynamic use of ultrasound can be conducted by a provider operating alone, or by two providers. In the one-provider method, the provider holds the ultrasound transducer with the non-dominant hand and the needle with the dominant hand. In the two-provider method, a sterile assistant will hold and control the probe while the provider performs the needle insertion under real-time ultrasound guidance. We recommend the one-provider method, as it not only allows for more flexibility and the ability to perform the procedure independently, but also enables the provider to make very small movements of the ultrasound probe in conjunction with the needle to enhance localization of the needle tip. In a small study among 44 cases focusing on the specific question of whether single- vs. two-provider technique was advantageous revealed no significant differences.[12,13]

Out-of-Plane vs. In-Plane Approach: Needle insertion can be performed in either in- plane (longitudinal) or out-of- plane (transverse) in relation to the ultrasound transducer. During the in-plane insertion, the needle is placed parallel to the transducer and the full length of the needle shaft and tip are visualized. In the out-of plane approach, the needle is placed perpendicular to the transducer and either the needle shaft or the tip is visualized as a hyperechoic dot on monitor. In this method, needle, vein, adjacent artery or vein and tissue movements are observed. The choice of these two methods depends on the location of the vessel, provider experience, and anatomic relationships. In a study by Blaivas et al. they reported that the technique utilizing a transverse, short-axis view of the needle in vascular access was easier for novices to learn than a technique using longitudinal scan.[11]

5. Ultrasound - guided catheter insertion techniques

5.1 Internal jugular vein

Anatomy and ultrasound technique: The internal jugular vein (IJ) is typically located anterior and lateral to the carotid artery; however, there is a significant anatomic variation where the vein can overly the artery and even be medial to the artery. As described above, the IJ vein and carotid artery can be differentiated by the fact that the vein is compressible, non-pulsatile, and distensible by the Trendelenberg position or the Valsalva maneuver.[14] (Figure 4A and 4B)

Contralateral rotation of the head significantly affects the relative anatomy of the IJ vein and carotid artery. Extreme contralateral head rotation can decrease IJ vein diameter and increase overlap on the carotid artery.[8,14]

In longitudinal view, the IJ vein can be followed inferiorly, down to the level of the sternoclavicular joint where it joins the subclavian vein on each side and drains into the superior vena cava.[8]

Positioning and preparation: Proper positioning of the patient significantly affects the likelihood of a successful procedure. For the IJ cannulation, patient's head should be rotated slightly contralaterally, with the neck extended. Extreme rotation of the neck may increase the amount of overlap of the carotid artery and IJ vein. The patient should be placed in Trendelenburg position in order to maximally distend the IJ vein. The ultrasound machine should be placed by the same side of the bed and directly in front of the provider to provide a direct line of vision that is ergonomic and efficient.

An initial examination of the surrounding areas and the target vessels should be performed to confirm the patency of the IJ vein and absence of thrombosis prior to applying the sterile probe cover and prepping the patient. Following this important step, the procedural areas of the neck and upper chest should then be prepared in the usual manner, and full barrier precautions should be used to maintain sterility of the procedure.[2,8,9] A sterile probe cover should be applied as discussed in Table 1. The CVC catheter should be set up per normal routine. The catheter ports should be flushed to remove air and to check for their patency. The equipment needed for catheter insertion, including the CVC kit should be set and place within an easy reach. Local anesthetic should be applied at the site of puncture.

Catheter Insertion: Provider should use the dominant hand to handle the needle and the non-dominant hand to hold and handle the transducer. If prefer to start with transverse view, the needle is placed perpendicular to the transducer directly underneath the middle of the transducer while jugular vein placed in the center of the screen. The needle insertion site should be 0.5-1 cm proximal to the transducer. In this approach, the needle tip and the shaft are visualized as a hyperechoic dot on monitor. If the needle tip cannot be visualized, indenting the tissue overlying the vein or moving the transducer along the axis of the vein while "agitating" the needle may enhance the image of the needle and tip. If consider longitudinal plane, the needle is placed inline with and parallel to the transducer in which the entire length of the needle and the tip are visualized as puncture the vein. Once the vessel has been successfully punctured, the transducer can be set aside and the procedure can proceed normally with wire and catheter placement. The wire should be advanced slowly with no pressure at the length of the needle plus 5-6 cm. considering the short distance of the puncture site and superior vena cava to the right jugular vein extreme precaution should be used not to advance the catheter too far to prevent right atrial or ventricular wire insertion. After wire placement, the needle is removed and a small incision is made around the wire insertion to facilitate dilator insertion. After removal of the dilator, the catheter is then advanced to the desired distance that is 4-5 cm shorter in the right jugular vein compare to the left IJ vein.[8,9] Once the line is in place, it should be properly flushed in all ports, secured, and dressed. Post procedure chest X ray is required to confirm proper catheter placement and the lack of complications including pneumothorax to start using the central catheter.

5.2 Subclavian vein

Anatomy and ultrasound technique: Subclavian vein is a continuation of the axillary vein at the lateral border of the first rib that crosses over the first rib and passes in front of the anterior scalene muscle that separates the vein from subclavian artery. The subclavian vein (SC) continues in main length behind the medial third of clavicle which makes it less available for ultrasound scanning. At the junction of Sternoclavicular joint in each side SC veins join to the IJ veins and form the innominate vein to the left and brachiocephalic vein to the right side.[15]

To visualize the Subclavian vein, the ultrasound transducer is placed at the supraclavicular space posterior to the long axis of clavicle to obtain a longitudinal view of the SC vein. At this level it is critical to differentiate SC vein from the SC artery as they pass in parallel along side of each other. The SC vein can be distinguished from the artery by the fact that the SC vein is in a more medial and superficial than artery and by following its path medially it can be traced to IJ vein. The SC vein is not pulsating and affected by Valsalva maneuver similar to IJ vein.

SC vein can be visualized at the infraclavicular region by placing transducer at the mid third of clavicle while the half of the footprint covering the cross section of the clavicle and the lower half investigating the infraclavicular region.

Catheter insertion: The SC vein access with ultrasound guidance can be performed through either supraclavicular or infraclavicular approach. In supraclavicular approach while the vein is visualized the probe will be adjusted toward the medial end of the vein near the junction of IJ vein to provide sufficient space for the needle placement under real time ultrasound guidance. Following the puncture site identification, the area is prepped and draped sterilely and the ultrasound transducer sterile cover should applied as described previously. Furthermore, the ipsilateral IJV area should be prepped in case of possible catheter misplacement required proper ultrasound guided repositioning. While the needle gains access to the SC vein the guide wire would advance and the transducer can be set aside and proceed with a normal procedural steps according to the Seldinger's technique.

Typically, the subclavian vein is more difficult to visualize by ultrasound due to its position under the clavicle, which requires significant angulations and manipulation of the transducer to acquire and maintain sufficient imaging during real time procedure. Therefore, it is less ideal procedure compare to ultrasound guided IJ CVC access.

5.3 Femoral vein

The proximal femoral vein is medial to the femoral artery, deep to the fascia iliaca and superficial to the iliopsoas muscle. At the lower level the vein gradually descend posterior to the femoral artery that would be deeper in ultrasound scanning. For the purpose of CVC placement provider should consider more proximal (cephalad) puncture site where the vein is medial to the artery. Minimal pressure on the vein can totally compress the vein confirming the lack of thrombosis. Often, inguinal lymph nodes also appear as hyperechoic structure in the region that need to be distinguished by scanning proximally and distally in this region. The femoral vein should be distinguished from the artery by the fact that the vein is in a more medial and deeper than artery and by examining its compressibility and lack of pulsatile doppler.

Catheter insertion: Before applying sterile procedures, we recommend to perform a systematic anatomical survey from medial to lateral and superficial to deep, distinguishing vein from artery and investigating the presence of thrombi. The groin area should be exposed while patient is in supine and the leg is in natural position. After area and transducer preparation in a sterile manner (table 1), transducer should be placed along the inguinal crease. If the femoral artery and nerve are deep, the machine imaging capability should be adjusted appropriately by increasing the depth and adjusting the gain. Starting with a short axis view will provide a sufficient image of adjacent structure and facilitate a proper needle insertion. However, transducer can be rotated 90 degree while the femoral vein image keep in the center of screen and it provide a longitudinal view of the vein. While the venous puncture confirmed, the procedure should be proceed identical to the SC and IJ vein access considering the Seldinger's technique.

6. Ultrasound - guided peripheral venous access

Intravenous (IV) access is a basic and critical procedure, which routinely performs, in medical community. IV access usually uses to administer medication, IV fluid, obtaining blood sample and it is one of the necessary actions for patients who need to be admitted in hospital. This procedure usually performs by medical technician or nurses, but sometimes they are unable to obtain access and this could delay patients' care. This section will discuss important key features regarding peripheral IV access and pitfalls to enhance success rate to insert IV access without any invasive procedure.

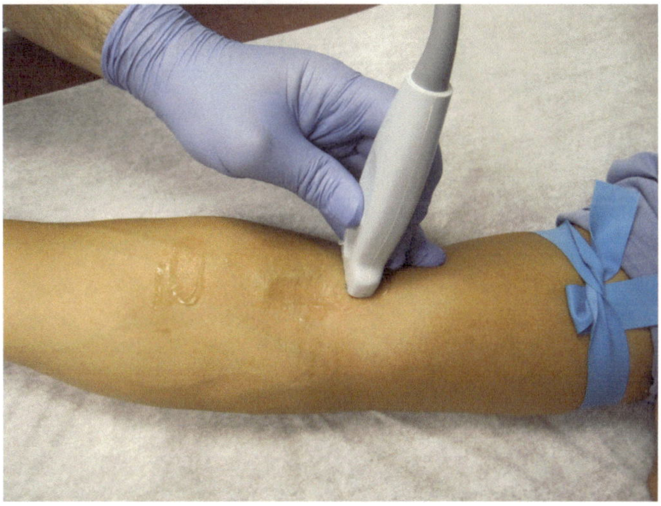

Fig. 5. Transverse probe position to approach peripheral IV access with orientation indicator toward to right side of patient

6.1 Anatomy

The upper extremity consists of two types of veins, superficial and deep. These 2 sets of veins have several communications, known as anastomose. The deep veins accompany the arteries. They are connected to the superficial system by perforating veins. The depth of vein is measured by distance from skin. The superficial veins start on the back of the hand as a dorsal arch. Cephalic and Basilic veins are example of superficial veins. Dorsal veins of the hand empty into the cephalic vein on the lateral aspect and into the basilic vein on the medial aspect of the forearm. The cephalic vein ascends in the radial (lateral) aspect of wrist and courses laterally upward around the anterior surface of the forearm. Under the front of the elbow it divides to some branches, which receives a communicating branch from the deep veins of the forearm and passes across to join the basilic vein. In the upper arm, the cephalic vein terminates in the infraclavicular fossa, and empty into the axillary vein. The

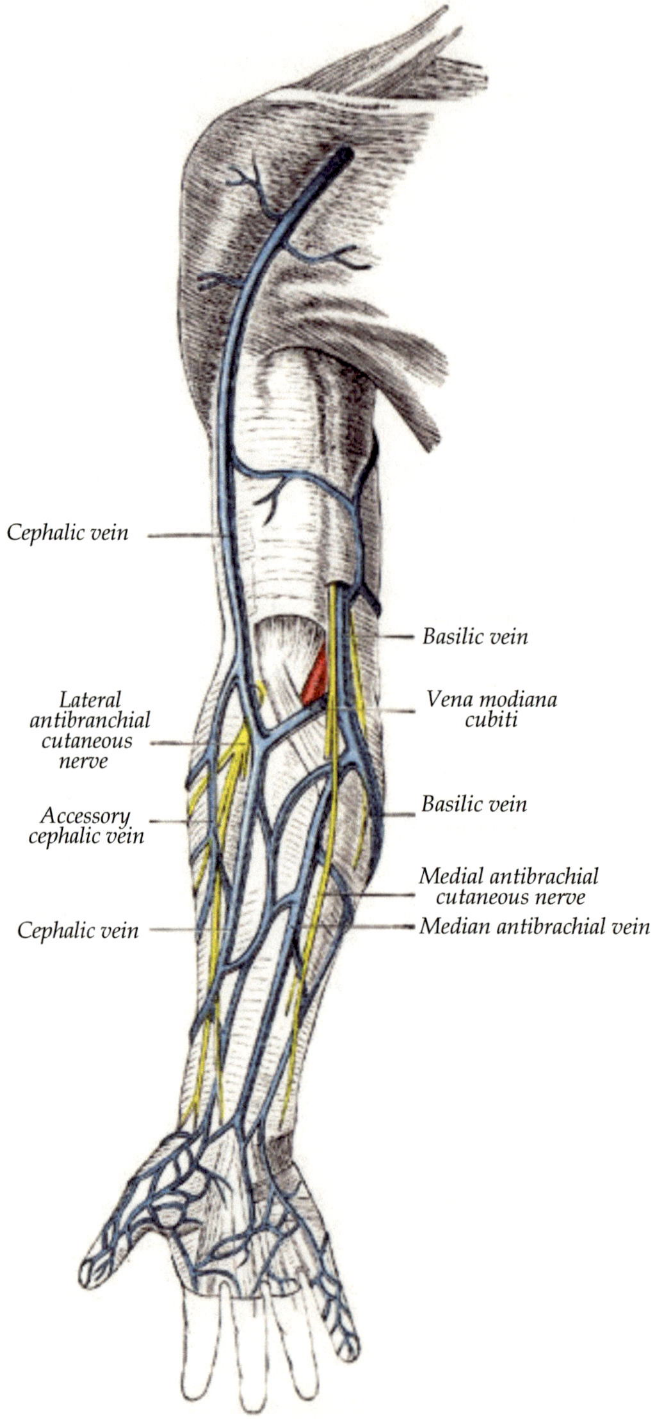
Cephalic vein
Basilic vein
Lateral antibranchial cutaneous nerve
Vena modiana cubiti
Basilic vein
Accessory cephalic vein
Medial antibrachial cutaneous nerve
Cephalic vein
Median antibrachial vein

Fig. 6.

basilic vein runs medially along the ulnar part of the forearm and penetrates the deep fascia as it courses past the elbow in the upper arm. It then joins with the deep brachial veins to become the axillary vein. The median cubital vein joins the cephalic and the basilic veins on the ventral surface of the elbow. The axillary vein becomes the subclavian vein at the lateral border of the first rib. At the medial border of the scalenus anterior muscle, the subclavian vein joins with the internal jugular vein to become the brachiocephalic vein, with the subclavian vein coursing anterior to the scalenus anterior muscle. The left and right brachiocephalic veins join to become the superior vena cava, which empties into the right atrium.[16,17]

6.2 Preparation

The ability to obtain US guided IV access is a skill that combines knowledge of peripheral IV access and US. Provider should collect necessary equipment prior to start the procedure at the bedside. Provider should consider contraindication to start IV access in upper extremities such as burn, cellulitis, end stage renal disease access, scar from previous trauma or surgery, and breast cancer on dependent arm. Provider should explain the procedure to patient and request permission to start IV access. Basic equipment at bedside should consist of appropriate angiocatheter size, tourniquet, skin cleaning instrument (alcohol or betadine swab), 2x2 gauze, tape, band-aid, sterile transparent dressing, blood tube, iv tubing and extensor, vaccutainer, normal saline flush, sharp container, biohazard bag, gloves, sterile lubricant and of course ultrasound machine.

6.3 Procedure

This procedure can be done as one or two person procedure. Usually one-person procedure is a routine and acceptable procedure. In this procedure provider can have a control of probe and can change angle, depth or approach instead of asking the second person to manage probe. The high frequency, linear probe is appropriate for peripheral IV access. Using high frequency probe will show superficial structure. The vascular structure consists of vein and artery. Veins will be anechoic structures and easily compressible with probe pressure. Arteries are anechoic structures, which they could be compressible but they have a pulse and will pulsate under probe pressure. There is another way to distinguish between veins and arteries using color Doppler flow. In this scenario, arteries will have central red color flow pulsating compare with veins that there is a blue non-pulsating color.

After having equipment ready for IV access and explain procedure to patient, skin needs to be clean with cleansing agents, and then tourniquet should be applied to upper arm. Ultrasound probe with orientation marker should be facing to right side of patient this will correlate with an indicator on the left side of US monitor and left side of probe. The next step is to use sterile gel to locate vascular structure. As mentioned above, veins are easily compressible with transducer pressure and should be located in the middle of screen. The depth key should be adjusted to make sure veins are in an approachable depth. Vascular structure on short axis should be circular versus long axis. Using short axis approach, the vein should be in the middle of screen. In this situation, middle of transducer is compatible with middle of US screen. Appropriate angiocatheter size should be use and clean 3cm above the antecubital area, then introduce angiocath with 45 degree and cannulate skin. You should see the tip of needle as a hyperechoic structure and you should approach the vein. You will stop advancing your needle as soon as you get blood flush back. Now remove introducer and advance plastic angiocatheter all the way in. You need to attach extensor and apply sterile dressing to accomplish your procedure. (Figure 5)

6.4 Complication

There are several complication related to peripheral IV access. These complications are divided to vascular, infectious, and neurological. Vascular complication include arterial puncture and formation of hematoma, local infiltration or extravasations of fluid, superficial or deep vein thrombosis. The most common infectious complications with US guided IV access are phlebitis and cellulitis. Soft tissue swelling and superficial vein thrombosis can mimic the infection at IV site. Paresthesia due to nerve irritation and local infiltration is the most common complication. There is no long-term nerve damage was reported.

7. US guided arterial line

The radial artery is the extension of the brachial artery. It is originating inferior to elbow along the lateral side of forearm along the radius bone. The main part of focus is radial artery in wrist.

Arterial line placement is an invasive procedure, which it requires skill and expertise to perform it. It is painful procedure and needs a lot of preparation. Preparation is already discussed in aforementioned section, but arterial line kit is additional equipment that we need for this procedure.

7.1 Indication

There are several indications for arterial line placement. Reliable and frequent blood pressure measurements in patients who are hemodynamically unstable, access to arterial blood for frequent acid-base, or blood gas sampling.[18]

7.2 Procedure

US guided arterial line requires fewer attempts and more success rate. After prep and drape in sterile fashion, and cover US probe with sterile cover, arterial line should be located. The characteristic of artery as mentioned above is pulsating in nature with special color Doppler and non compressible. US probe should be in radial side of wrist with orientation indicator facing to right side of patient. After anterior surface of the artery is punctured with the bevel of the angiocatheter facing up and pulsatile blood return, this indicates an intra-arterial position. The rest of procedure is the same as described in peripheral IV access.

The arterial line complications include arterial puncture and hematoma, thrombosis, and infection.

8. References

[1] McGee DC, Gould MK. Preventing complications of central venous catheterization. NEJM 2003;348(12):1123-33

[2] Hind DH, Calvert N, McWilliams R, et al. Ultrasonic locating devices for central venous cannulation: meta-analysis. BMJ 2003;327:361

[3] Denys BG, Uretsky BF, Reddy PS. Ultrasound-assisted cannulation of the internal jugular vein, A prospective comparison to the external landmark-guided technique; Circulation 1993;87 (5):1557-62

[4] Brannam L, Blaivas M, Lyon M, Flake M. Emergency nurses' utilization of ultrasound guidance for placement of peripheral intravenous lines in difficult-access patients. Academic Emergency Medicine 2004;11(12):1361-3

[5] Schoenfeld E, Boniface K, Shokoohi H. ED technicians can successfully place ultrasound-guided intravenous catheters in patients with poor vascular access. American Journal of Emergency Medicine 2011;29(5):496-501

[6] Constantino TG, Parikh AK, Satz WA, Fojtik JA. Ultrasonography-guided peripheral intravenous access versus traditional approaches in patients with difficult intravenous access. Ann Emerg Med 2005;46(5):456-461

[7] Resnick JR, Cydulka R, Jones R., Comparison of two transducers for ultrasound-guided vascular access in long axis. J Emerg Med. 2007 Oct;33(3):273-6

[8] Leung J, Duffy M, Finckh A. ,Real-time ultrasonographically-guided internal jugular vein catheterization in the emergency department increases success rates and reduces complications: a randomized, prospective study. Ann Emerg Med. 2006 Nov;48(5):540-7

[9] Khoo SW, Han DC., The use of ultrasound in vascular procedures. Surg Clin North Am. 2011 Feb;91(1):173-84

[10] Stone MB, Moon C, Sutijono D, Blaivas M , Needle tip visualization during ultrasound-guided vascular access: short-axis vs long-axis approach. Am J Emerg Med. 2010 Mar;28(3):343-7

[11] Blaivas M, Brannam L, Fernandez E: Short axis versus long-axis approaches for teaching ultrasound-guided vascular access on a new inanimate model. Acad Emerg Med 2003; 10:1307–13116

[12] Milling T, Holden C, Melniker L, et al: Randomized controlled trial of single-operator vs. two-operator ultrasound guidance for internal jugular central venous cannulation. Acad Emerg Med 2006; 13:245–247

[13] Rose JS, Norbutas CM. , A randomized controlled trial comparing one-operator versus two-operator technique in ultrasound-guided basilic vein cannulation. J Emerg Med. 2008 Nov;35(4):431-5

[14] Maecken T, Marcon C, Bomas S, Zenz M, Grau T., Relationship of the internal jugular vein to the common carotid artery: implications for ultrasound-guided vascular access. Eur J Anaesthesiol. 2011 May;28(5):351-5

[15] Mallin M, Louis H, Madsen T, A novel technique for ultrasound-guided supraclavicular subclavian cannulation. Am J Emerg Med. 2010 Oct;28(8):966

[16] Gregg SC, Murthi SB, Sisley AC, Stein DM, Scalea TM., Ultrasound-guided peripheral intravenous access in the intensive care unit. J Crit Care. 2010 Sep;25(3):514-9

[17] Costantino TG, Kirtz JF, Satz WA., Ultrasound-guided peripheral venous access vs. the external jugular vein as the initial approach to the patient with difficult vascular access. J Emerg Med. 2010 Oct;39(4):462-7
[18] Shiloh AL, Savel RH, Paulin LM, Eisen LA., Ultrasound-guided catheterization of the radial artery: a systematic review and meta-analysis of randomized controlled trials. Chest. 2011 Mar;139(3):524-9

10

Rheumatoid Arthritis Assessment with Ultrasonography

Thierry Marhadour and Alain Saraux
Rheumatology, CHU and University Hospital,
La Cavale Blanche, Brest
France

1. Introduction

Musculoskeletal ultrasound is a rapidly growing imaging modality used for the investigation and management of musculoskeletal disorders. The first report of musculoskeletal ultrasonography was published in 1958 by K. T. Dussik who measured the acoustic attenuation of articular and periarticular tissues including skin, adipose tissue, muscle, tendon, articular capsule, articular cartilage and bone (Dussik et al., 1958). It was first used in rheumatoid arthritis by Cooperberg in 1978 for the assessment of synovitis in the knee. (Cooperberg et al., 1978). De Flaviis made the first report of ultrasonography in the hand in rheumatoid arthritis in 1988, describing synovitis, tenosynovitis, and erosions (De Flaviis et al., 1988).

The first application of power Doppler in demonstrating soft tissue hyperaemia in musculoskeletal disease was reported in 1994 by J. S. Newman (Newman et al., 1994). Since, power Doppler has started to replace gray-scale ultrasonography as an indicator of inflammatory joint disease.

Ultrasonography has a number of advantages, including good patient tolerability and ability to scan multiple joints in a short period of time. Thanks to smaller high-frequency transducers that were better suited for superficial structures such as the small joints, many reports and studies have been published. However, there are scarce data regarding its validity, reproducibility, and responsiveness to change, making interpretation and comparison of studies difficult. In particular, there are limited data describing standardized scanning methodology and standardized definitions of ultrasonography pathologies.

2. Generalities

2.1 Technique

In contrast to conventional radiography, musculoskeletal ultrasonography can provide multiplanar images of cortical bone, synovium, tendons, muscles, ligaments, and nerves. It is a safe, portable and relatively inexpensive technique. Rheumatoid arthritis is the most studied inflammatory disease in rheumatologic ultrasonography.

Equipment is widely available and comparatively flexible. Examinations can be performed at the bedside. The mean price to acquire a machine is nowadays about 40 000 euros, but costs are decreasing.

In B mode ultrasound, a linear array of transducers simultaneously scans a plane through the body that can be viewed as a two-dimensional image on screen. It allows getting pictures of joints and periarticular structures. The higher the frequency is, the greater both the axial and the lateral resolution of image will be, but at the cost of reduced tissue penetration. Therefore, a higher-frequency transducer is best used for superficial structures, such as the small joints of the hand and feet (e.g. 7–18 MHz), and a low frequency transducer is used for deeper joints, such as the hip (e.g. 3–5 MHz).

Doppler mode makes use of the Doppler effect in measuring and visualizing blood flow. Power Doppler denotes only the amplitude of the Doppler signal, which is determined by the volume of blood present so it is better suited to the assessment of low-velocity flow in small vessels (e.g. synovium). This would be a way to assess joint inflammation.

Learning is quite short: D'agostino evaluated that five hours of theory and three months of practice (around 70 exams) are needed. The concordance between learners and teachers is good, approximately about 80 % (D'agostino et al., 2004).

2.2 Elementary lesions in rheumatoid arthritis

OMERACT stands for Outcome Measures in Rheumatology. It is an informal international network of working groups and gatherings interested in outcome measurement across the spectrum of rheumatology intervention studies. Thanks to Omeract, there is consensus on ultrasonography definitions for common pathological lesions seen in patients with inflammatory arthritis (Wakefield et al., 2006).

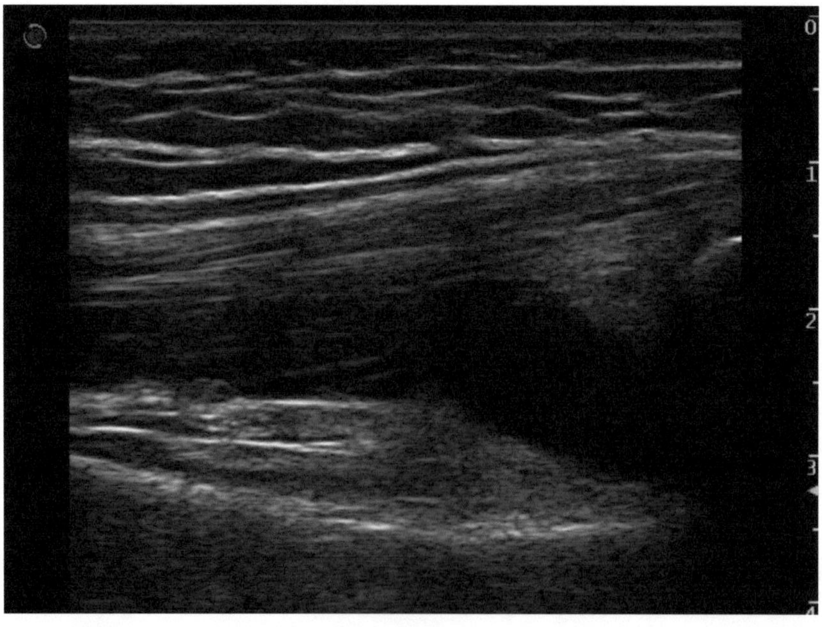

Fig. 1. Effusion of knee

Synovial fluid

Abnormal hypoechoic or anechoic (relative to subdermal fat, but sometimes may be isoechoic or hyperechoic) intraarticular material that is displaceable and compressible, but does not exhibit Doppler signal (Fig. 1).

Synovial hypertrophy

Abnormal hypoechoic (relative to subdermal fat, but sometimes may be isoechoic or hyperechoic) intraarticular tissue that is nondisplaceable and poorly compressible and which may exhibit Doppler signal (Figs. 2, 3).

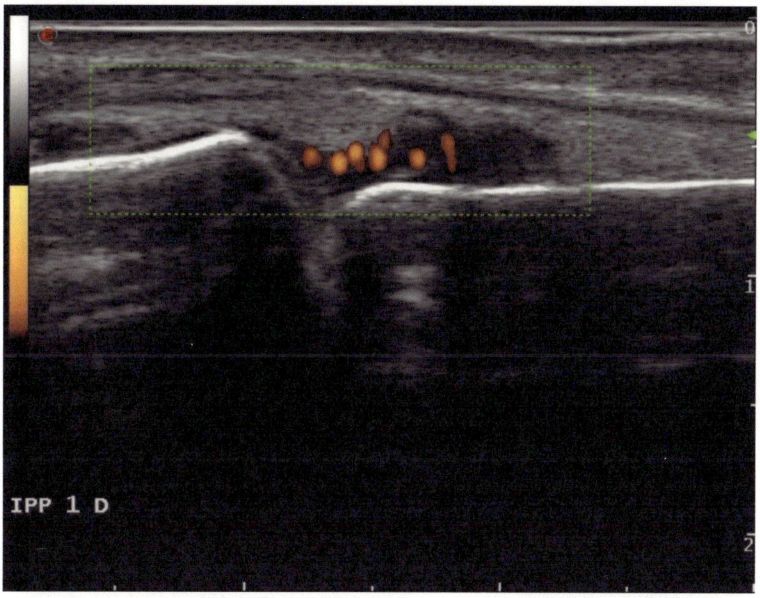

Fig. 2. MCP synovitis with power Doppler signal

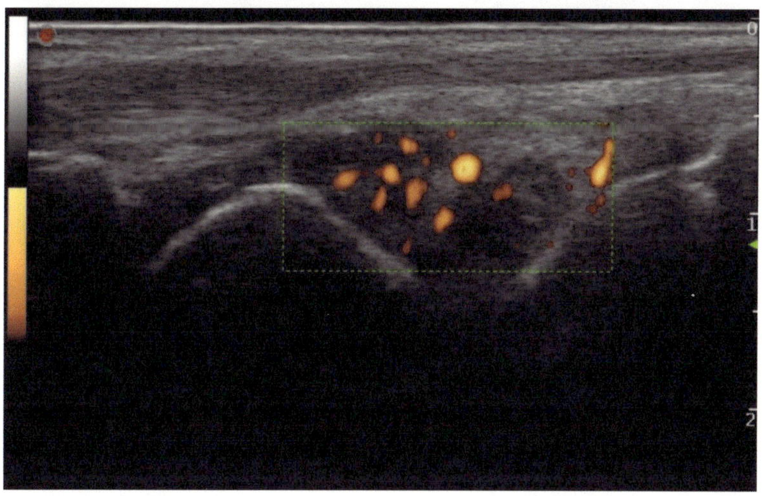

Fig. 3. Arthritis of the wrist

Tenosynovitis

Hypoechoic or anechoic thickened tissue with or without fluid within the tendon sheath, which is seen in 2 perpendicular planes and which may exhibit Doppler Signal (Fig. 4).

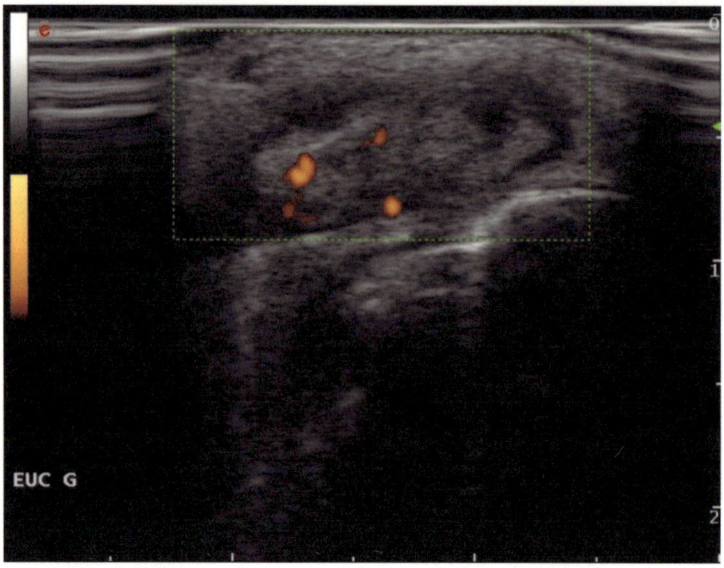

Fig. 4. Tenosynovitis of the left extensor carpi ulnaris tendon with power Doppler signal

Bone erosion

An intraarticular discontinuity of the bone surface that is visible in 2 perpendicular planes (Fig. 5).

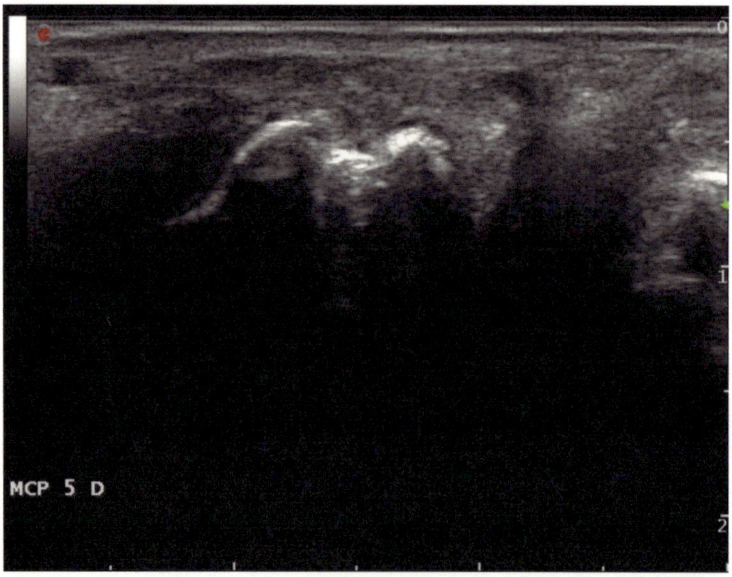

Fig. 5. Bone erosion in the head of the right fifth metacarpal (transversal plane)

2.3 Classification

Joint assessment can be binary (synovitis present or absent) or semi-quantitative. The first one is easily applicable in routine practice whereas the second is mostly used in trials. Szkudlarek described semi-quantitative scales for synovial hypertrophy, effusion Doppler signal and erosions (Szkudlarek et al., 2003).

Joint effusion was defined as a compressible anechoic intracapsular area (0=no effusion, 1=minimal amount of joint effusion, 2=moderate amount of joint effusion [without distension of the joint capsule], 3=extensive amount of joint effusion [with distension of the joint capsule]).

Synovitis was defined as a noncompressible hypoechoic intracapsular area (synovial thickening) (0=no synovial thickening, 1=minimal synovial thickening [filling the angle between the periarticular bones, without bulging over the line linking tops of the bones], 2=synovial thickening bulging over the line linking tops of the periarticular bones but without extension along the bone diaphysis, 3=synovial thickening bulging over the line linking tops of the periarticular bones and with extension to at least one of the bone diaphyses).

Bone erosions were defined as changes in the bone surface of the area adjacent to the joint (0=regular bone surface, 1=irregularity of the bone surface without formation of a defect seen in 2 planes, 2=formation of a defect in the surface of the bone seen in 2 planes, 3=bone defect creating extensive bone destruction).

Power Doppler signal was used to display flow signal in the synovium (0=no flow in the synovium, 1=single vessel signals, 2=confluent vessel signals in less than half of the area of the synovium, 3=vessel signals in more than half of the area of the synovium)

Omeract developed a semi-quantitative scale to assess synovitis in B Mode and power Doppler (Wakefield et al., 2005) (table 1). This score is also based on the assessment of effusion, synovial hypertrophy and Doppler flow.

B Mode	- Grade 0: Normal joint (no synovial hyperthrophy, no joint effusion) - Grade 1: Minimal synovitis (minimal synovial hyperthrophy, with or without minimal joint effusion) - Grade 2: Moderate synovitis (moderate synovial hyperthrophy with or without minimal or moderate joint effusion) - Grade 3: Severe synovitis (severe synovial hypertrophy, with or without severe joint effusion)
Power Doppler	- Grade 0: no vessel in the synovium; - Grade 1: up to 3 single spots signals or 1 confluent spot + up to 2 single spots - Grade 2: vessel signals in less than half of the area of the synovium (< 50%) - Grade 3: vessel signals in more than half of the area of the synovium (> 50%)

Table 1. Omeract semi-quantitative scale for joint assessment

2.4 Scores

For the time being, there is no consensus on ultrasound score. There are comprehensive scores, which integrate the 44 joints of the Disease Activity Score (Wakefield et al., 2005);

there are reduced scores, like the one developed by Backhaus which assess only 7 joints (Backhaus et al., 2009). Actually, Omeract is working on a consensus score, which will be called Gloss (Global Omeract Sonography Scoring). It should be feasible, whereas bringing more information than clinical examination (D'Agostino et al., 2009).

2.5 Artefacts

Some artefacts have to be known:

Anisotropy: This is the effect that makes a tendon appear bright when it runs at 90 degrees to the ultrasound beam, but dark when the angle is changed.

Enhancement: Some structures however allow sound to pass through them more easily than others. The most dramatic example is watery fluid, such as in an effusion, or in a cyst. These are described as being translucent. Because only a minimal amount of energy is absorbed by the fluid, the region that lies behind will receive more sound than the processor expects for that depth. This area will therefore appear uniformly brighter.

Attenuation or **Shadowing** is the reverse effect, where some tissues absorb relatively more of the sound. The area of the image deep to this will appear darker. In the extreme almost no sound is transmitted, leaving a dark shadow behind the structure. This can be caused by a calcification for example.

3. Contribution of ultrasonography in the monitoring of rheumatoid arthritis

3.1 Synovitis

Ultrasound synovitis is not specific of rheumatoid arthritis. Synovial hypertrophy or effusion can be seen in other inflammatory rheumatism, and even in osteoarthritis (Rosenberg et al., 2009). Consequently, the interest for diagnosis of rheumatoid arthritis is poor, but it can help in presence of polyarthralgia. Van de Stadt studied 192 patients with polyarthralgia who had rheumatoid factor and / or CCP antibodies. Subclinical ultrasound anomaly of a joint was predictive of evolution toward authentic arthritis at joint level, but this wasn't true at patient level (Van de Stadt et al., 2010). Nevertheless, the topography of swollen joints and the other signs (like tenosynovitis and obviously erosions) may guide the diagnosis.

Actually, ultrasonography is important for rheumatoid arthritis monitoring. There are several studies that prove that ultrasonography is more sensitive than clinical examination for synovitis assessment. Szkudlarek studied small joints (Metacarpophalangeal MCP 2 and 3, Proximal Interphalangeal PIP 2, and Metatarsophalangeal MTP 1 and 2) in 30 rheumatoid arthritis patients and found approximately 50 % more synovitis with ultrasonography in B mode than with clinical assessment (Szkudlarek et al., 2003).

In other studies, by comparison with MRI, ultrasonography was found to be markedly more sensitive and accurate than clinical examination to search synovitis on the ten MTP joints (sensibility respectively 0.87 versus 0.43) (Szkudlarek et al., 2004) and on the second to fifth MCP and IPP of the dominant hand (sensibility respectively 0.7 versus 0.4) (Szkudlarek et al., 2006).

Ultrasonography is also more sensitive in early rheumatoid arthritis. In 44 patients whose rheumatoid arthritis duration was less than 2 years, Salaffi found a mean swollen joint count of 19.1 (+/-4.1) with ultrasonography and 12.6 (+/-3.6) with clinical examination. Power Doppler signal in the synovium was present in 43 joints, of which 60% showed clinical signs of inflammation (swelling and/or tenderness). Power Doppler signal in the synovium was absent in 107 joints, of which 36% presented clinical signs of inflammation (Salaffi et al., 2008).

Power Doppler permits assessment of low-velocity flow in small vessels and is considered to reflect disease acute inflammatory activity. In the Sea study, the use of Power Doppler dramatically reduced the number of arthritis in rheumatoid arthritis considered as active by clinicians (Marhadour et al., 2010). If the swollen joint count was based on ultrasonography result, disease activity index was lower than if based on clinician assessment.

3.2 Erosions

The detection of radiographic erosions in early disease is associated with a poor outcome (Van der Heijde et al., 1992) and may influence the timing and choice of disease-modifying antirheumatic drug therapy.

Erosion of hand in ultrasonography was first described in 1988, in 20 rheumatoid arthritis patients (De Flaviis et al., 1988) and then Grassi confirmed the ability of ultrasonography to show erosions in a controlled trial with 20 rheumatoid arthritis patients and 20 controls (Grassi et al., 1993).

Ultrasonography is more sensitive than X-Ray to detect erosion in rheumatoid arthritis. In 2000, Wakefield was the first to demonstrate that sonography detects more erosion on the MCP joints of rheumatoid arthritis patients than does conventional radiography, especially in early disease. He compared ultrasonography and X-Ray for erosion detection in the MCP joints of rheumatoid arthritis patients and studied its reliability. There were 100 rheumatoid arthritis patients who were split according to their disease duration. Those with disease duration of less than 12 months with no prior DMARD therapy were classified as having early disease, while those with disease duration of more than 2 months were classified as having late disease. The control group included 20 patients. In the early rheumatoid arthritis group, sonography detected a 6.5-fold increase in the number of erosions detected by sonography over that detected by radiography (P=0.0001), in 7.5-fold the number of patients. In the group with late rheumatoid arthritis, sonography detected a 3.4-fold increase (P=0.0001), in 2.7 fold the number of patients. Sonography detected more erosions than radiography in all MCP joints except the fourth, where it detected fewer (sonography detected proportionately more erosions where the transducer had good access, in particular, the first, second, and fifth joints). Significantly fewer of the small sonographic erosions (less than 2 mm) were visible on radiography (P=0.0001). In this study, MRI was used to validate the additional sonographic lesions not seen on radiography, giving some evidence of their pathologic specificity. Wakefield explained that there were two reasons why sonography detected more erosions than radiography in this study: first, the 3-dimensional capability of sonography allowed joints to be examined in several different planes; second, sonography was able to detect smaller erosions. Erosions were most frequently seen on either the radial or the ulnar aspect of the MCP joint, with relatively few occurring on the volar or dorsal surfaces (Wakefield et al., 2000).

Alasaarela assessed the value of ultrasonography, magnetic resonance imaging, computed tomography (CT) and plain radiography (PR) in detecting bone erosions on the humeral in 26 rheumatoid arthritis patients. MRI depicted humeral erosions in 25 (96%), ultrasonography in 24 (92%), CT in 20 (77%) and PR in 19 (73%) of the 26 shoulders. MRI and ultrasonography were superior to CT in detecting small erosions. Ultrasonography was the most sensitive method to show surface erosions on the greater tuberosity (Alasaarela et al., 1998).

Conventional radiography is based on attenuation of X-rays, and calcified tissues such as bone are readily depicted because of their markedly greater attenuation in comparison with the surrounding soft tissues. Because imaging with ultrasonography does not depend on X-rays, it has been speculated to which extent erosions detected using these modalities reflects true loss of calcified tissue, that is, are true erosions. Therefore, ultrasonography has been compared to computed tomography, which is considered as a gold standard. On 17 rheumatoid arthritis patients, ultrasonography exhibited high specificities (91 %) in detecting bone erosions in MCP joints, even in the radiographically non-erosive joints (92%). Although, sensitivity was moderate (42%) (Døhn et al., 2006).

Nevertheless, a recent study which evaluated bone erosion in 127 healthy subjects matched with a cohort of patients with early arthritis (the ESPOIR cohort) detected bone erosion in 11% of healthy subjects at metacarpo and metatarsophalangeal joint of both hands and feet. However, the combination of power Doppler signal plus bone erosion, on the same joint, was never seen in healthy subjects. A single case of bone erosion or synovial thickening in B-mode is common in healthy subjects. However, more than 1 case of synovial thickening in B-mode or bone erosion is a strong argument for the diagnosis of early inflammatory arthritis (Millot et al., 2010).

4. Outcome assessment validation strategy in rheumatoid arthritis

4.1 Generalities

Scientific rules must be respected when developing a measurement tool. Since ninety's, some consensus are growing in rheumatoid arthritis metrology, especially thanks to OMERACT, which developed a filter of 3 criteria:

1. *Truth*: is the measure truthful, does it measure what it intends to measure? Is the result unbiased and relevant? This criterion captures the issues of face, content, construct and criterion validity.
   Face validity: It is the validity of a test at face value. In other words, a test can be said to have face validity if it "looks like" it is going to measure what it is supposed to measure
   Content validity: Refers to the extent to which a measure represents all facets of a given phenomena.
   Criterion validity: Criterion or concrete validity is the extent to which the measures are demonstrably related to concrete criteria in the "real" world, ie gold standard. For ultrasonography, gold standards are histology or surgical macroscopic findings.
   Construct validity is achieved when measures agree with other measures that evaluate the same phenomenon. For ultrasonography, this can be other imaging techniques or laboratory and clinical data.
2. *Discrimination*: Does the measure discriminate between situations that are of interest? The situations can be states at one time (for classification or prognosis) or states at

different times (to measure change). This criterion captures the issues of reliability and sensitivity to change.

3. *Feasibility*: Can the measure be applied easily, given constraints of time, money, and interpretability? This criterion addresses the pragmatic reality of the use of the measure, one that may be decisive in determining a measure's success.

4.2 Application to ultrasonography

Despite increasing interest in ultrasonography, widespread application has been impeded by a perception that its use is unproven and unreliable. There was limited data describing standardized scanning methodology and standardized definitions of ultrasonography pathologies in addition to how to quantify these abnormalities.

Reliability of a test result is its ability to be reproduced. There are various ways of expressing reliability: Cohen's Kappa (the more the result is near from 1, the best is the agreement), intraclass correlation coefficient (ICC), coefficient of variation, overall agreement, and Kendall's W coefficient. In ultrasonography, it can be divided into the acquisition and the reading phases, as well as the reliability of one observer (intra observer) and multiple observers (interobserver) to reproduce the result. The scanning technique for each joints needs to be standardized, that's why position statements have been developed through consensus meetings (Backhaus, 2001). It is important to test the acquisition reliability of ultrasonography because of its multiplanar capability, and because the sonographer chooses the images he wants to save (even with standard imaging protocols).

Responsiveness is the ability of the tool to demonstrate change. Ultrasonography will be considered sensitive to change if it detects small variation in disease activity. This can be useful to demonstrate the action of a new treatment.

5. Is ultrasonography reliable for the monitoring of rheumatoid arthritis ?

5.1 Synovitis

A first systematic review was performed in 2007 by the Omeract Ultrasound Group on the metric properties of ultrasonography for the detection of synovitis in inflammatory arthritis (the major inflammatory condition studied was rheumatoid arthritis). The major joints assessed were the hand and knee. Few comparisons were done versus histology or surgical findings. Reliability was evaluated with a filter including intra/inter observer acquisition, intra/inter observer reading, sensitivity to change, criterion validity and construct validity. The authors concluded that there were major gaps in the reliability testing, primarily in the assessment of acquisition, and Omeract encouraged rheumatologists to perform more studies on reliability (Joshua et al., 2007).

A way to increase the quality of a reliability study is to multiply the number of examiners. The Sea study was realised in this purpose (Jousse-Joulin et al., 2010). 7 patients with rheumatoid arthritis were examined by 7 clinicians and then 7 sonographers examined each of the 7 patients twice, using B Mode and power Doppler OMERACT grading. The clinical reference standard was the presence of synovitis according to at least 50% of clinical examiners. Different standards were used for sonography (the sonographer with the best reliability, the presence of synovitis according to at least 50% of sonographers) using different grade to define sonographic abnormalities [at least grade 1 (ALG1) or at least grade 2 (ALG2)]. Agreement was assessed by Cohen's kappa. Concerning intraobserver acquisition reliability for B mode, it was relatively good but varied upon the grade defining synovitis. In ALG1 the results varied to poor (for one sonographer) to fair agreement in 3 sonographers and good for 3 whereas using ALG2, the intraobserver reliability was better with a good agreement for 6:7 sonographers in B mode. The results were slightly lower using power Doppler in both ALG1 and ALG2, as only 2 of 7 sonographers had a good agreement. Interobserver acquisition reliability was also evaluated. The results of the detection of synovitis in B mode with ALG1 showed a fair agreement for 5 of 6 sonographers and only one sonographer has a good agreement. For ALG2, results were better as 4 of 6 sonographers had a good agreement. Using power Doppler with ALG1 we observed a poor agreement for 3 sonographers and a fair agreement for 3. Using ALG2, the power Doppler kappa values were quite similar with one good agreement, 3 fair, and one poor agreement. When we used grade 2 in B mode or in power Doppler, the intra and inter reliability was better. In our study, the reliability was not clearly different between the different sites.

Another systematic review was performed in 2010, focusing exclusively on rheumatoid arthritis (Cheung et al., 2010). 35 studies with a total of 1415 patients were analyzed. Intra and inter observer reliability for still images in B mode and power Doppler was high (k=0.5-1 for intraobserver in B mode; k=0.59-1 for intra observer in power Doppler; k=0.49-1 for inter observer in B mode; k=0.66-1 for inter observer in power Doppler). It appeared that still-image interpretation was more reliable than image acquisition. However, results of acquisition reliability were variable and sometimes poor with kappa values reaching 0.2, and very few studies assessed intraobserver acquisition reliability in either B-mode or power Doppler. Differences in the scanning technique and the lack of familiarity of the ultrasonography machine may also explain the poor results in reliability studies. In this review, few studies looked at the image acquisition reliability. Intraobserver reliability in this domain has been the least studied, and the time interval for retesting was as short as 30 minutes. Power Doppler interobserver reliability was higher than B-mode in still-image interpretation. This may be due to the fact that grading and detection of signal flow on still images would be less liable to variation than identification of hypoechoicstructures. Presence or absence of color signal is also easier to differentiate.

In his 2003's study, Szkudlarek evaluated interobserver agreement between ultrasonography investigators. For the detection of synovitis, the ICC and unweighted kappa estimations for the examined parameters showed a moderate-to-good correlation (0.61–0.81 and 0.48–0.68, respectively) between the ultrasonography investigators. The overall agreement was high (79–91%) (Szkudlarek et al., 2003).

The most important study to evaluate different scoring systems on three main groups of joints (20, 28 and 38) using both a count and a score (comparing the clinical, ultrasonography B mode and ultrasonography power Doppler techniques of acquisition resulting in 18 different global scoring systems) have been published in 2010 (Dougados et al., 2010). A systematic evaluation of the main psychometric/methodological properties in accordance to the OMERACT filter permitted an overview of the performances of these different scoring systems (intra-observer reliability using the intra-class coefficient of correlation, validity on 76 enrolled patients, face validity using the alpha Cronbach test and external validity using the level of correlation between the scoring system and CRP, sensitivity to change was using the Standardized Response Mean in the 66 patients who completed 4 months of the study and discriminating capacity was using the Standardized Mean Differences in the patients considered by the physician as significantly improved or not at the end of the study). The obtained data suggest that the ultrasonography scoring systems are at least as valid as the conventional clinical ones. Moreover, the ultrasonography acquisition of synovitis appeared to be more objective and can be easily documented. Other studies are required in order to achieve an optimal ultrasonography scoring system endorsed by international societies for monitoring rheumatoid arthritis patients both in clinical trials and in daily practice.

5.2 Erosions

Because of the discrepancy between magnetic resonance and computed tomography concerning erosions, some authors noted that the absolute numbers and sizes of the erosions on the bone surface are not known. To resolve this problem, Koski assessed the ability of ultrasound imaging to detect erosions in a bone phantom model (Koski et al., 2010). 21 bovine lower leg bones were prepared and then were examined by 4 sonographers. The mean correlation coefficient for a correct result in terms of the number of erosions detected was 0.88 (0.75 - 0.75). The overall Cohen's kappa coefficient for interobserver agreement was 0.683 in terms of discrimination between healthy bones and bones with erosions. Ultrasound can be considered as a valid and reliable to detect cortical bone erosions in vitro, when the round erosion is at least 1 mm deep and 1.5 mm wide.

When Wakefield compared ultrasonography to X-rays for the detection of erosion, he assessed intra and inter observer agreement. The intraobserver kappa value for agreement for the detection of cortical bone erosions on the second MCP joint of 55 rheumatoid arthritis patients was 0.75. The interobserver kappa value for agreement between 2 observers for the detection of cortical bone erosions on MCP joints 2–5 in 40 rheumatoid arthritis patients (160 joints) was 0.76. These good results confirmed that ultrasonography is a reliable technique for detecting MCP joint erosions (Wakefield 2000).

Rahmani compared ultrasonography to X-rays and MRI in early rheumatoid arthritis. In 12 patients, 120 first to fifth metacarpophalangeal joints and 96 second to fifth proximal interphalangeal joints were examined. The overall sensitivity and specificity of ultrasonography compared to MRI in detecting bone erosion were 0.63 and 0.98, respectively with a considerable agreement (kappa = 0.68, $p < 0.001$). In patients with more active disease, the sensitivity and specificity were 0.67 and 0.99 (kappa = 0.74, $p < 0.001$) compared to 0.59 and 0.97 (kappa = 0.61, $p < 0.001$) for the rest of patients according to DAS28. Therefore, ultrasonography might be considered as a valuable tool for early detection of bone erosion. (Rahmani et al., 2010).

Not only can ultrasonograpy be seen as reliable for bone erosion, but also for cartilage damage assessment, as Filippucci demonstrated. Two rheumatologists performed ultrasonograpy examination on 80 MCP joints of 20 rheumatoid arthritis patients. There was moderate to good interobserver reproducibility, using a semiquantitative scoring. Unweighted k values were 0.561, 0.366 and 0.766 at dorsal, lateral and volar quadrants respectively (Filippucci et al, 2010).

6. Conclusion

Ultrasonography is a powerful tool to assess rheumatoid arthritis activity. It is widely available, can be performed at the bedside, is not expansive and non ionizing. It is more sensitive than clinical examination to detect synovitis and more sensitive than x-rays to detect erosions. Even though more and more studies have been published to prove its reliability, more consensuses are needed for images acquisition. The next step will be to assess its sensitivity to change, which will expand its use for treatment monitoring.

7. References

Alasaarela E, Suramo I, Tervonen O, Lähde S, Takalo R, & Hakala M. Evaluation of humeral head erosions in rheumatoid arthritis: a comparison of ultrasonography, magnetic resonance imaging, computed tomography and plain radiography. *Br J Rheumatol.* 1998 Nov;37(11):1152-6

Backhaus M, Burmester GR, Gerber T, Grassi W, Machold KP, Swen WA, Wakefield RJ, & Manger B; Working Group for Musculoskeletal Ultrasound in the EULAR Standing Committee on International Clinical Studies including Therapeutic Trials. Guidelines for musculoskeletal ultrasound in rheumatology. *Ann Rheum Dis.* 2001 Jul;60(7):641-9.

Backhaus M, Ohrndorf S, Kellner H, Strunk J, Backhaus TM, Hartung W, Sattler H, Albrecht K, Kaufmann J, Becker K, Sörensen H, Meier L, Burmester GR, & Schmidt WA. Evaluation of a novel 7-joint ultrasound score in daily rheumatologic practice: a pilot project. *Arthritis Rheum.* 2009

Cheung PP, Dougados M, & Gossec L. Reliability of ultrasonography to detect synovitis in rheumatoid arthritis: a systematic literature review of 35 studies (1,415 patients). *Arthritis Care Res* (Hoboken). 2010 Mar;62(3):323-34

Cooperberg PL, Tsang I, Truelove L, & Knickerbocker WJ. Gray scale ultrasound in the evaluation of rheumatoid arthritis of the knee. *Radiology.* 1978 Mar;126(3):759-63

D'Agostino MA, Maillefert JF, Said-Nahal R, Breban M, Ravaud P, & Dougados M. Detection of small joint synovitis by ultrasonography: the learning curve of rheumatologists. *Ann Rheum Dis.* 2004 Oct;63(10):1284-7

D'Agostino MA, Conaghan PG, Naredo E, Aegerter P, Iagnocco A, Freeston JE, Filippucci E, Moller I, Pineda C, Joshua F, Backhaus M, Keen HI, Kaeley G, Ziswiler HR, Schmidt WA, Balint PV, Bruyn GA, Jousse-Joulin S, Kane D, Moller I, Szkudlarek M, Terslev L, & Wakefield RJ. The OMERACT ultrasound task force -- Advances and priorities. J Rheumatol. 2009 Aug;36(8):1829-32. Erratum in: *J Rheumatol.* 2009 Nov;36(11):2625. Zisweiler, Hans-Rudolf [corrected to Ziswiler, Hans-Rudolf]

De Flaviis L, Scaglione P, Nessi R, Ventura R, & Calori G. Ultrasonography of the hand in rheumatoid arthritis. *Acta Radiol.* 1988 Jul-Aug;29(4):457-60

Døhn UM, Ejbjerg BJ, Court-Payen M, Hasselquist M, Narvestad E, Szkudlarek M, Møller JM, Thomsen HS, & Østergaard M. Are bone erosions detected by magnetic resonance imaging and ultrasonography true erosions? A comparison with computed tomography in rheumatoid arthritis metacarpophalangeal joints. *Arthritis Res Ther.* 2006;8(4):R110

Dougados M, Jousse-Joulin S, Mistretta F, d'Agostino MA, Backhaus M, Bentin J, Chalès G, Chary-Valckenaere I, Conaghan P, Etchepare F, Gaudin P, Grassi W, van der

Heijde D, Sellam J, Naredo E, Szkudlarek M, Wakefield R, & Saraux A. Evaluation of several ultrasonography scoring systems for synovitis and comparison to clinical examination: results from a prospective multicentre study of rheumatoid arthritis. *Ann Rheum Dis.* 2010 May;69(5):828-33.

Dussik KT, Fritch DJ, Kyriazidou M, & Sear RS. Measurements of articular tissues with ultrasound. Am J Phys Med. 1958 Jun;37(3):160-5Grassi W, Tittarelli E, Pirani O, Avaltroni D, Cervini C. Ultrasound examination of metacarpophalangeal joints in rheumatoid arthritis. *Scand J Rheumatol.* 1993;22(5):243-7

Filippucci E, da Luz KR, Di Geso L, Salaffi F, Tardella M, Carotti M, Natour J, & Grassi W. Interobserver reliability of ultrasonography in the assessment of cartilage damage in rheumatoid arthritis. *Ann Rheum Dis.* 2010 Oct; 69(10):1845-8.

Joshua F, Lassere M, Bruyn GA, Szkudlarek M, Naredo E, Schmidt WA, Balint P, Filippucci E, Backhaus M, Iagnocco A, Scheel AK, Kane D, Grassi W, Conaghan PG, Wakefield RJ, & D'Agostino MA. Summary findings of a systematic review of the ultrasound assessment of synovitis. *J Rheumatol.* 2007 Apr;34(4):839-47

Jousse-Joulin S, d'Agostino MA, Marhadour T, Albert JD, Bentin J, Chary Valckenaere I, Etchepare F, Gaudin P, Hudry C, Chalès G, Grange L, Hacquard C, Loeuille D, Sellam J, Dougados M, & Saraux A. Reproducibility of joint swelling assessment by sonography in patients with long-lasting rheumatoid arthritis (SEA-Repro study part II). *J Rheumatol.* 2010 May;37(5):938-45

Koski JM, Alasaarela E, Soini I, Kemppainen K, Hakulinen U, Heikkinen JO, Laasanen MS, & Saarakkala S. Ability of ultrasound imaging to detect erosions in a bone phantom model. *Ann Rheum Dis.* 2010 Sep;69(9):1618-22.

Marhadour T, Jousse-Joulin S, Chalès G, Grange L, Hacquard C, Loeuille D, Sellam J, Albert JD, Bentin J, Chary Valckenaere I, d'Agostino MA, Etchepare F, Gaudin P, Hudry C, Dougados M, & Saraux A. Reproducibility of joint swelling assessments in long-lasting rheumatoid arthritis: influence on Disease Activity Score-28 values (SEA-Repro study part I). *J Rheumatol.* 2010 May;37(5):932-7

Millot F, Clavel G, Etchepare F, Gandjbakhch F, Grados F, Saraux A, Rat AC, Fautrel B, Bourgeois P, & Fardellone P; Investigators of the French Early Arthritis Cohort ESPOIR. Musculoskeletal ultrasonography in healthy subjects and ultrasound criteria for early arthritis (the ESPOIR cohort). *J Rheumatol.* 2011 Apr; 38(4):613-20.

Newman JS, Adler RS, Bude RO, & Rubin JM. Detection of soft-tissue hyperemia: value of power Doppler sonography. *AJR Am J Roentgenol.* 1994 Aug;163(2):385-9

Rahmani M, Chegini H, Najafizadeh SR, Azimi M, Habibollahi P, & Shakiba M. Detection of bone erosion in early rheumatoid arthritis: ultrasonography and conventional radiography versus non-contrast magnetic resonance imaging. *Clin Rheumatol.* 2010 Aug;29(8):883-91

Rosenberg C, Arrestier S, Etchepare F, Fautrel B, Rozenberg S, & Bourgeois P. High frequency of ultrasonographic effusion in interphalangeal joints of healthy subjects: a descriptive study. *Joint Bone Spine.* 2009 May;76(3):265-7. Epub 2009 Mar 14.

Salaffi F, Filippucci E, Carotti M, Naredo E, Meenagh G, Ciapetti A, Savic V, & Grassi W. Inter-observer agreement of standard joint counts in early rheumatoid arthritis: a comparison with grey scale ultrasonography--a preliminary study. *Rheumatology* (Oxford). 2008 Jan;47(1):54-8

Szkudlarek M, Court-Payen M, Jacobsen S, Klarlund M, Thomsen HS, & Østergaard M. Interobserver agreement in ultrasonography of the finger and toe joints in rheumatoid arthritis. *Arthritis Rheum.* 2003 Apr;48(4):955-62

Szkudlarek M, Narvestad E, Klarlund M, Court-Payen M, Thomsen HS, & Østergaard M. Ultrasonography of the metatarsophalangeal joints in rheumatoid arthritis: comparison with magnetic resonance imaging, conventional radiography, and clinical examination. *Arthritis Rheum.* 2004 Jul;50(7):2103-12

Szkudlarek M, Klarlund M, Narvestad E, Court-Payen M, Strandberg C, Jensen KE, Thomsen HS, & Østergaard M. Ultrasonography of the metacarpophalangeal and proximal interphalangeal joints in rheumatoid arthritis: a comparison with magnetic resonance imaging, conventional radiography and clinical examination. *Arthritis Res Ther.* 2006;8(2):R52

Van der Heijde DM, van Leeuwen MA, van Riel PL, Koster AM, van 't Hof MA, van Rijswijk MH, & van de Putte LB. Biannual radiographic assessments of hands and feet in a three-year prospective followup of patients with early rheumatoid arthritis. *Arthritis Rheum.* 1992 Jan;35(1):26-34

van de Stadt LA, Bos WH, Meursinge Reynders M, Wieringa H, Turkstra F, van der Laken CJ, & van Schaardenburg D. The value of ultrasonography in predicting arthritis in auto-antibody positive arthralgia patients: a prospective cohort study. *Arthritis Res Ther.* 2010;12(3):R98

Wakefield RJ, Gibbon WW, Conaghan PG, O'Connor P, McGonagle D, Pease C, Green MJ, Veale DJ, Isaacs JD, & Emery P. The value of sonography in the detection of bone erosions in patients with rheumatoid arthritis: a comparison with conventional radiography. *Arthritis Rheum.* 2000 Dec;43(12):2762-70

Wakefield RJ, Balint PV, Szkudlarek M, Filippucci E, Backhaus M, D'Agostino MA, Sanchez EN, Iagnocco A, Schmidt WA, Bruyn GA, Kane D, O'Connor PJ, Manger B, Joshua F, Koski J, Grassi W, Lassere MN, Swen N, Kainberger F, Klauser A, Ostergaard M, Brown AK, Machold KP, & Conaghan PG; OMERACT 7 Special Interest Group. Musculoskeletal ultrasound including definitions for ultrasonographic pathology. J Rheumatol. 2005 Dec;32(12):2485-7. Erratum in: *J Rheumatol.* 2006 Feb;33(2):440.

11

Sonogram of Biliary Dilatation in Children

Hung-Chang Lee, Chuen-Bin Jiang, Wai-Tao Chan, Chun-Yan Yeung
Division of Pediatric Gastroenterology and Nutrition,
Department of Pediatrics, Mackay Memorial Hospital, Taipei
Taiwan

1. Introduction

The biliary trees descend from the canaliculi at the hepatocytes in the liver. Bile drains from this level into intrahepatic ducts, smaller ducts combine to form the segmental bile ducts which within the liver gradually enlarge and merge to the right and left hepatic ducts. The right and left hepatic ducts join together to form the common hepatic duct (CHD) at porta hepatis. The common bile duct (CBD) is formed by the junction of the cystic duct with the CHD. The CBD traverses through the head of the pancreas entering the duodenum through the Sphincter of Oddi at the Ampulla of Vater. Prior to draining into the duodenum, the CBD is joined by the pancreatic duct. A smaller accessory pancreatic duct and sphincter is usually present (but rarely visible by sonography) from the dorsal pancreatic embryologic rotation. (Fig. 1)

2. Scanning technique and normal findings of biliary tree

A standard commercial purpose ultrasound machine can perform the typical biliary system study of children in routine examinations of the gallbladder and the bile ducts. Curvilinear abdominal probes with the frequency range of 3–5 MHz are ideal for examination of the biliary tree, thus enabling the detection of the gallbladder and bile ducts from a wide range of body sizes (from obese children to small infants).

To perform the examination of the biliary tree sonography, the child is usually in the supine position. All children prepared for ideal ultrasound examination of the gallbladder and bile ducts should fast for at least 4-6 hours prior to the examination. Adequate fasting distends the gallbladder and bile ducts for optimal investigation of the lumen and the wall. Since the duodenum is in close proximity to both the gallbladder and the extrahepatic ducts, fasting also reduces the contents of the stomach and duodenum which very often obscure the common bile duct.

The gallbladder is a pear-shaped structure with thin white walls surrounding a black fluid lying in a fossa formed by the junction of the right and left main lobes of the liver. The most effective window to scan the gallbladder is to sweep the transducer over the right subcostal area. The maneuver starts with the probe in longitudinal orientation and the probe-indicator oriented toward the patient's head. By sweeping the probe, the gallbladder is identified and makes small adjustments to create the best long-axis view. After the long-axis is thoroughly examined, rotate the probe 90 degrees and demonstrate the short-axis view (Fig. 2).

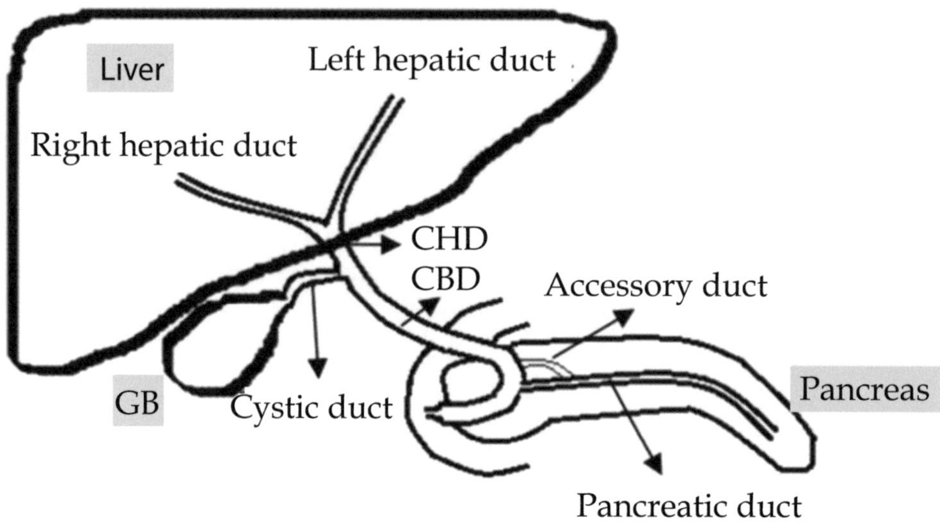

Fig. 1. The anatomy of the biliary tree. (GB: gallbladder, CHD: common hepatic duct, CBD: common bile duct)

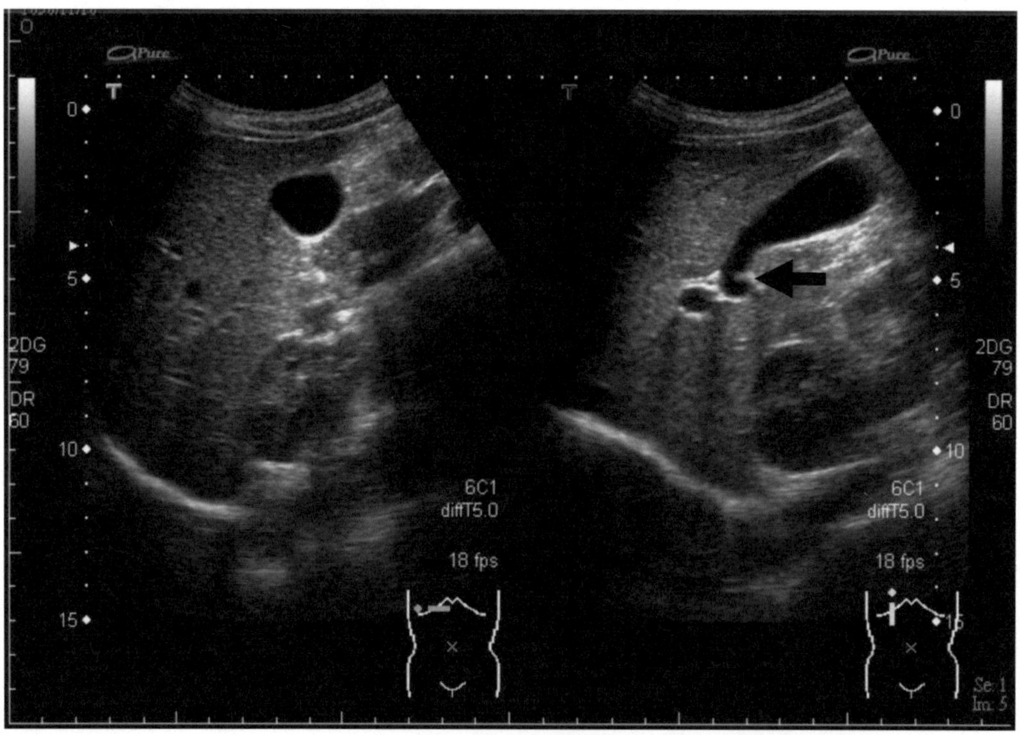

Fig. 2. Normal presentation of gallbladder. Left: the short-axis view. The gallbladder appears spherical. The narrowest portion of the wall is proper to measure the wall of gallbladder. Right: the long-axis view. The gallbladder will usually appear as a pear-shaped, hypoechoic structure with a hyperechoic wall. There is no acoustic shadowing posterior to the gallbladder. The wall folds one time upon itself may falsely present a septum (arrow)

In the short-axis view, the gallbladder will appear spherical. The whole gallbladder should be demonstrated from the neck to the fundus. The normal length of gallbladder is 1.5 to 3.0 cm in neonates and young infants, and approximately 1 cm in normal width. In older children and adolescents, the gallbladder length is 3 to 8 cm and the width is less than 3.5 cm.[1] Sometimes the gallbladder wall may falsely present a septum because the wall folds one or several times upon itself. The size of normal and pathological gallbladder shows a great variability from a normal large to a small slender gallbladder. It depends on the fasting condition, the degree of the distention and the possible underlying disease. Similarly, the wall thickness is variable and depends on the same conditions. Evaluation from the short-axis view is the gold standard to measure the wall thickness of gallbladder and at its most narrow point is the best reliable place to measure the anterior wall. The normal wall of gallbladder is thin and hyperechoic with mild posterior enhancement. The upper limit of wall thickness is 3 mm in the fasting state.[2] The neck of the gallbladder joins the cystic duct and locates near the hilar region of the liver. Generally there is no acoustic shadowing posterior to the gallbladder.

The cystic duct is a folded tubular structure, and it joins the common hepatic duct to create the common bile duct. It lies posterior to the common bile duct in 95 percent and anterior to the common bile duct in 5 percent of individuals.[3] The cystic duct in children is not routinely seen unless it is dilated.[4] It is usually seen only the distal part of the duct near its insertion into the common bile duct.

The CBD is easily identified through its association with the portal vein. In the long axis view of the gallbladder, adjust the probe from the neck of the gallbladder to the porta hepatis and the portal vein will appear as a hypoechoic with echogenic walls. The CBD presents just anterior to the portal vein and three echogenic lines will be seen (Fig. 3). The first line closest to the probe will be the anterior wall of the common bile duct. The second line is the shared wall of the CBD and portal vein. Finally, the third line is the posterior wall of the portal vein. The differentiation between the CBD and portal vein can be easily done by color Doppler technique if there is confusion to distinguish. The portal vein will demonstrate flow and the CBD does not. The diameter of the common duct should be measured on the sagittal scan to confirm the presence or absence of ductal dilatation. Measurement of the caliper of CBD is usually done between the interior margin of the anterior and the posterior wall. The distal portion of the common duct is typically larger than the proximal portion.[4] It is very difficult to follow the CBD once it passes posterior to the second portion of the duodenum.

3. How dilated is dilated?

Because ultrasonography is easy to perform and does not expose the patient to radiation or contrast agents, it is being used more often in children to diagnose disorders of the biliary tract and gallbladder.[5-7] Measurement of the extrahepatic bile duct (CBD) is usually taken at the level where paralleled with the portal vein. The upper limit of normal for the CBD of infants and children has been estimated in several studies. Hernanz-Schulman et al[1] reported an upper limit of 1.2mm in infants <3 months old, less than 1.6 mm in infancy and less than 3mm in childhood. Carroll et al[8] stated that a normal common bile duct should not exceed 1mm in infants <3 months old. E. Fitzpatrick et al[9] stated that bile duct dilatation <3mm (non-fasting ultrasound) with neonatal cholestasis is unlikely to be of significance whereas >4mm is likely to be associated with choledochal malformation or need for intervention. Siegel[10] stated that the sonographic findings of a visible intrahepatic biliary duct and/or CBD diameter wider than 2mm in infancy, greater than 4 mm in childhood, and greater than 7 mm after adolescence were abnormal. However, the differentiation between choledochal malformation and variation within the normal limit is still difficult.[11, 12]

We had evaluated sonographically 162 children who met the Siegel's criteria for biliary tract dilatation. In our 18 years study, all cases of intrahepatic biliary tree dilatation and those with both intra- and extrahepatic duct dilatations were anomalous. However, in cases of extrahepatic biliary tract dilatation, 73% of patients with extrahepatic biliary dilatation had biliary anomalies. Thirty one children who had no clinical symptoms /signs as well as normal laboratory data during the follow-up period were thought to be normal variants. The mean diameters of them were 4.4 ± 1.2 mm.[13]

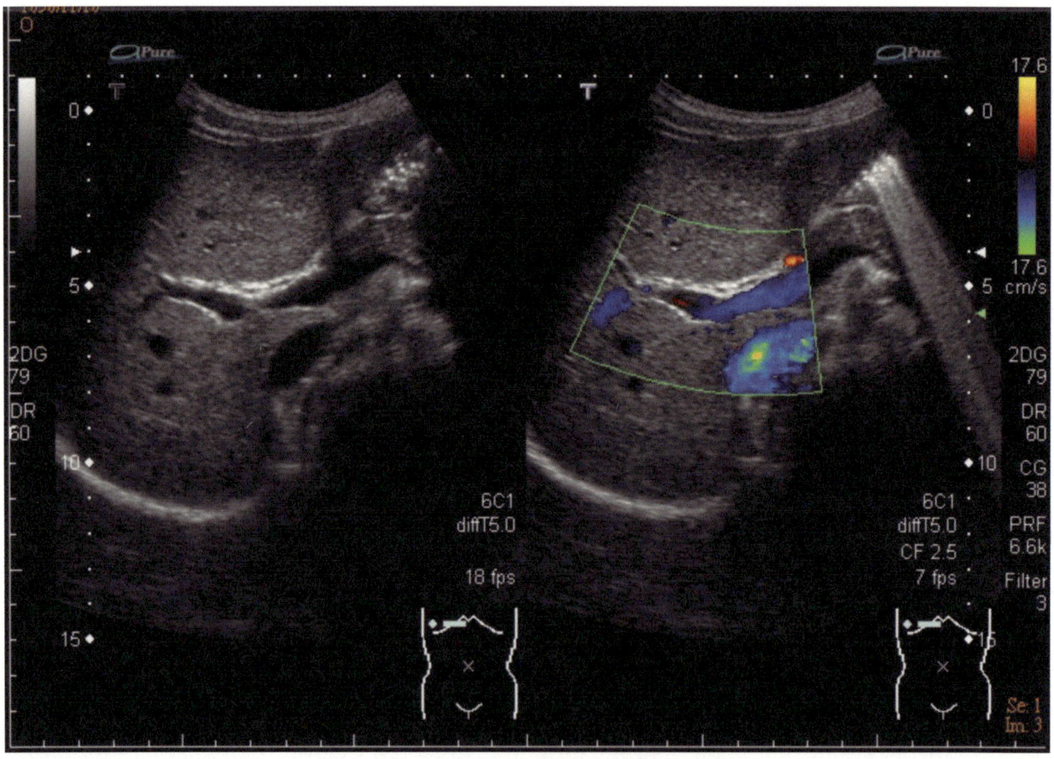

Fig. 3. Normal presentation of CBD Left: The CBD lies just anterior to the portal vein in porta hepatis and three echogenic lines will be seen. The first line closest to the probe will be the anterior wall of the CBD. The second line is the shared wall of the CBD and portal vein. And the third line is the posterior wall of the portal vein. Measurement of the caliper of CBD is usually done between the interior margin of the anterior and the posterior wall. Right: The CBD and portal vein can be easily differentiated by color Doppler. The portal vein will demonstrate flow and the CBD will not. (CBD: common bile duct)

4. Differential diagnosis of biliary dilatation in children

Anomalous biliary tract dilatation, also namely biliary cysts, may be congenital or acquired. Most congenital lesions are found in the common bile duct, thus referred as choledochal cyst (CC). The anatomic classification of CC most commonly used was defined by Todani who divided CC into 5 types.[14-,16] The most common type (Type I) is a congenital cystic dilatation of the common bile duct without associated intrahepatic ductal dilatation (Fig. 4 & 5). Type II is a diverticular malformation of the common bile duct, and Type III is a choledochocele associated with an ampullary obstruction. The Type IV malformation has multiple cysts of the intrahepatic or extrahepatic ducts, or both (Fig. 6). Type V has single or multiple intrahepatic cysts (Fig. 7).

In our study,[13] excluding cases associated with biliary atresia, the accuracy of diagnosing choledochal cysts in extrahepatic biliary tract dilatation was 71% and 97% using cutoffs of 7 mm and 10 mm as the minimum diameter respectively.

We also reported 158 pediatric patients with biliary cysts seen between June 1981 and July 2004.[17] Patients were divided into three groups: biliary atresia-associated biliary cyst (BABC), non-biliary atresia-associated choledochal cyst (NBACC) in infancy, and late NBACC (> 1 year of age). The mean diameter in BABC (7.9 ± 1.5 mm) was significantly less than that in infantile NBACC (16.0 ± 3.7mm, $p < 0.001$) and late NBACC (21.5 ± 5.6 mm, $p < 0.001$). In NBACC, older age at diagnosis was associated with greater cyst diameter ($r = 0.7$, $p < 0.001$).

BABC had been reported and had names synonymously as biliary duct dilatation with biliary atresia (BDBA),[13] choledochal cyst associated with extrahepatic biliary atresia (CCBA),[18] and type I cyst of BA.19 A survey by the American Academy of Pediatric Surgery Section found that 13% of patients with cystic dilatation of the CBD had extrahepatic biliary atresia.[20] In our study, there was a higher incidence that BABC accounted for 36.2% of the infantile biliary cysts.[17]

The type V CC was also termed Caroli disease.[14,16] It involves dilatation of one or more segments of the intrahepatic ducts. Typically the intrahepatic ducts show marked saccular enlargement with communication between the cysts under sonography (Fig. 7). Caroli disease may be one part of ADPKD (Autosomal Dominant Polycystic Kidney Disease) or ARPKD (Autosomal Recessive Polycystic Kidney Disease) if intrahepatic dilatation located peripherally in the liver, namely type II Caroli disease.[21] It can be differentiated from autosomal dominant polycystic liver disease which showed isolated intrahepatic cysts with no tubular connections between them.[22,23]

Several reports described that anomaly of pancreatic fusion[24,25] or pancreatic heterotopias[26] might cause congenital biliary dilatation.

Acquired cases usually appear as fusiform dilatations, which can be seen in those with tumors, lithiasis, and inflammation of the biliary tract (Fig. 8). External compression due to vascular malformation of the portal vein may also cause biliary tract dilatation. Tumor of biliary tract is extremely uncommon in children. Sludge and stone may be seen in those with hemolytic disease such as congenital spherocytosis, prolonged fasting, medications and total parenteral nutrition use. Cholangitis may induce biliary dilatation (BD) and mimic choledochal cyst.[17] Other conditions have been reported to be related to BD, including

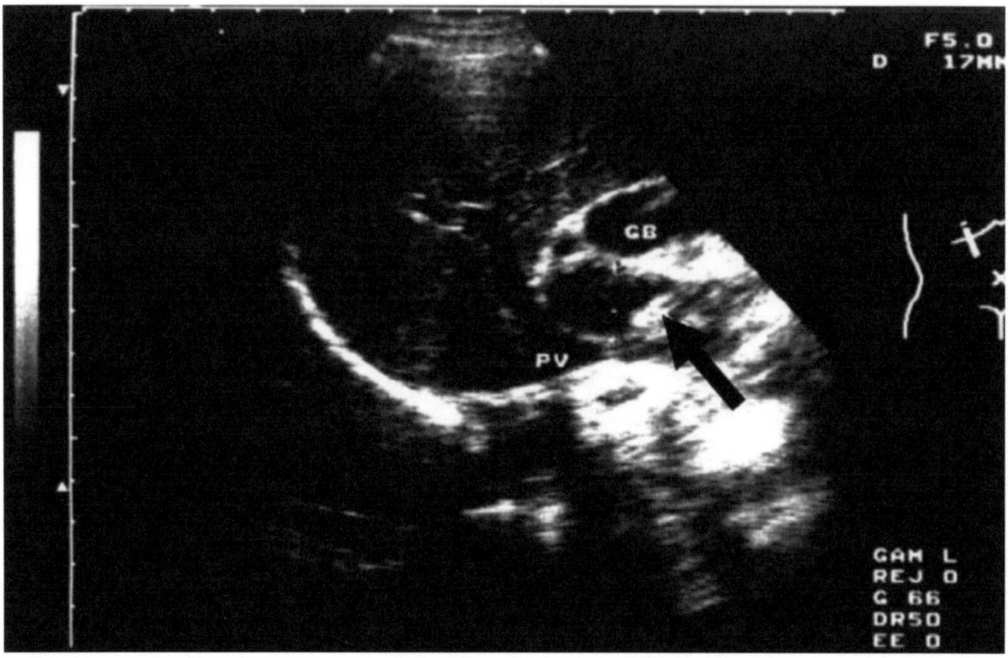

Fig. 4. Choledochal cyst Type Ia: cystic dilatation in the common bile duct with stone formation (arrow). PV = portal vein, GB = gallbladder. (From Lee HC: *J Med Ultrasound* 2007;15(3):191–196.)

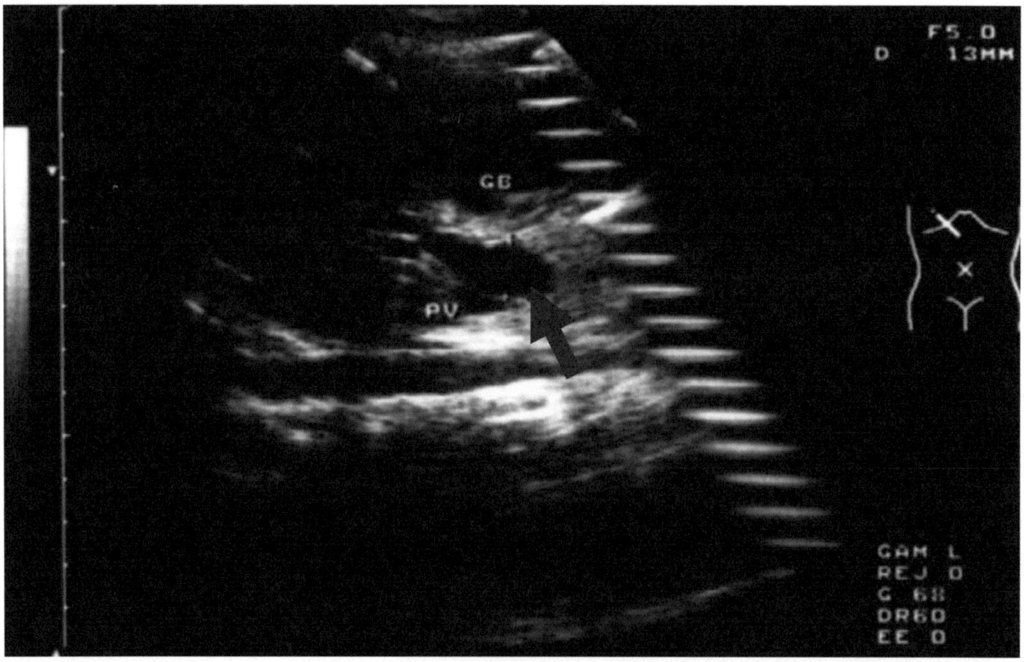

Fig. 5. Choledochal cyst Type Ic: a fusiform dilatation (arrow) in the common bile duct. PV = portal vein; GB = gallbladder. (From Lee HC: *J Med Ultrasound* 2007;15(3):191–196.)

pancreatitis, gastrointestinal graft-versus-host disease, infections other than intra-abdominal sites, neonatal sepsis.[27]

Some sonographic findings may be mistaken as biliary tract dilatation, such as an elongation or folding of gallbladder neck, a dilated main hepatic artery anterior to the main portal vein, and a marked concentric, hypoechoic thickening of the walls of the CBD. However, a dilated CBD may be mistaken as normal-sized, such as a partially obscured dilated CBD by sludge or blood clot with only the residual lumen visualized.[23] Careful and thorough examination to explore the lesions and the association with the surrounding structures should be undertaken. Looking for any special characteristic findings may help to avoid misdiagnosis.

Under sonography, a thin walled cystic or fusiform mass can be seen in the right upper quadrant of abdomen at subhepatic area or porta hepatis. The gall bladder must be visualized separately to make a diagnosis of choledochal cyst. The bile duct(s) can be seen communicating to the lesion.[28] The lesion has been described "tear drop" in shape with a sharp proximal end connected to the biliary tree. Stasis of bile may result in sludge or stone within the lesion. Septa are seldom found.

Any cystic lesions which are seen in the right upper quadrant sonographically must be differentiated. These include enteric duplication cyst, especially duodenal origin, hepatic cyst, pancreatic pseudocyst, mesenteric or omental cyst, renal cyst, and aneurysm of vessel at porta hepatis etc.

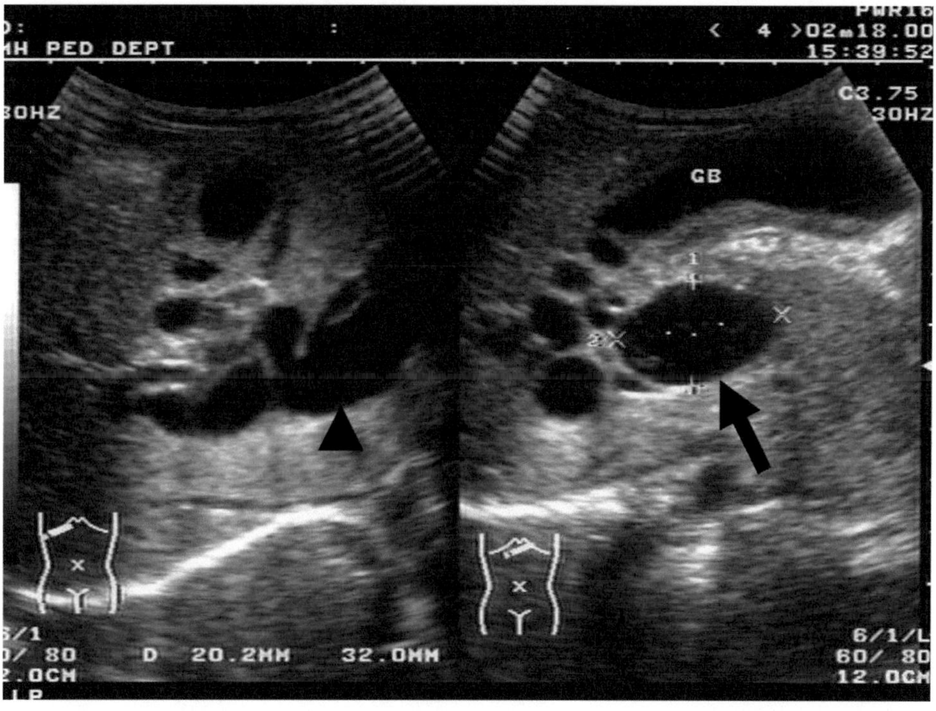

Fig. 6. Choledochal cyst Type IVa: a common bile duct cyst (arrow) with intrahepatic duct dilatation (arrowhead). GB=gallbladder. (From Lee HC: *J Med Ultrasound* 2007;15(3):191-196.)

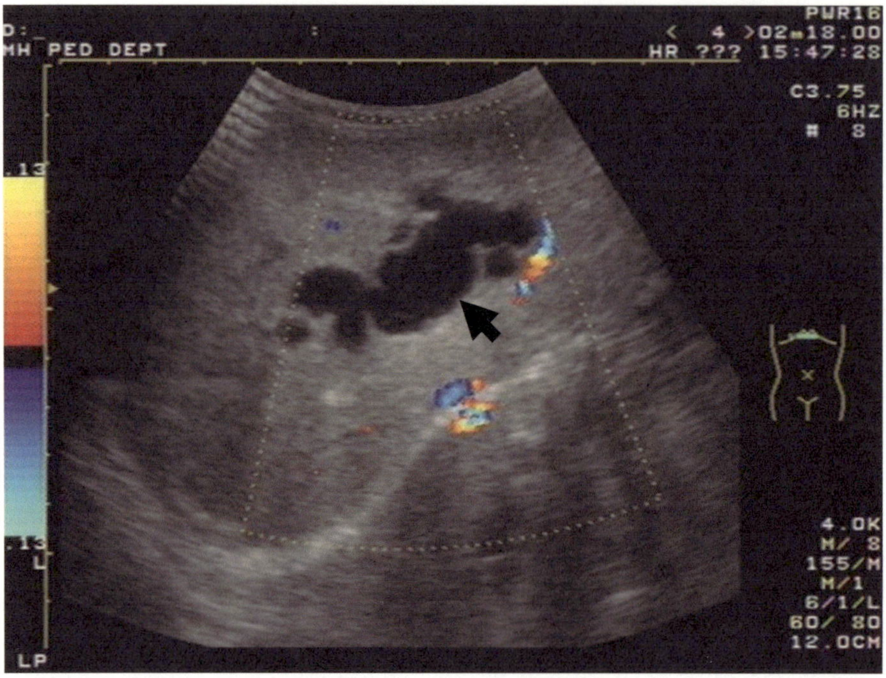

Fig. 7. Choledochal cyst Type V: saccular dilatation of the intrahepatic ducts (arrow). (From Lee HC: *J Med Ultrasound* 2007;15(3):191–196.)

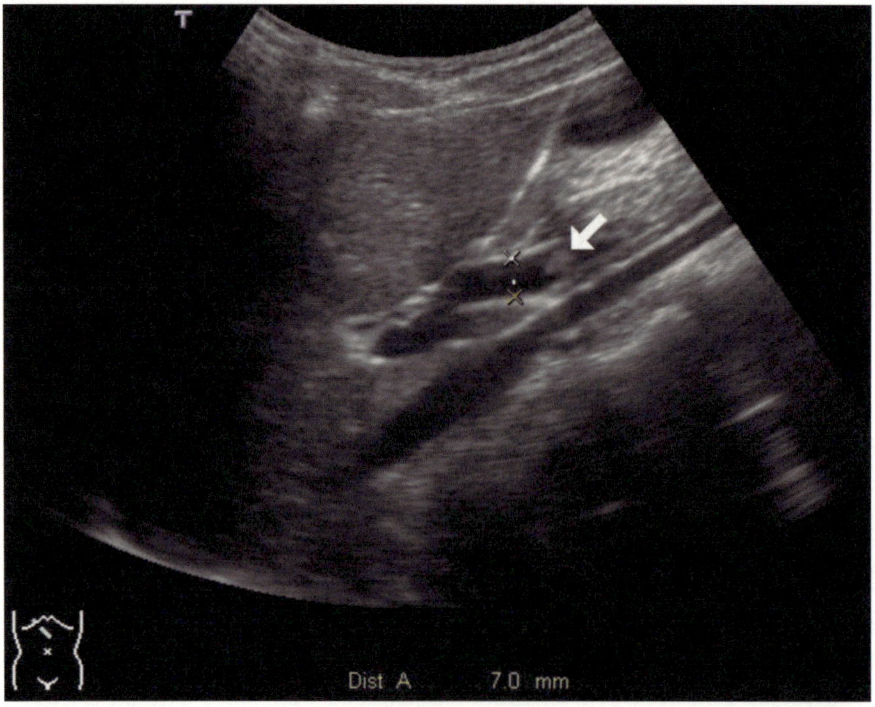

Fig. 8. Dilated common bile duct (7.0mm) with a stone (arrow) and acoustic shadow

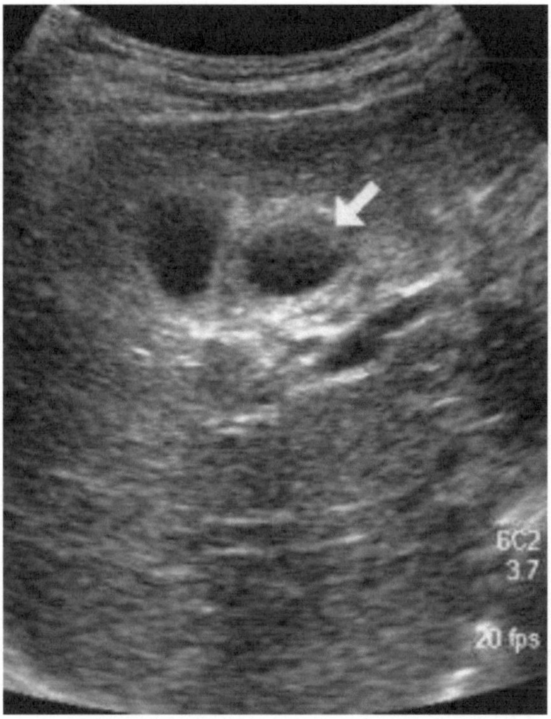

Fig. 9. A duodenal duplication cyst nearby gall bladder with the appearance of "rim sign" (arrow)

Enteric duplication cysts are mostly found in ileum and stomach.[29] Several reports described duplication cyst originated from duodenum.[30] Abdominal pain and intestinal obstruction are the most common clinical manifestations.[31,32] Duodenal duplication cysts frequently associate with pancreatitis.[30] Enteric duplication cysts consist of enteric wall in structure.[29] Mucosa and muscular layer of enteric duplication cysts give raise to an inner echogenic rim and an outer hypoechoic rim respectively when they are examined by sonography. The appearance is recognized as "rim sign" (Fig. 9) which is identified in the dependent portion of the cyst.[31]

Congenital hepatic cysts (Fig. 10) are rare and usually are found incidentally. Most hepatic cysts located under anterior surface of the liver. They are usually anechoic with acoustic enhancement noted under sonography. They may show internal echo due to hemorrhage or infection, septa etc. Viewing the lesion through various scanning windows and angles helps differentiate it from choledochal cyst.

Mesenteric or omental cyst, now known as cystic lymphatic malformations, arises from non-communicating ectopic lymphatic structures in the abdomen. On ultrasound, the lesion presents as a thin wall cyst with multiple thin septa inside.[33-35] Usually, mesenteric or omental cyst is large in size and may mimic ascites, so called "pseudo-ascites".[36] Clinically, abdominal distension with or without a palpable mass is the most frequent presentation.[36] Small cyst may occur less commonly. The content of the cyst may be anechoic, or shows internal echo from hemorrhage, debris, chylous fluid or infection.[34,35] Progressive

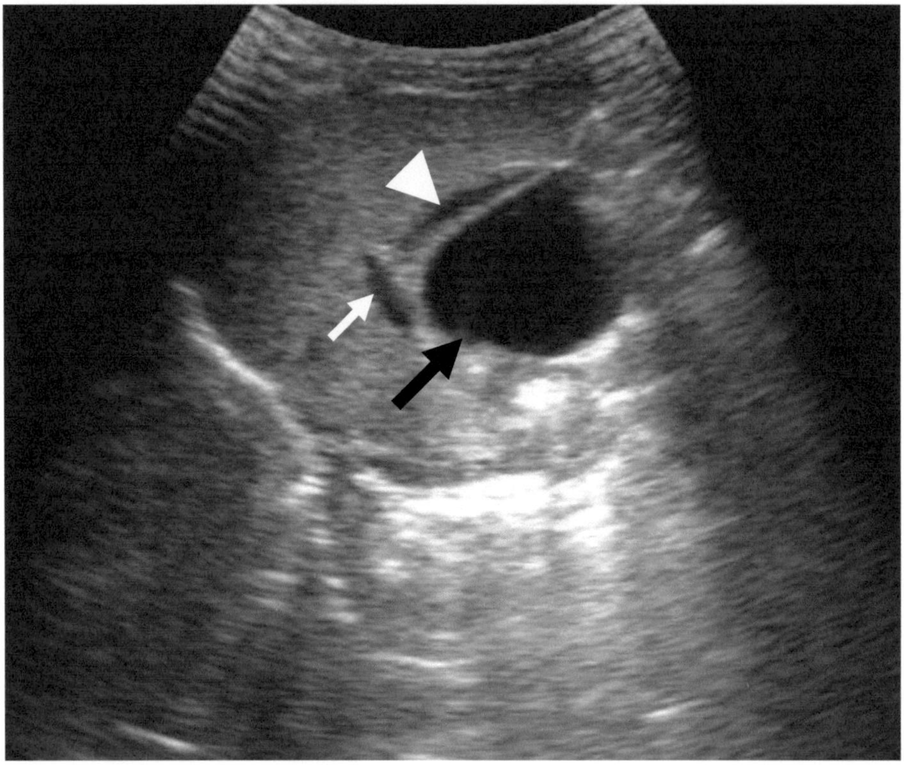

Fig. 10. A cystic mass (black arrow) at the porta hepatis compressing gall bladder (white arrow head) and portal vein (white arrow). Further study demonstrated the lesion to be a hepatic cyst

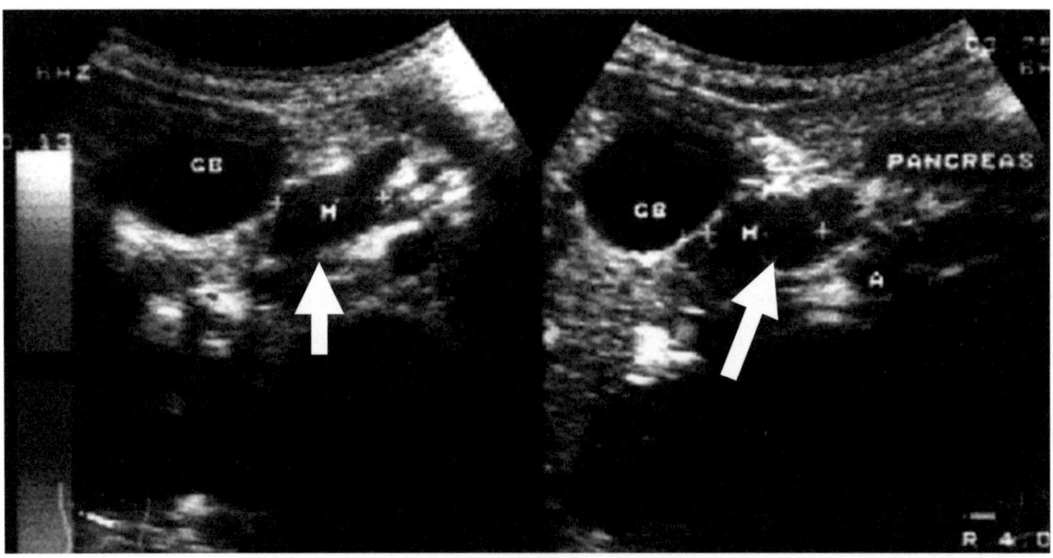

Fig. 11. A pseudocyst of pancreas (M, arrow) between the gallbladder (GB) and pancreas at the epigastrium 5 days after blunt abdominal injury. A: aorta

enlargement, increase in fluid echogenicity, thickening of wall and septa and multiplication of septa may be seen by sequential sonography.[34]

Two-thirds of childhood pancreatic pseudocysts (Fig. 11) arise from the body or tail of the pancreas, mostly unilocular.[37] Most of them are secondary to pancreatitis or blunt abdominal trauma. Pseudocyst is associated to the pancreas. The borders are usually echogenic and thicker than that of simple cyst.

Vascular malformations, though uncommon, simulate cystic lesions at the porta hepatis, may be mistaken as choledochal cyst. These include portal vein aneurysm (Fig. 12) and hepatic artery aneurysm. Most of the lesions are found incidentally when having a sonographic examination and appear as an anechoic fusiform or saccular structure. Sometimes these lesions may contain thrombus inside and give an echogenic image. These lesions can be distinguished readily by Doppler technique which demonstrates blood flow inside the cystic mass.[38,39]

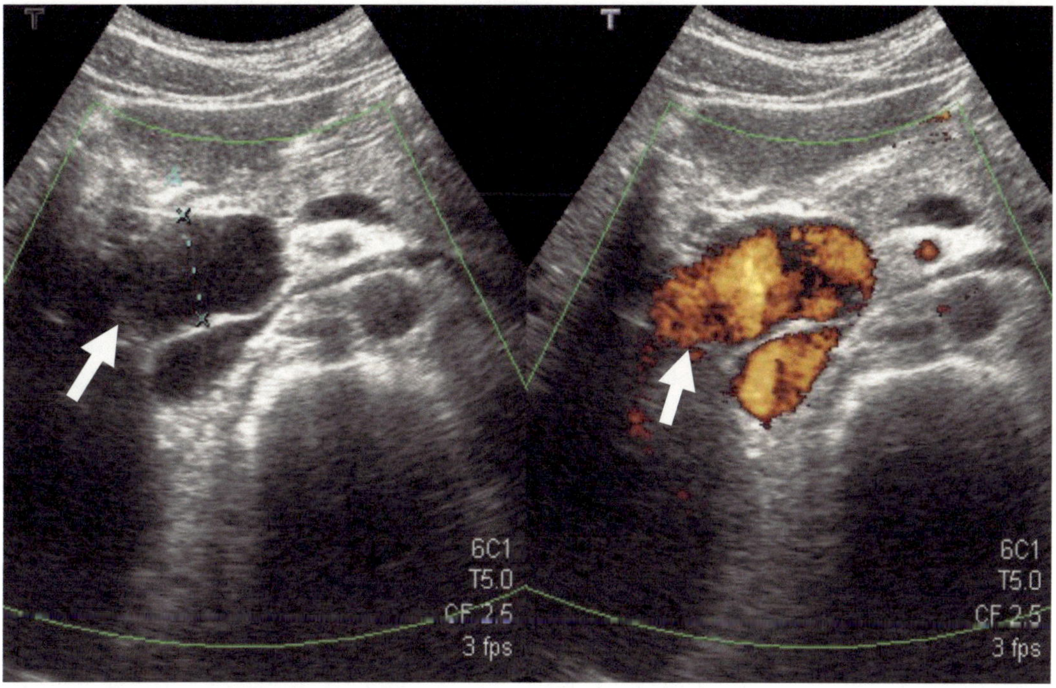

Fig. 12. A large cystic mass (arrow) at the porta hepatis with blood flow shown in the lesion (R't). Further imaging study revealed portal vein aneurysm

5. References

[1] Hernanz-Schulman M, Ambrosino MM, Freeman PC, et al: Common bile duct in children: Sonographic dimensions. *Radiology* 1995; 195:193.

[2] Wolson AH. Ultrasound measurements of the gallbladder. In: Goldberg BB, Kurtz AB, editors. *Atlas of ultrasound measurements*. Chicago: Year Book Publishers, Inc.; 1990. p.108–12.

[3] R. A. L. Bissett, A. N. Khan: *Differential Diagnosis in Abdominal Ultrasound*, 3/e; 2002

[4] Marilyn J. Siegel, Jaundice in Infants and Children. *Ultrasound Clin* 1: 2006;1:431-441.

[5] Akhan O, Demirkazik FB, Özmen MN, et al: Choledochal cysts: Ultrasonographic findings and correlation with other imaging modalities. *Abdom Imaging* 1994;19:243.

[6] Sringer MD, Dhawan A, Davenport M, et al: Choledochal cysts: Lessons from a 20 year experience. *Arch Dis Child* 1995;73:528.

[7] Young W, Blane C, White SJ, et al: Congenital biliary dilatation: A spectrum of disease detailed by ultrasound. *Br J Radiol* 1990;63:333.

[8] Carroll BA, Oppenheimer DA, Muller HH. High-frequency real-time ultrasound of the neonatal biliary system. *Radiology* 1982;145:437–40.

[9] E. Fitzpatrick, R. Jardine, P. Farrant, et al. Predictive value of bile duct dimensions measured by ultrasound in neonates presenting with cholestasis, *J Pediatr Gastroenterol Nutr* 2010;51:55–60.

[10] Siegel MJ. Liver and biliary tract. In: Siegel MJ, ed. *Pediatric Sonography*. New York: Raven Press, 1995:171.

[11] Grosfeld JL, Rescorla FJ, Skinner MA, et al. The spectrum of biliary tract disorders in infants and children. Experience with 300 cases. *Arch Surg* 1994;129:513–8.

[12] Lee SS, Min PC, Kim GS, et al. Choledochal cyst. A report of nine cases and review of the literature. *Arch Surg* 1969;99:19–28.

[13] Lee HC, Yeung CY, Chang PY, et al. Dilatation of the biliary tree in children: sonographic diagnosis and its clinical significance. *Journal of Ultrasound in Medicine.* 2000;19:177-182.

[14] Todani T, Watanabe Y, Narusue M, Tabuchi K, Okajima K. Congenital bile duct cysts: Classification, operative procedures, and review of thirty-seven cases including cancer arising from choledochal cyst. *American Journal of Surgery.* 1977;134(2):263-269.

[15] Todani T, Narusue M, Watanabe Y, Tabuchi K, Okajima K. Management of congenital choledochal cyst with intrahepatic involvement. *Ann Surg.* 1978;187(3):272-280.

[16] Crittenden SL, McKinley MJ. Choledochal cyst--clinical features and classification. *American Journal of Gastroenterology.* Aug 1985;80(8):643-647.

[17] Lee HC, Yeung CY, Fang SB, Jiang CB, Sheu JC, Wang NL. Biliary Cysts in Children - Long-term Follow-up in Taiwan. *Journal of the Formosan Medical Association.* 2006;105(2):118-124.

[18] Kim WS, Kim IO, Yeon KM, Park KW, Seo JK, Kim CJ. Choledochal cyst with or without biliary atresia in neonates and young infants: US differentiation. *Radiology.* 1998;209(2):465-469.

[19] Tsuchida Y, Kawarasaki H, Iwanaka T, Uchida H, Nakanishi H, Uno K. Antenatal diagnosis of biliary atresia (type I cyst) at 19 weeks' gestation: differential diagnosis and etiologic implications. *Journal of Pediatric Surgery.* May 1995;30(5):697-699.

[20] Bancroft JD, Bucuvalas JC, Ryckman FC, Dudgeon DL, Saunders RC, Schwarz KB. Antenatal diagnosis of choledochal cyst. *Journal of Pediatric Gastroenterology & Nutrition.* Feb 1994;18(2):142-145.

[21] Nakanuma Y, Terada T, Ohta G, Kurachi M, Matsubara F. Caroli's disease in congenital hepatic fibrosis and infantile polycystic disease. *Liver.* Dec 1982;2(4):346-354.

[22] Rosenthal SJ, Cox GG, Wetzel LH, Batnitzky S. Pitfalls and differential diagnosis in biliary sonography. *RadioGraphics.* 1990;10:285-311.

[23] Parulekar SG. Transabdominal Sonography of Bile Ducts. *Ultrasound Quarterly.* 2002;18(3):187-202.

[24] Tadokoro H, Suyama M, Kubokawa Y, Sai JK. Persistence of the Left Part of the Ventral Pancreas May Cause Congenital Biliary Dilatation. *Pancreas.* 2003;27(1):47-51.

[25] Nomura T, Shirai Y, Wakai T, Yokoyama N, Sakata J, Hatakeyama K. Narrow portion of the terminal choledochus is a cause of upstream biliary dilatation in patients with anomalous union of the pancreatic and biliary ducts. *World Journal of Gastroenterology.* 2005;11(41):6503-6507.

[26] Kattepura S, Nanjegowda NB, Babu MK, Das K. Macroscopic pancreatic heterotopia on a congenital biliary dilatation. *Pediatric Surgery International.* 2010;26:847-849.

[27] Shaoul R, Sukhotnik I, Toubi A. Neonatal sepsis presenting as a choledochal cyst. *Acta Paediatrica.* 2008;97:246-249.

[28] Kim OH, Chung HJ, Choi BG. Imaging of the choledochal cyst. *RadioGraphics.* 1995;15:69-88.

[29] Swischuk L. Alimentary tract. In: Swischuk L, ed. *Imaging of the Newborn, Infant and Young Child.* 4 ed. Baltimore: William and Wilkins; 1997:426.

[30] Chen JJ, Lee HC, Yeung CY, Chan WT, Jiang CB, Sheu JC. Meta-analysis: the clinical features of the duodenal duplication cyst. *Journal of Pediatric Surgery.* 2010;45(8):1598-1606.

[31] Pinter AB, Schubert W, Szemledy F, Gobel P, Schafer J, Kustos G. Alimentary tract duplications in infants and children. *European Journal of Pediatric Surgery.* Feb 1992;2(1):8-12.

[32] Segal SR, Sherman NH, Rosenberg HK, et al. Ultrasonographic features of gastrointestinal duplications. *Journal of Ultrasound in Medicine.* Nov 1994;13(11):863-870.

[33] Chateil JF, Brun M, Vergnes P, Andrieu de Lewis P, Perel Y, Diard F. Abdominal cystic lymphangiomas in children: presurgical evaluation with imaging. *European Journal of Pediatric Surgery.* Feb 2002;12(1):13-18.

[34] Konen O, Rathaus V, Dlugy E, et al. Childhood abdominal cystic lymphangioma. *Pediatric Radiology.* Feb 2002;32(2):88-94.

[35] Ros PR, Olmsted WW, Moser RP, Jr., Dachman AH, Hjermstad BH, Sobin LH. Mesenteric and omental cysts: histologic classification with imaging correlation. *Radiology.* Aug 1987;164(2):327-332.

[36] Lin J, Fisher J, Caty M. Newborn intraabdominal cystic lymphatic malformations. *Seminars in Pediatric Surgery.* 2000;9:141-145.

[37] Wootton-Gorges SL, Thomas KB, Harned RK, Wu SR, Stein-Wexler R, D. Strain J. Giant cystic abdominal masses in children. *Pediatric Radiology.* 2005;35:1277-1288.

[38] Lee HC, Yang YC, Shih SL, Chiang HJ. Aneurysmal dilatation of the portal vein. *Journal of Pediatric Gastroenterology & Nutrition.* Apr 1989;8(3):387-389.

[39] Athey PA, Sax SL, Lamki N, Cadavid G. Sonography in the diagnosis of hepatic artery aneurysms. *American Journal of Roentgenology.* 1986;147:725-727.

Part 2

New and Advanced Applications in Sonography

12

Application of Orbital Sonography in Neurology

Michael Ertl[1], Maria-Andreea Gamulescu[2] and Felix Schlachetzki[1]
[1]*Department of Neurology, University of Regensburg, Bezirksklinikum Regensburg*
[2]*Department of Ophthalmology, Regensburg University Medical Center*
Germany

1. Introduction

Color-coded duplex sonography is a well established non-invasive method for vascular and parenchymal examination in a wide range of neurological disorders including stroke, cerebral venous thrombosis and degenerative diseases, amongst others. Considering development, cell types and vascular structures as well as pathology and pathophysiology, high similarities and interactions exist between the central nervous system (CNS) and the eye.

When applied to the eye and the orbit, high-resolution color-coded duplex sonography (OCCS) may depict a variety of pathologic alterations such as papilledema or central retinal artery occlusion, that represent manifestation of CNS disorders (i.e. raised intracranial pressure) or systemic diseases (i.e. atherothrombotic/ thrombembolic occlusions), respectively. Although easily accessible, OCCS has not yet gained widespread use in daily neurological practice despite the fact that most modern ultrasound systems are capable of performing such an endeavor. However, this technique may be a very helpful, fast and powerful diagnostic procedure in addition to the diagnostic battery needed for unraveling specific CNS or systemic diseases.

In this book chapter article we highlight different aspects of OCCS and concentrate on methods and diseases relevant for neurologists. The differential diagnosis of orbital tumors (e.g. lymphoma, optic sheath meningeoma, pseudotumor orbitae, myositis, and others) or vascular abnormalities (e.g. varicosis, superior orbital venous dilatation in arterio-venous-fistula) will not be discussed. The first part introduces the reader to the technical requirements, restraints and safety for performing sonography of the eye. Normal relevant anatomy as well as normal values will be given. The second part focuses on common vascular pathologies such as central retinal artery occlusion in the context of suspected giant cell arteritis as well as swelling of the optic nerve and papilledema linked to raised intracranial pressure. Being a fairly young technique, few studies employing OCCS exist, yet a large variety of interesting pathology and variations may be found as exemplified in the third and final part of the chapter.

Ocular color-coded duplex sonography is a fascinating technique with high potential for neurologists in differential diagnosis and therapy of an expanding variety of acute and chronic CNS disease.

2. Technique and safety considerations

Orbital sonography can be easily performed using most color duplex ultrasound systems equipped with high frequency linear array transducers. Since the optic lens as well as the vitreous do not absorb significant ultrasound energy and make near field artifacts virtually impossible, commonly used transmit frequencies in neurology from 7 to 15 MHz may be used. According to the physics of wave propagation in tissue and the resulting axial and lateral resolutions, the general aim is to apply high frequencies up to 14 MHz or more. The acoustic output of the ultrasound systems needs to be adjusted to the requirements of orbital sonography according to the ALARA principle (‚as low as reasonable achievable') in order to avoid damage to the lens and retina (Toms 2006). The main biological effects would be cavitation and temperature increase, the latter being dependent from the insonation time. In animal experiments harmful effects of ultrasound acoustic power to ocular structures (esp. lens and choroid) could be demonstrated (Lizzi et al. 1978). Therefore, current guidelines released by the FDA limit the acoustic output to temporal average intensities of up to 50mW/cm^2 and a mechanical index (MI) of up to 0.23 (Food and Drug Administration 2008). An on-screen indicator of ultrasonic output, the MI is a measure of the likelihood that a clinically important non-thermal biological effect may occur during a diagnostic examination (American Institute of Ultrasound in Medicine 2000). However, most examinations last less than 5 minutes for each eye, hereby limiting the possibility of thermal damage. In order to prevent cavitation effects, the settings for orbital sonography may be as follows:

- B-mode – transmit frequency 14 MHz, mechanical index (MI) = 0.23, single focal zone at 2.5 cm, bandwidth 74 dB;
- C-mode – transmit frequency 10 MHz, MI = 0.23, color scale optimized for low velocities, no wall filter;
- pw-Mode – transmit frequency 2 MHz, MI = <0.23 (<0.44*) (Tab. 1).

	B-mode	C-mode	pw-mode
transmit frequency	14MHz	10MHz	2MHz
mechanical index (MI)	<0.23	<0.23	0.23 (<0.44*)
single focal zone	2.5cm		
bandwidth	74dB		
Special recommendations		color scale optimized for low velocities no wall filter	

Table 1. Machine parameters in B-mode, C-mode and pw-mode, *often the lowest output value

It needs to be kept in mind that most color-duplex machines require reduction of the acoustic output in each mode, that is the B-mode, color-mode and spectral Doppler-mode (the latter might not display values below 0.44).

During the examination the patient lies in supine position with the eyes closed (Fig. 1a). A layer of acoustic gel is applied to the closed lids, the transducer is placed on the upper and slightly lateral eye-lids with the examiner's hand resting on the orbital margin to minimize pressure on the globe (Fig. 1b/c). To optimize the display of anatomical stuctures, esp. the optic nerve, the transducer is positioned a little on the temporal side and the patient is asked to try to look straight even with the eyes closed. Pressure on the globe should be as low as possible as this might result in a decrease in blood flow velocity of retro-orbital vessels (Tranquart et al. 2003). The optic nerve presents as a hypoechogenic structure beyond the globe in this horizontal scanning plane and the optic disc and provides an anatomical landmark for the ultrasound examination (Fig. 2).

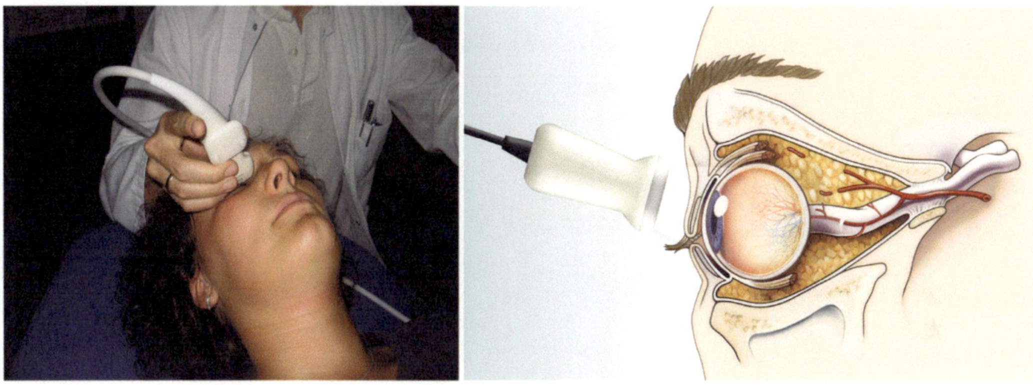

(a) (b)

Fig. 1. Standard examination parameters. (a) Patient lies in supine position with the eyes closed. (b) The transducer is placed on the upper eye-lids (slightly lateral) with the examiner's hand resting on the orbital margin. (c) Illustration of correct transducer positioning and anatomical overview. Copyright ® M.Ertl, with permission

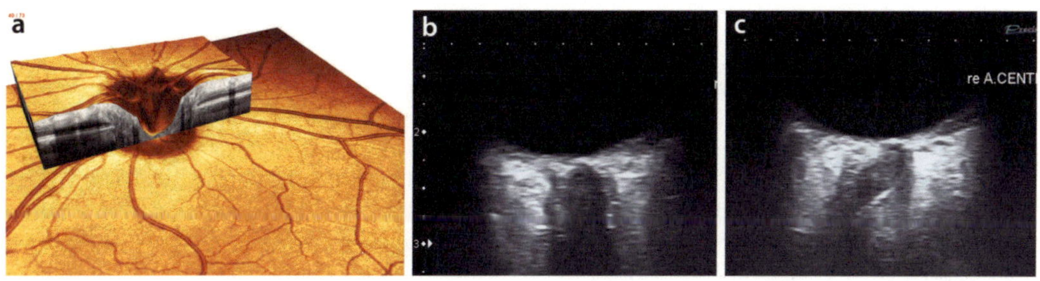

Fig. 2. Anatomical landmarks for ultrasound examination (a) Ocular coherence tomography (Spectralis ®, Heidelberg Engineering, Germany) excellently demonstrating the retinal vasculature and layers of the retina. However, inlay demonstrates limited penetration beyond the level of the retina. (b) High resolution B-mode sonography in the horizontal and lateral scanning plane presenting the optic nerve as a hypoechogenic structure beyond the retina surrounded by the hyperechoic subarachnoid space and the hypoechoic dura mater. The optic nerve provides an anatomical landmark for the ultrasound examination. For anatomical correlates see Figure 3. (c) In a strictly axial horizontal image plane, the optic nerve appears curved limiting the diagnostic accuracy of optic nerve diameter measurements

In order to enable side-to-side comparison, the left side on the monitor pictures the nasal orbit.

3. Vascular diagnostics

The central retinal artery (CRA), a distal branch of the ophthalmic artery, enters the optic nerve approximately 1-1,5 cm distal from the globe coming from the dorsolateral direction (Fig. 3). It supplies the retina and can be identified together with its parallel running central retinal vein (CRV) using the color-mode.

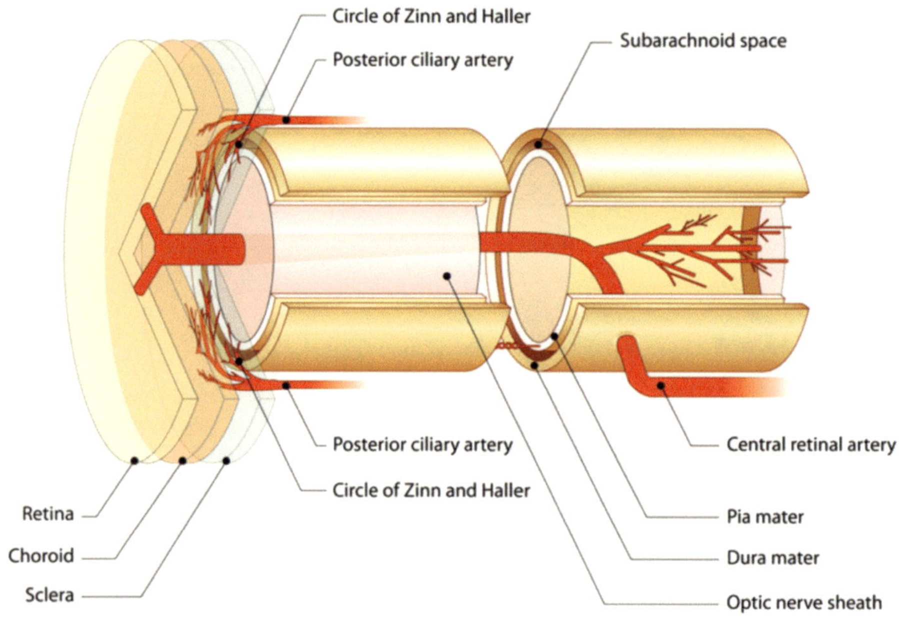

Fig. 3. Anatomy of retrobulbar structures: vascular supply of the retina and the optic nerve and sorrounding structures. Copyright ® M.Ertl, with permission

Normal values were first established by Lieb et al. 1991 and are summarized in Table 2 (Lieb et al. 1991). For best visualization, the probe should be positioned as described above with a good view of the optic nerve in the axial plane. The focus zone should be set in at the level of the optic disc. In color-mode the pulse-repetition-frequency should be adjusted to register low-flow signals of the central retinal artery and the central retinal vein. Color gain has to be adapted according to the flow velocities as well as to reduce background noise and color signals generated by minimal eye movements (movement artifacts) (Fig. 4).

Orbital vessel	Mean ± SD Blood Flow, cm/s (Range)
Central retinal artery	10.3 ± 2.1 (6.4-17.2)
Central retinal vein	2.9 ± 0.73 (1.9-5.4)
Ophthalmic artery	31.4 ± 4.2 (23.5-39.8)
Posterior ciliary artery	12.4 ± 4.8 (1.4-22.7)

Table 2. Maximum systolic blood flow velocities in orbital vessels

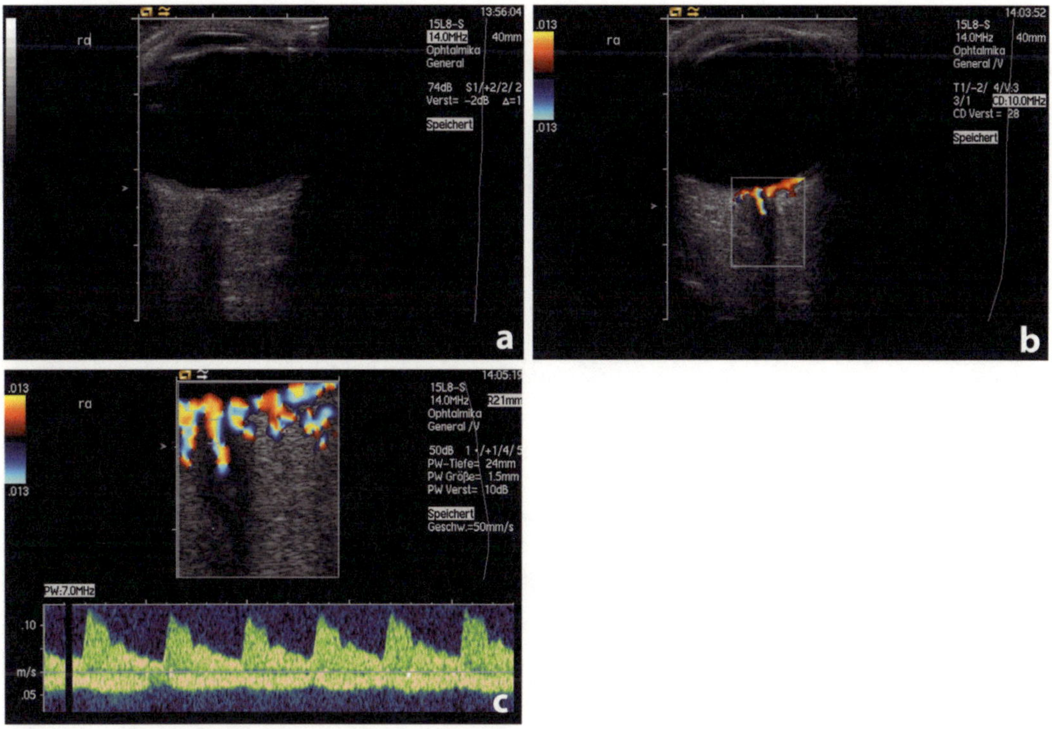

Fig. 4. Normal retrobulbar findings using high-resolution ultrasound in B-mode, Color-mode and spectral Doppler: B-mode: (a) The optic nerve presents as a hypoechogenic structure beyond the retina and the optic disc (b) Color-coded Duplex mode: central retinal artery (CRA) accompanying the optic nerve; section of retinal vessels from the posterior ciliary artery and the Circle of Zinn and Haller (c) Spectral-Doppler with Duplex-mode: normal spectrum of the CRA with peak-systolic velocity of 10.3 ± 2.1 cm/s and the underlying central retinal vein with peak-systolic velocity of 2.9 ± 0.73 cm/s (see also Table 2)

Alterations of flow in the CRA can occur in a variety of circumstances causing decreased visual acuity. In elderly patients this is mainly due to hypoperfusion or occlusion of the CRA caused by thrombo-embolic events (Brown and Magargal 1982; Gold 1977) or as CRA involvement in temporal arteritis (TA) (McFadzean 1998). In case of a central retinal artery occlusion (CRAO) a hyperechoic structure might be depicted in the optic nerve head, representing a fresh cholesterol embolus (Pfaffenbach and Hollenhorst 1972), which was termed "spot sign" by Schlachetzki and colleagues (Schlachetzki et al. 2010) (Fig. 5a). This finding is accompanied by absent flow in the CRA, whereas flow in the CRV is still detectable (Fig. 5b). The incidence of this phenomenon was first investigated by Foroozan et al. (Foroozan et al. 2002). In their retrospective study a "spot sign" occurred in 31% of cases of sudden ocular blindness. However, in an ongoing prospective study we found an incidence of up to 90% in patients with CRAO (Ertl et al., submitted).

In patients with TA, either reduced (Fig. 6a) or absent flow in CRA (Fig. 6c) was evident. The diagnosis of TA can by firmly supported by hypoechoic vasculitic vessel wall changes in the temporal arteries (so called "halo"-sign) (Arida et al. 2010), but the negative predictive

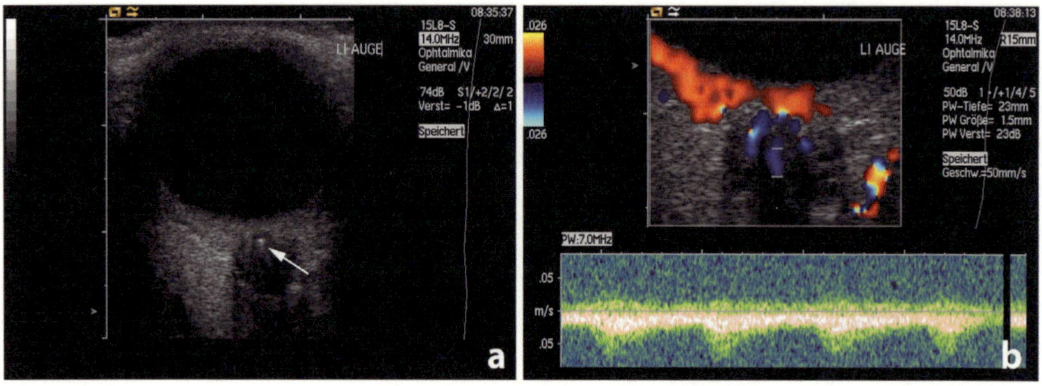

Fig. 5. Ultrasound findings in a patient with embolic central retinal artery occlusion. (a) B-mode: Hyperechogenic „spot sign“ in the optic nerve head (arrow), representing an embolus in the distal CRA. (b) Color-Duplex- and spectral Doppler-mode: absent flow in the CRA with persistant perfusion of the central retinal vein

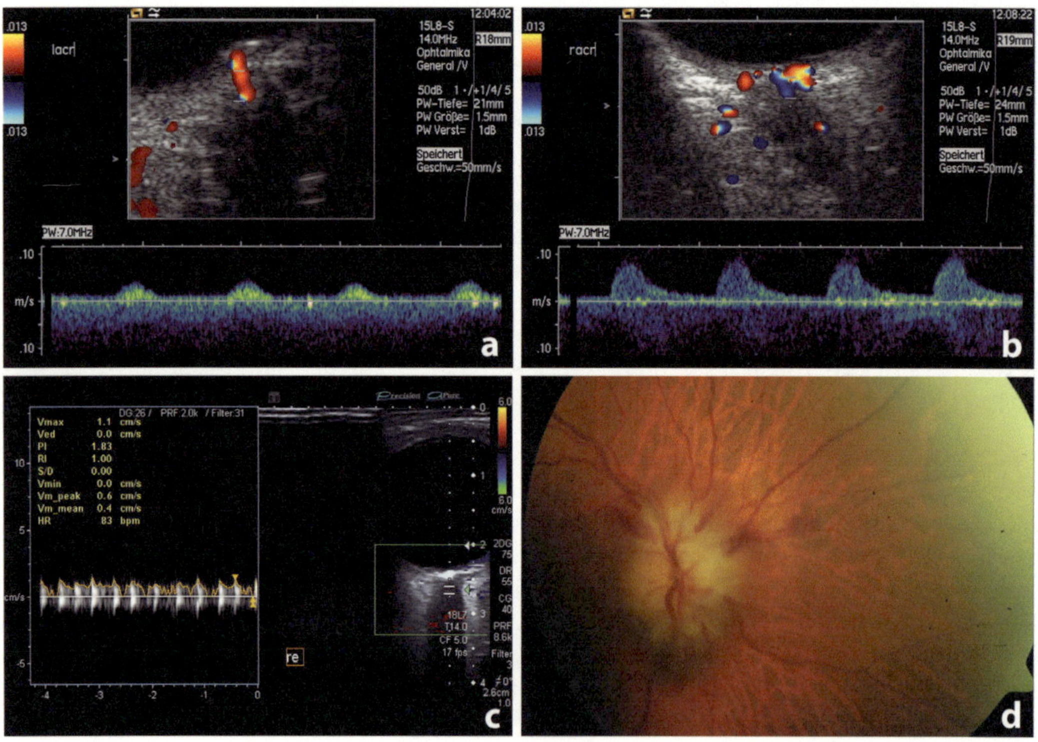

Fig. 6. Ultrasound and funduscopic findings in patients with central retinal artery occlusion due to temporal arteritis. (a) Patient 1: Color-Duplex- and spectral Doppler-mode: Pseudovenous flow in the affected CRA. (b) Patient 1: Color-Duplex- and spectral Doppler-mode: normal flow in the unaffected contralateral CRA. (c) Patient 2: Color-Duplex- and spectral Doppler-mode: zero-flow in the affected CRA. (d) Patient 2: fundoscopy: blurred rim of optic disc, optic disc edema and hyperemia, small splinter hemorrhage

value is only 68% and thus far not sufficient to rule out that disease. In patients with sudden retinal blindness and borderline symptoms for TA (only 2-3 positive ACR-criteria), a visible "spot sign" could be very helpful to rule out vasculitis, as could be demonstrated in the above-mentioned prospective study (Ertl et al., submitted).

Quick and sound differentiation of both etiologies is important for the initiation of specific treatments: thrombo-embolic occlusions need to be treated with platelet-inhibitors and high doses of cholesterol-lowering drugs, among control of additional cerebrovascular risk factors, whereas TA requires a sufficient and long-lasting steroid therapy to prevent secondary blindness of the unaffected eye.

Absent or reduced flow in the central retinal artery should lead to detailed workup looking for sources of cardiac emboli (ECG, cardiac echo, long term ECG, holter monitoring) and artherosclerosis (IMT using carotid ultrasound, presence of hemodynamically relevant carotid stenoses, etc.). Muller et al. found that in the majority of patients with ocular syndromes and ICA-stenosis greater than 50% (according to the NASCET-classification (Arning et al. 2010)), the ICA-stenosis was located on the ipsilateral side (Muller et al. 1993). Reversely, other studies could show a significant flow reduction in the ophthalmic artery and the central retinal artery in patients with ICA-stenosis of 70% or more (NASCET-classification) (Paivansalo et al. 1999). Consequently peak systolic velocity in the CRA and the posterior ciliary artery improved after carotid endarterectomy (Mawn et al. 1997).

A major advantage of OCCS is the visualization of structures lying behind the retina. Indirect fundoscopy and photodocumentation, common tools for ophthalmic investigations, are excellent methods to display pathologies up to the level of the retina or the choroid. Unfortunately, these techniques lack sensitivity or depth penetration beyond the choroid, and thus cannot elicitate the underlying cause of CRAO. Conventional A- and B-mode ultrasound systems for visualization of the globe and orbit used in opthmalmology have transmit frequencies between 10 to 20MHz. The last mentioned very high frequency has difficulties to penetrate beyond the choroid, and often these equipment lack Doppler or color-coded Doppler capabilities.

4. Assessment of intracranial pressure

Elevation of intracranial pressure (ICP) is a common phenomenon caused by a variety of neurological disorders as brain tumors, intracranial bleedings, or head trauma. Elevated ICP can be associated with life threatening conditions, e. g. brainstem herniation. Therefore these critically ill patients need to be monitored regularly to an extend of several times a day. Neuroimaging techniques as computed tomography (CT) and magnet resonance imaging (MRI) can help to assess raised ICP but have their diagnostic limitations as well (Hiler et al. 2006; Winkler et al. 2002) and require a potentially harmful patient transport. The gold standard for ICP measurement remain to be invasive intracranial devices: in addition to the need for neurosurgical operation and contraindications (e.g. thrombocytopenia) these methods are associated with certain complications as hemmorhage, infections and shunt malfunction (Brain Trauma Foundation 2000).

OCCS might be an interesting bedside alternative for follow-up examination of these critically ill patients. Several studies investigated the utility of measurements of the optic nerve sheath diameter (ONSD) as an indicator for ICP measurement and management (Antonelli et al. 2009; Galetta et al. 1989; Hansen and Helmke 1997). The optic nerve as part of the central nervous system (CNS) is surrounded by cerebrospinal fluid (CSF), and thus communicates with the inner and outer subarachnoid space. Therefore, elevation of ICP can be assessed by measuring the ONSD, but also the intraocular prominence of the papilla.

The transducer is positioned as described in the technical segment, the beam is focused on the area behind the papilla and the optic nerve should be depicted in the axial plane. The optic nerve sheath is demonstrated as a thin bilateral hyperechogenic line surrounding the hypoechogenic optic nerve (Fig. 7). Due to trabecular structures in this compartment the optic nerve sheat (ONS) reflects a high fraction of ultrasonic energy, while the optic nerve runs in line with the ultrasound beam without reflection. The ONSD is measured 3 mm behind the optic disc by measuring the distance between the hyperechogenic borders of the ONS (Fig. 7). Most authors suggest normal values < 5,0 mm for patients > 1 year (Ballantyne et al. 2002; Blaivas et al. 2003; Girisgin et al. 2007; Helmke and Hansen 1996; Newman et al. 2002; Tayal et al. 2007; Tsung et al. 2005). A reliable cut-off value to predict an ICP > 20cmH_2O seems to be 5,7-6,0 mm with a sensitivity of 87-95% and a specificity of 79-100% (Geeraerts et al. 2007; Geeraerts et al. 2008; Soldatos et al. 2008; Watanabe et al. 2008). A meta-analysis of six studies having compared the reliability ONSD-measurements with classical invasive ICP monitoring in patients with intracranial hemorrhage and traumatic

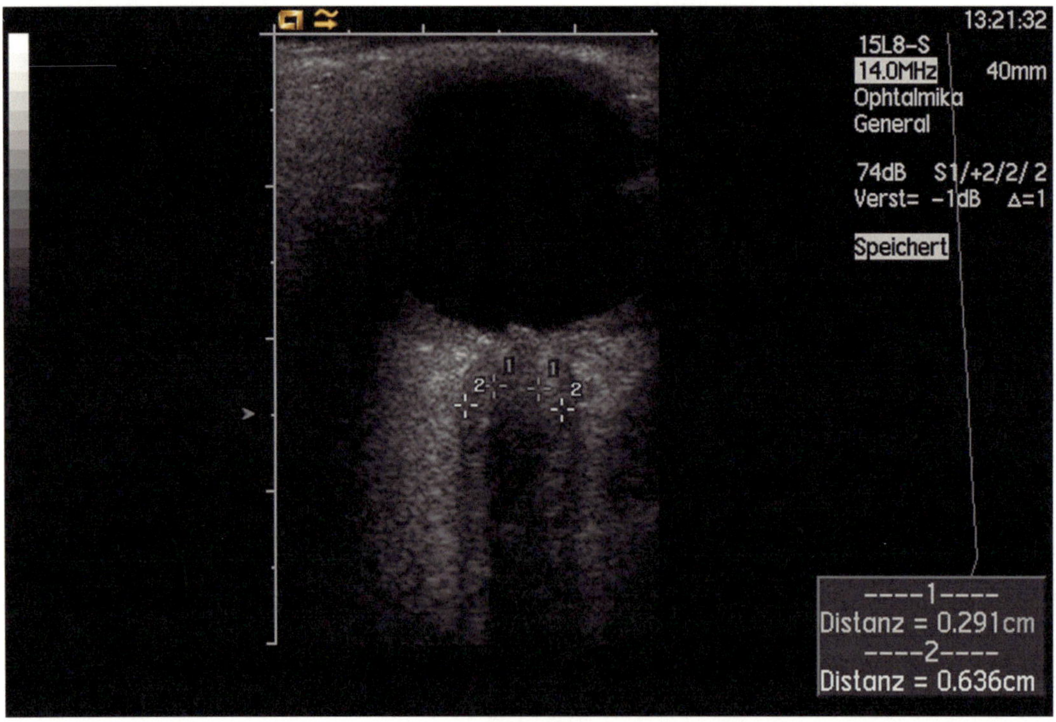

Fig. 7. Measurement of optic nerve sheath diameter using ultrasound: the optic nerve sheath is demonstrated as a thin bilateral hyperechogenic line surrounding the hypoechogenic optic nerve. The diameter is calculated by the distance of the two cursors named "2". Normal values range from 5,7-6,0 mm with a definitely pathologic diameter in this patient

brain injury also showed a good accuracy of the ultrasound technique. The pooled sensitivity for the detection of raised ICP was 90% (Dubourg et al. 2011). In the hands of experienced sonographers and standardized examination procedures several studies demonstrated a high intra- and interoberserver reliability (Ballantyne et al. 2002; Helmke and Hansen 1996).

Apart from the above mentioned symptomatic causes of raised ICP in idiopathic intracranial hypertension (IIH), also often referred to as pseudotumor cerebri, the mechanism of ICP increase are still not well understood. Classically patients, often obese women during childbearing age, present with headache and loss of visual acuity or visual field deficits (Degnan and Levy 2011). Though not being a life threatening condition it is still associated with permanent, and partly severe, visual deficits (Friedman 2001; Lueck and McIlwaine 2002; Rowe and Sarkies 1998; Wall 2010). Visual symptoms are thought to be due to transient or permanent ischemic damage to the optic nerve caused by pressure (Jaggi et al. 2010; Wall 2010). Regular ophthalmologic follow-up examinations with visual acuity tests and fundoscopy are recommended, and patients often need to reduce weight and need to be treated with diuretic drugs (esp. acetazolamide), regular lumbar punctures or even operative shunt techniques.

Bäuerle et al. performed a prospective study to evaluate the immediate correlation of optic nerve diameter (OND), ONSD and papilledema with CSF-pressure reduction caused by therapeutic lumbar puncture in patients with IIH. Patients with IIH showed a significantly enlarged ONSD (6.4 ± 0.6 mm bilaterally) compared with healthy individuals (5.4 ± 0.5 mm) and a significant decrease in ONSD (right ONSD 5.8 ± 0.7 mm, $p < 0.004$; left ONSD 5.9 ± 0.7 mm, $p < 0.043$) 24 hours after lumbar puncture (Bauerle and Nedelmann 2011). In some patients with IIH, though, the ONSD did not change at all after lumbar puncture. This could be an effect of a postulated optic nerve compartment syndrome, an idea which first came up with persistent papilledema and visual disturbance in IIH-patients despite a functioning lumbo-peritoneal shunt (Kelman et al. 1991). Pathologic changes in trabecular structures of the ONS might interfere with the physiologic bidirectional flow of the CSF to the basal cisterns leading to persistent optic disc swelling (Killer et al. 2007). Years ago, Ossoinig suggested the use of the stretch-test (originally called the "30 degrees-test"): in widened optic nerve patterns due to fluid around the optic nerve parenchyma, a decreased optic nerve thickness was observed after performing the stretch-test (positive test result), whereas in solid lesions of the optic nerve no change of optic nerve thickness was found (negative test result) (Haritoglou et al. 2002). In patients with increased ICP due to any cause, either ophthalmoscopic evaluation or bilateral retrobulbar ultrasound is mandatory, as asymmetric and unilateral papilledemae in patients with IIH are well described (Seggia and De Menezes 1993). In addition, Bäuerle et al. did not find any correlation of papilledema and OND with CSF reduction in the short-term follow-up. Due to anatomic reasons the anterior segment of the ONSD responds quickly to changes of CSF pressure. This is a particular advantage of retrobulbar ultrasound compared to funduscopic re-evaluations, as changes behind the level of the optic disc cannot be visualized by the latter technique.

Although papilledema does not quickly respond to changes in CSF-pressure it is a manifestation of chronic ICP-increase (Villa et al. 1997) and other diseases as optic neuritis (Ashurst et al. 2010) for example.

To find a proper scanning plane, the probe is set as described above, with a good view on the optic nerve in the axial plane. The plane with the maximum disc elevation or excavation is selected, the measurements are performed in the "freeze" mode: disc elevation is quantified by putting the first caliper on the uppermost part of the swollen disc, the second caliper is positioned on the strongly reflecting line representing the lamina cribrosa (Fig. 8).

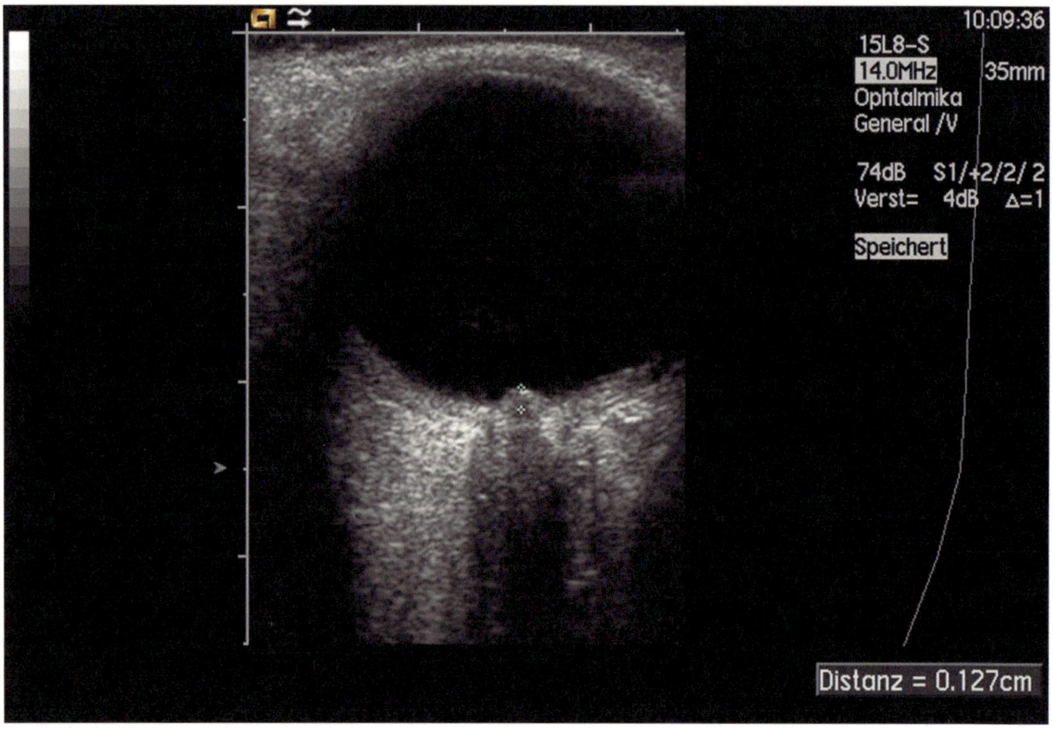

Fig. 8. Measurement of papilledema using ultrasound: disc elevation is quantified by putting the first caliper on the uppermost part of the swollen disc, the second caliper is positioned on the strongly reflecting line representing the lamina cribrosa

In patients with IIH the severity of disc swelling seems to have prognostic implications as well: in a combined retrospective and prospective study Wall et al. found a significant correlation of the severity of papilledema in patients with asymmetric papilledema and IIH, and their visual deficits (Wall and White 1998). This underlies the importance of regular follow-up quantification of optic disc swelling in these patients. Quantification of optic disc swelling is a reliable and reproducible technique, which was demonstrated by Tamburelli et al (Tamburrelli et al. 2000). In their study, data from patients with IIH taken by a confocal scanning laser ophthalmoscope were compared to ultrasound measurements demonstrating a good correlation. The mean depth measurements ranged from 0.68 to 2.01 mm (1.17 +/- 0.38 mm) and were comparable to those quantified by a confocal scanning laser ophthalmoscope (0.45 to 1.23 mm (0.93 +/- 0.24 mm)) (Tamburrelli et al. 2000).

Retrobulbar sonography is an inexpensive, quick, safe and reliable tool to monitor ICP changes. It is relatively easy to learn compared to transcranial duplex sonography, which improves inter-observer reliability. Still, in critically ill patients, invasive ICP measurement techniques remain the gold standard but can be complemented by using orbital ultrasound. In IIH ONSD measurements are a suitable alternative to funduscopy for non-ophthalmologists in the long-term follow up.

5. Miscellaneous

In clinical practice the neurologist is sometimes faced with the problem to discriminate between papilledema and pseudopapilledema. Papilledema is a correlate for raised ICP. A complete diagnostic workup to find the underlying cause is mandatory.

A common cause for pseudopapilledema are optic disc drusen. They can be an incidental finding in routine ophthalmologic exams. Most optic disc drusen remain asymptomatic (Davis and Jay 2003), but upon thorough investigation visual field defects can be detected in up to 90% (Gaynes and Towle 1967; Savino et al. 1979). The funduscopic discrimination between papilledema and pseudopapilledema is not trivial, as the term "pseudopapilledema" already indicates. Typical signs of true papilledema in funduscopy are cotton wool spots, multiple hemorrhages around the disc, hyperemia, venous congestion, and exudates.

Drusen consist of calcific dispositions in the optic nerve head and can be depicted as high-reflectance spots in the anterior optic nerve, especially after lowering the gain. Therefore retrobulbar b-mode-sonography can help to confirm the diagnosis of optic disc drusen if the fundoscopy is not decisive (Fig. 9).

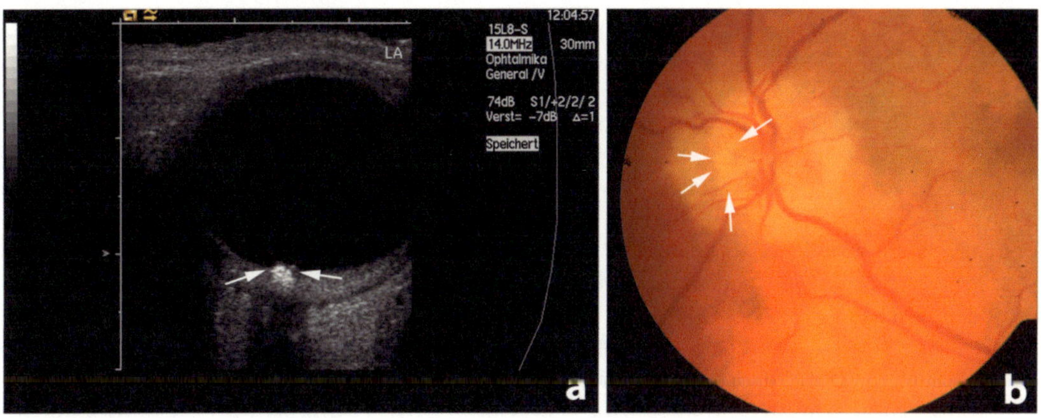

Fig. 9. Optic disc drusen seen in funduscopy and high-resolution ultrasound: (a) B-mode sonography: calcific dispositions in the optic nerve head representing optic disc drusen. (b) Fundoscopy: nasally located superficial drusen, blurred rim of optic disc, optic disc edema and hyperemia

6. References

American Institute of Ultrasound in Medicine (2000). "Section 7--discussion of the mechanical index and other exposure parameters. American Institute of Ultrasound in Medicine." *J Ultrasound Med* 19(2): 143-148, 154-168.

Antonelli, M., E. Azoulay, M. Bonten, J. Chastre, G. Citerio, G. Conti, D. De Backer, F. Lemaire, H. Gerlach, J. Groeneveld, G. Hedenstierna, D. Macrae, J. Mancebo, S. M. Maggiore, A. Mebazaa, P. Metnitz, J. Pugin, J. Wernerman and H. Zhang (2009). "Year in review in Intensive Care Medicine, 2008: I. Brain injury and neurology, renal failure and endocrinology, metabolism and nutrition, sepsis, infections and pneumonia." *Intensive Care Med* 35(1): 30-44.

Arida, A., M. Kyprianou, M. Kanakis and P. P. Sfikakis (2010). "The diagnostic value of ultrasonography-derived edema of the temporal artery wall in giant cell arteritis: a second meta-analysis." *BMC Musculoskelet Disord* 11: 44.

Arning, C., B. Widder, G. M. von Reutern, H. Stiegler and M. Gortler (2010). "[Revision of DEGUM ultrasound criteria for grading internal carotid artery stenoses and transfer to NASCET measurement]." *Ultraschall Med* 31(3): 251-257.

Ashurst, J., J. Schofer and P. Sierzenski (2010). "Unilateral papilledema: a case of optic neuritis diagnosed with bedside ocular sonography." *Del Med J* 82(4): 137-139.

Ballantyne, S. A., G. O'Neill, R. Hamilton and A. S. Hollman (2002). "Observer variation in the sonographic measurement of optic nerve sheath diameter in normal adults." *Eur J Ultrasound* 15(3): 145-149.

Bauerle, J. and M. Nedelmann (2011). "Sonographic assessment of the optic nerve sheath in idiopathic intracranial hypertension." *J Neurol.*

Blaivas, M., D. Theodoro and P. R. Sierzenski (2003). "Elevated intracranial pressure detected by bedside emergency ultrasonography of the optic nerve sheath." *Acad Emerg Med* 10(4): 376-381.

Brain Trauma Foundation (2000). "The Brain Trauma Foundation. The American Association of Neurological Surgeons. The Joint Section on Neurotrauma and Critical Care. Recommendations for intracranial pressure monitoring technology." *J Neurotrauma* 17(6-7): 497-506.

Brown, G. C. and L. E. Magargal (1982). "Central retinal artery obstruction and visual acuity." *Ophthalmology* 89(1): 14-19.

Davis, P. L. and W. M. Jay (2003). "Optic nerve head drusen." *Semin Ophthalmol* 18(4): 222-242.

Degnan, A. J. and L. M. Levy (2011). "Pseudotumor Cerebri: Brief Review of Clinical Syndrome and Imaging Findings." *AJNR Am J Neuroradiol.*

Dubourg, J., E. Javouhey, T. Geeraerts, M. Messerer and B. Kassai (2011). "Ultrasonography of optic nerve sheath diameter for detection of raised intracranial pressure: a systematic review and meta-analysis." *Intensive Care Med.*

Food and Drug Administration (2008). "Food and Drug Administration: Information for Manufacturers Seeking Clearance of Diagnostic Ultrasound Systems and Transducers."

Foroozan, R., P. J. Savino and R. C. Sergott (2002). "Embolic central retinal artery occlusion detected by orbital color Doppler imaging." *Ophthalmology* 109(4): 744-747; discussion 747-748.

Friedman, D. I. (2001). "Papilledema and pseudotumor cerebri." *Ophthalmol Clin North Am* 14(1): 129-147, ix.

Galetta, S., S. F. Byrne and J. L. Smith (1989). "Echographic correlation of optic nerve sheath size and cerebrospinal fluid pressure." *J Clin Neuroophthalmol* 9(2): 79-82.

Gaynes, P. M. and P. A. Towle (1967). "Hemorrhage in hyaline bodies (drusen) of the optic disc during an attack of migraine." *Am J Ophthalmol* 63(6): 1693-1696.

Geeraerts, T., Y. Launey, L. Martin, J. Pottecher, B. Vigue, J. Duranteau and D. Benhamou (2007). "Ultrasonography of the optic nerve sheath may be useful for detecting raised intracranial pressure after severe brain injury." *Intensive Care Med* 33(10): 1704-1711.

Geeraerts, T., S. Merceron, D. Benhamou, B. Vigue and J. Duranteau (2008). "Non-invasive assessment of intracranial pressure using ocular sonography in neurocritical care patients." *Intensive Care Med* 34(11): 2062-2067.

Girisgin, A. S., E. Kalkan, S. Kocak, B. Cander, M. Gul and M. Semiz (2007). "The role of optic nerve ultrasonography in the diagnosis of elevated intracranial pressure." *Emerg Med J* 24(4): 251-254.

Gold, D. (1977). "Retinal arterial occlusion." *Trans Sect Ophthalmol Am Acad Ophthalmol Otolaryngol* 83(3 Pt 1): OP392-408.

Hansen, H. C. and K. Helmke (1997). "Validation of the optic nerve sheath response to changing cerebrospinal fluid pressure: ultrasound findings during intrathecal infusion tests." *J Neurosurg* 87(1): 34-40.

Haritoglou, C., H. Herzum, O. Ehrt, K. C. Ossoinig and A. Kampik (2002). "[Echographic differential diagnosis of optic nerve widening]." *Ophthalmologe* 99(7): 559-565.

Helmke, K. and H. C. Hansen (1996). "Fundamentals of transorbital sonographic evaluation of optic nerve sheath expansion under intracranial hypertension II. Patient study." *Pediatr Radiol* 26(10): 706-710.

Hiler, M., M. Czosnyka, P. Hutchinson, M. Balestreri, P. Smielewski, B. Matta and J. D. Pickard (2006). "Predictive value of initial computerized tomography scan, intracranial pressure, and state of autoregulation in patients with traumatic brain injury." *J Neurosurg* 104(5): 731-737.

Jaggi, G. P., M. Harlev, U. Ziegler, S. Dotan, N. R. Miller and H. E. Killer (2010). "Cerebrospinal fluid segregation optic neuropathy: an experimental model and a hypothesis." *Br J Ophthalmol* 94(8): 1088-1093.

Kelman, S. E., R. C. Sergott, G. A. Cioffi, P. J. Savino, T. M. Bosley and M. J. Elman (1991). "Modified optic nerve decompression in patients with functioning lumboperitoneal shunts and progressive visual loss." *Ophthalmology* 98(9): 1449-1453.

Killer, H. E., G. P. Jaggi, J. Flammer, N. R. Miller, A. R. Huber and A. Mironov (2007). "Cerebrospinal fluid dynamics between the intracranial and the subarachnoid space of the optic nerve. Is it always bidirectional?" *Brain* 130(Pt 2): 514-520.

Lieb, W. E., S. M. Cohen, D. A. Merton, J. A. Shields, D. G. Mitchell and B. B. Goldberg (1991). "Color Doppler imaging of the eye and orbit. Technique and normal vascular anatomy." *Arch Ophthalmol* 109(4): 527-531.

Lizzi, F. L., A. J. Packer and D. J. Coleman (1978). "Experimental cataract production by high frequency ultrasound." *Ann Ophthalmol* 10(7): 934-942.

Lueck, C. and G. McIlwaine (2002). "Interventions for idiopathic intracranial hypertension." *Cochrane Database Syst Rev*(3): CD003434.

Mawn, L. A., T. R. Hedges, 3rd, W. Rand and P. A. Heggerick (1997). "Orbital color Doppler imaging in carotid occlusive disease." *Arch Ophthalmol* 115(4): 492-496.

McFadzean, R. M. (1998). "Ischemic optic neuropathy and giant cell arteritis." *Curr Opin Ophthalmol* 9(6): 10-17.

Muller, M., K. Wessel, E. Mehdorn, D. Kompf and C. M. Kessler (1993). "Carotid artery disease in vascular ocular syndromes." *J Clin Neuroophthalmol* 13(3): 175-180.

Newman, W. D., A. S. Hollman, G. N. Dutton and R. Carachi (2002). "Measurement of optic nerve sheath diameter by ultrasound: a means of detecting acute raised intracranial pressure in hydrocephalus." *Br J Ophthalmol* 86(10): 1109-1113.

Paivansalo, M., K. Riihelainen, T. Rissanen, I. Suramo and L. Laatikainen (1999). "Effect of an internal carotid stenosis on orbital blood velocity." *Acta Radiol* 40(3): 270-275.

Pfaffenbach, D. D. and R. W. Hollenhorst (1972). "Morbidity and survivorship of patients with embolic cholesterol crystals in the ocular fundus." *Trans Am Ophthalmol Soc* 70: 337-349.

Rowe, F. J. and N. J. Sarkies (1998). "Assessment of visual function in idiopathic intracranial hypertension: a prospective study." *Eye (Lond)* 12 (Pt 1): 111-118.

Savino, P. J., J. S. Glaser and M. A. Rosenberg (1979). "A clinical analysis of pseudopapilledema. II. Visual field defects." *Arch Ophthalmol* 97(1): 71-75.

Schlachetzki, F., S. Boy, U. Bogdahn, H. Helbig and M. A. Gamulescu (2010). "The Retrobulbar "Spot Sign" - Ocular Sonography for the Differential Diagnosis of Temporal Arteritis and Sudden Blindness." *Ultraschall Med.*

Seggia, J. C. and M. L. De Menezes (1993). "[Pseudotumor cerebri without optic papilledema]." *Arq Neuropsiquiatr* 51(4): 511-518.

Soldatos, T., D. Karakitsos, K. Chatzimichail, M. Papathanasiou, A. Gouliamos and A. Karabinis (2008). "Optic nerve sonography in the diagnostic evaluation of adult brain injury." *Crit Care* 12(3): R67.

Tamburrelli, C., T. Salgarello, C. G. Caputo, A. Giudiceandrea and L. Scullica (2000). "Ultrasonographic evaluation of optic disc swelling: comparison with CSLO in idiopathic intracranial hypertension." *Invest Ophthalmol Vis Sci* 41(10): 2960-2966.

Tayal, V. S., M. Neulander, H. J. Norton, T. Foster, T. Saunders and M. Blaivas (2007). "Emergency department sonographic measurement of optic nerve sheath diameter to detect findings of increased intracranial pressure in adult head injury patients." *Ann Emerg Med* 49(4): 508-514.

Toms, D. A. (2006). "The mechanical index, ultrasound practices, and the ALARA principle." *J Ultrasound Med* 25(4): 560-561; author reply 561-562.

Tranquart, F. O., O. Bergès, P. Koskas, S. Arsene, C. Rossazza, P.-J. Pisella and L. a. Pourcelot (2003). "Color doppler imaging of orbital vessels: Personal experience and literature review." *Journal of Clinical Ultrasound* 31(5): 258-273.

Tsung, J. W., M. Blaivas, A. Cooper and N. R. Levick (2005). "A rapid noninvasive method of detecting elevated intracranial pressure using bedside ocular ultrasound: application to 3 cases of head trauma in the pediatric emergency department." *Pediatr Emerg Care* 21(2): 94-98.

Villa, A. M., S. F. Anderson and R. E. Abundo (1997). "Bilateral disc edema in retinitis pigmentosa." *Optom Vis Sci* 74(3): 132-137.

Wall, M. (2010). "Idiopathic intracranial hypertension." *Neurol Clin* 28(3): 593-617.

Wall, M. and W. N. White, 2nd (1998). "Asymmetric papilledema in idiopathic intracranial hypertension: prospective interocular comparison of sensory visual function." *Invest Ophthalmol Vis Sci* 39(1): 134-142.

Watanabe, A., H. Kinouchi, T. Horikoshi, M. Uchida and K. Ishigame (2008). "Effect of intracranial pressure on the diameter of the optic nerve sheath." *J Neurosurg* 109(2): 255-258.

Winkler, F., S. Kastenbauer, T. A. Yousry, U. Maerz and H. W. Pfister (2002). "Discrepancies between brain CT imaging and severely raised intracranial pressure proven by ventriculostomy in adults with pneumococcal meningitis." *J Neurol* 249(9): 1292-1297.

13

The Role of TCCS in the Assessment of the Main Anatomical Patterns of the M1 Segment of the Middle Cerebral Artery

Fabrice Vuillier[1,3], Laurent Tatu[1,3],
Paola Montiel[1], Françoise Cattin[2] and Thierry Moulin[1]
[1]Department of Neurology,
[2]Department of Neuroradiology
[3]Department of Anatomy,
Jean Minjoz CHU, University of Franche-Comté Medical School, Besançon, France

1. Introduction

Since the first use of transcranial Doppler sonography by Aaslid et al. in 1982 (Aaslid, R. et al, 1982), ultrasound exploration of intracranial arteries has become highly advanced. The introduction of transcranial color-coded sonography (TCCS) made it possible to use real-time B-mode imaging and Doppler-signal color coding along with conventional transcranial Doppler (TCD) sonography (Bogdahn, U. et al, 1982).

Thus, with B-mode imaging and color coding of the Doppler, vessels can be reliably identified. Theoretically, TCCS studies of the anatomy of the M1 segment of the middle cerebral artery (MCA) could have an impact on the precise localization of a blood clot site, on the potentialization of thrombolysis using ultrasound, and on the morphological profile of recanalization. Thus, TCCS morphological findings provide fundamental information that is complementary to that obtained using 3D time-of-flight (TOF) magnetic resonance angiography (MRA), which is considered to be the reference standard.

2. The M1 segment of the middle cerebral artery

2.1 Anatomical patterns

The princeps anatomical descriptions of the MCA still represent the basis of current knowledge (Duret, H., 1874; Foix, C. and Lévy, M., 1927). Later, microdissection on human cadavers led to a better understanding of the anatomical patterns of the MCA (Gibo, H. et al, 1981; Tanriover, N. et al, 2003; Umansky, F. et al, 1984; Yasargil, M.G., 1984). The proximal part of the MCA is commonly known as the M1 segment (Gibo, H. et al, 1981) although other terms, such as the horizontal segment (Herman, L.H. et al, 1963) or the sphenoidal segment (Gibo, H. et al, 1981), have also been used. The M1 segment may be defined in relation to the references to brain structures found nearby, from its origin to its end (Gibo, H. et al, 1981). As such, its origin is situated laterally in relation to the optic chiasm, at the level of the medial end of the lateral fissure. Its course then leads laterally, behind the anterior perforated substance and towards the insula. Leaving aside the parenchyma, a definition based on angiographic references has been suggested and has often been used (Krayenbuhl, H.A. and Yasargil, M.G., 1968). The origin of the M1 segment is then located at the division of the internal carotid artery (ICA), at the same level as the anterior cerebral artery (ACA). Its diameter and direction make the M1 segment appear to be a lateral extension of the ICA. According to this definition, the M1 segment ends when the artery curves sharply back and up, at the point known as the genu of the M1 segment (Fig. 1).

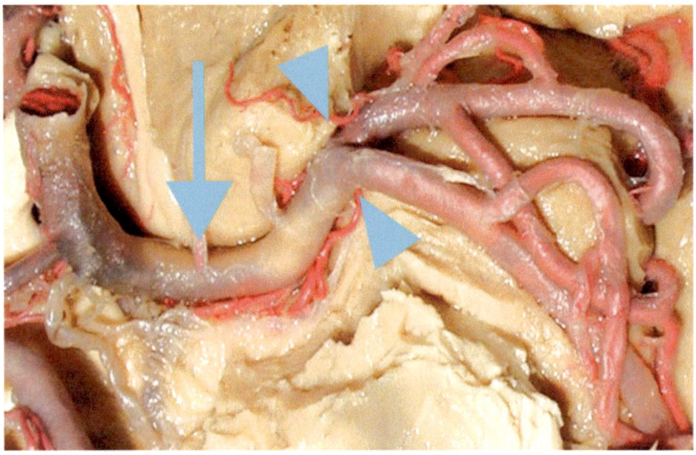

Fig. 1. Inferior view of the left middle cerebral artery. Its course is straight (c.f. arrow) up to the point where the artery curves sharply back and up at the genu where it divides into two branches, defined as a bipode division (c.f. arrow heads)

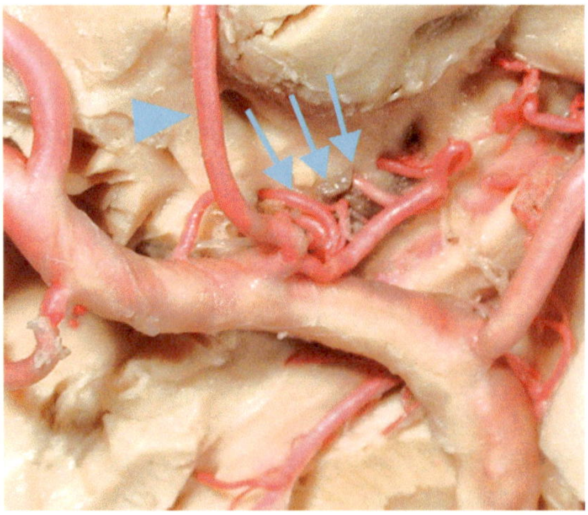

Fig. 2. Deep perforating branches of the M1 segment (c.f. arrows) arising from an early cortical branch (c.f. arrow head)

In most cases, close to the genu, the M1 segment divides into two branches, defined as a bipode division (anterior and posterior divisions). An absence of division, defined as the monopode type, or an M1 segment trifurcation with superior, middle and inferior divisions, are observed less frequently. The early cortical branches (ECB) are defined as small diameter arteries that usually arise almost at a right angle to the M1 segment and that run toward the cortex. The type of branch can be defined using anatomical criteria from microdissection studies, based on the diameter and direction of the branches in relation to the M1 segment (Tanriover, N. et al, 2003). Although these criteria allow us to distinguish the main division branches from the ECB in most cases, they may not be entirely accurate, particularly with regard to early proximal cortical branches that may be taken for early bifurcations (Foix, C. and Lévy, M., 1927).

The deep perforating branches of the M1 segment, defined as the lenticulostriate arteries, arise proximal to the M1 segment division. Usually, deep perforating branches are divided into medial, intermediate and lateral groups (Fig. 2).

2.2 Technical approach of the M1 segment

The use of conventional angiography, which was considered for a long time to be the gold standard in the diagnosis of intracranial arterial anomalies, has also been the source of a number of anatomical descriptions (Newton, T.H. and Potts, D.G. 1974; Nomura, T., 1970). Most of these studies have been carried out from a neurosurgical perspective with a view to contributing to improvements in the treatment of aneurysms and intracranial arteriovenous malformations. With the development of high-field-strength MR imaging, it is now possible to carry out, in vivo, a precise visualization of the intracranial arteries and, in particular, the M1 segment of the MCA, using 3D TOF MRA (Fig.3). However, 3T MRA has not been widely used, particularly in stroke patients (Choi, C.G et al, 2007). Thus, 3T MRA could help neurologists to better understand the angioarchitecture of intracranial arteries in order to optimize stroke management.

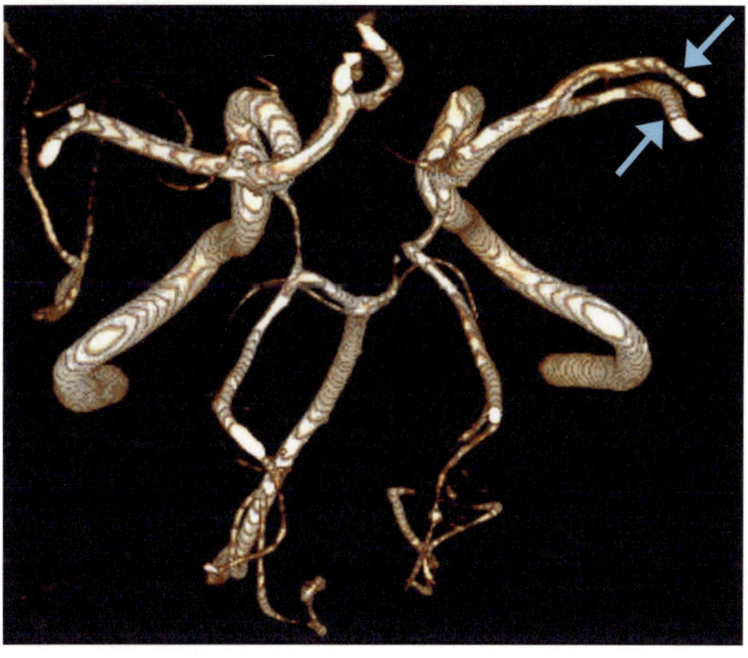

Fig. 3. MRA of the circle of Willis showing a bipode division of the right MCA (c.f. arrows)

In the field of ultrasound application, B-mode imaging and Doppler-signal color coding are used only to measure the angle of insonation in order to obtain absolute flow velocities more accurately than is possible with TCD (Martin, P.J. et al, 1995; Kimura, K. et al, 1998). Consequently, even if TCCS presents certain advantages, its main clinical applications in the assessment of cerebrovascular diseases are similar to those of TCD. Prior to our study, the ability of TCCS to provide a visualization of the intracranial arteries using a morphological approach, especially in the distal part of the M1 segment, had not been properly evaluated.

3. TCCS examination of the M1 segment

3.1 General procedure

TCCS is carried out through the left and right temporal bone window with a 2-MHz probe and can be performed at the bedside in the stroke unit within the first 48 hours of hospitalization. To achieve the best possible visualization of the M1 segment, the investigation should be carried out using power-Doppler (Fig. 4). This is the most angle-independent imaging technique and is more appropriate than color-Doppler for morphological studies on arteries (Griewing, B. et al, 1998; Postert, T. et al, 1997).

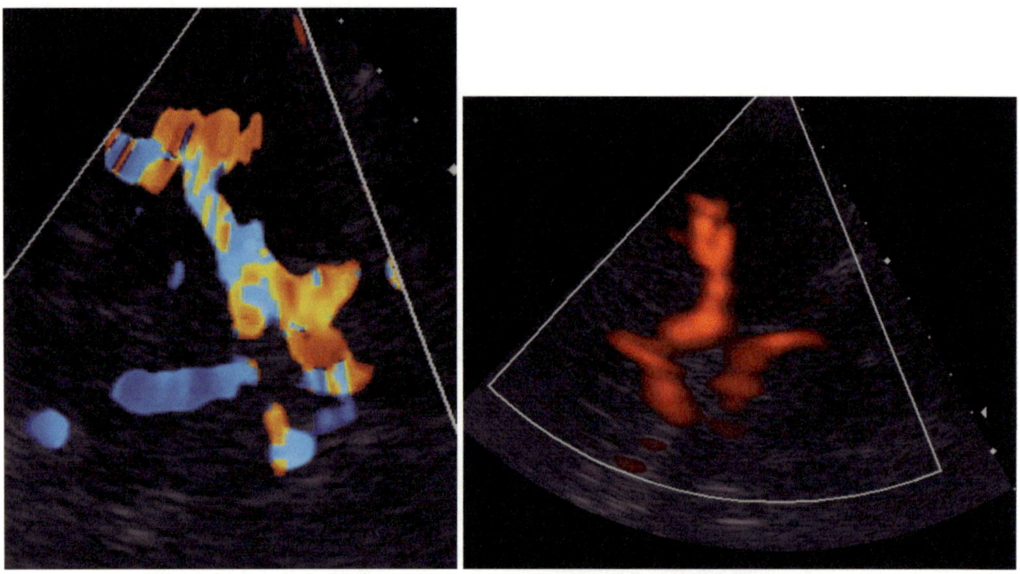

Fig. 4. M1 segment using color-Doppler (a) and power-Doppler (b)

Power-Doppler is used taking particular care to obtain a long-axis view of the M1 segment and several images of its course, end and division. This is done by tilting, rotating and shifting the transducer (Fig. 5).

For a long time, because the acoustic temporal bone window is more restricted in the elderly, and notably in women, TCCS was usually carried out on patients aged under 55 years (Itoh, T. et al, 1993). Thanks to the use of contrast enhancement, the sensitivity and specificity of diagnostic ultrasound imaging have been considerably improved (Droste,

D.W. et al, 2002). Usually, contrast enhancement (Sonovue TM) is administered, as necessary, via continuous infusion up to a total dose over 8 minutes. The temporal bone window is considered as absent when no part of the M1 segment can be detected and as insufficient when it is not possible to view the entire course of the M1 segment. In good conditions, the course and division patterns of the M1 segment can be defined and compared to the MRA results. Thus, it is now possible to carry out TCCS in the conditions encountered in most stroke patients.

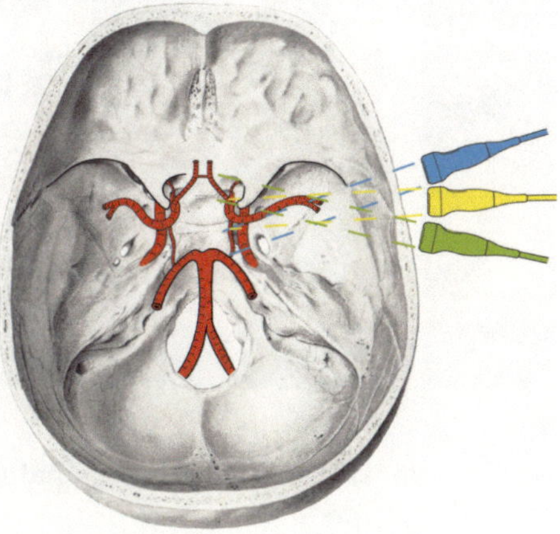

Fig. 5. Directions of the probe through the temporal bone window to obtain a long-axis view of the M1 segment and several images of its course, end and division

3.2 TCCS anatomical capacity

Using TCCS, the main anatomical features, such as the type of course and division of the M1 segment, can be determined.

As shown in Figure 6, the precise direction in the horizontal plane and the length of the M1 segment can be defined. In the majority of cases, the M1 segment is straight, which facilitates its exploration using TCCS. In some cases, however, the course of the M1 segment curves and does not always follow the same concavity direction. This type of course, and in particular a curve with a posterior concavity, has already been reported, when the M1 segment is described as being parallel to the large sphenoid ridge (Gibo, H. et al, 1981). A tendency towards an anterior concavity has been reported, although less frequently (Nomura, T., 1970). In these cases, TCCS exploration can be more difficult, requiring more complicated manipulations of the probe. The length of the M1 segment, which is usually approximately 20mm, can provide the neurologist with important information in order to identify the precise location of the clot in relation to the collateral branches and to evaluate the gradual recanalization of the M1 segment. Evaluations of the diameter of the M1 segment are usually used to judge the severity of stenosis in conventional arteriography, angio-CT or MRA. In TCCS, stenosis is usually evaluated using velocity values. The advent of ultrasound technology could enable us to evaluate the diameter of certain intracranial arteries, such as the distal part of the ICA or of the basilar artery.

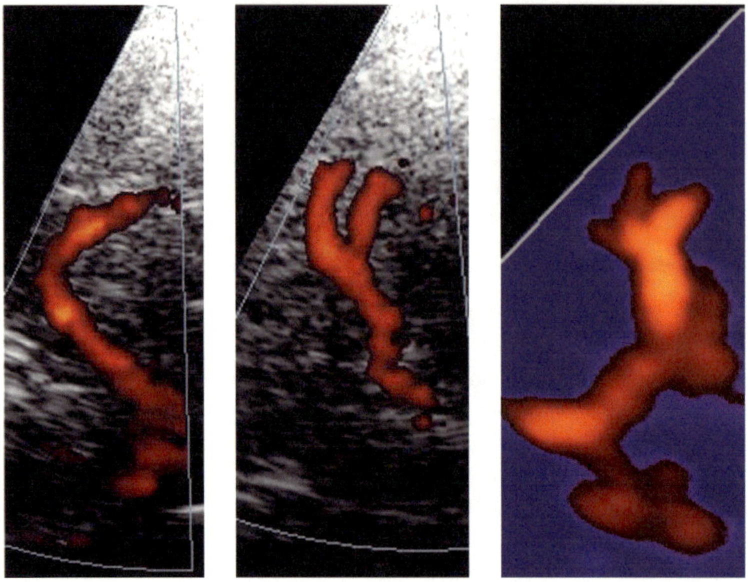

(a) (b) (c)

Fig. 6. TCCS using power-Doppler showing the division patterns of the M1 segment: (a) monopode, (b) bipode and (c) tripode

TCCS is a useful tool in defining the type of M1 segment division. As in our study, TCCS was able to show that the division was monopode in 16/68 cases (23.5%; Fig. 6a), bipode in 50/68 cases (73.5%; Fig. 6b) and tripode in 2/68 cases (3%; Fig. 6c), confirming the classic data (Gibo, H. et al, 1981; Tanriover, N. et al, 2003). The type of division could not be defined in the remaining 17/85 cases (20%).

In our study, TCCS anatomical patterns of the M1 segment were compared to 3D TOF-MRA at 3 T, which is the gold standard technique used to depict the normal anatomy of the intracranial artery (Willinek, W.A. et al, 2003). Our comparisons between TCCS and MRA findings indicated concordance in most cases (67%), especially when the division was bipode (Fig. 7).

The fact that false-positive results were uncommon (positive predictive value = 87%) indicates the efficacy of TCCS in depicting bipode division. Nevertheless, in all false-negative cases, the division was taken to be monopode, whereas it was bipode on MRA. These facts illustrate the difficulty of identifying certain division branches, confirming a classic limitation of TCCS. Our results demonstrate that if TCCS is performed with care, it can provide anatomical information on the whole M1 segment. Our results also highlighted the ability of TCCS to analyze the distal part of the M1 segment, despite potential difficulties such as the insonation angle and a more superficial situation (Itoh, T. et al, 1993; Zunker, P. et al, 2002). The main technical limitation that we encountered (in 11/23 cases) was an unfavourable angle between the ultrasound beam and the division branches of the M1 segment, which led to an unfavourable insonation angle. As for the anatomical causes of discordance, we observed that the anatomical criteria could not be applied accurately in 12/23 cases. This can be explained by the difficulty of accurately evaluating the diameter of the branch and its angle of origin, because contrast enhancement creates color artefacts

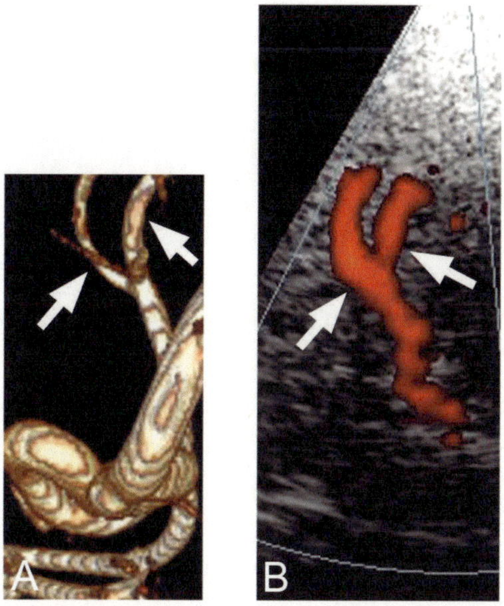

Fig. 7. MRA (a) and TCCS (b) showing a bipode division with a good correlation between the two techniques

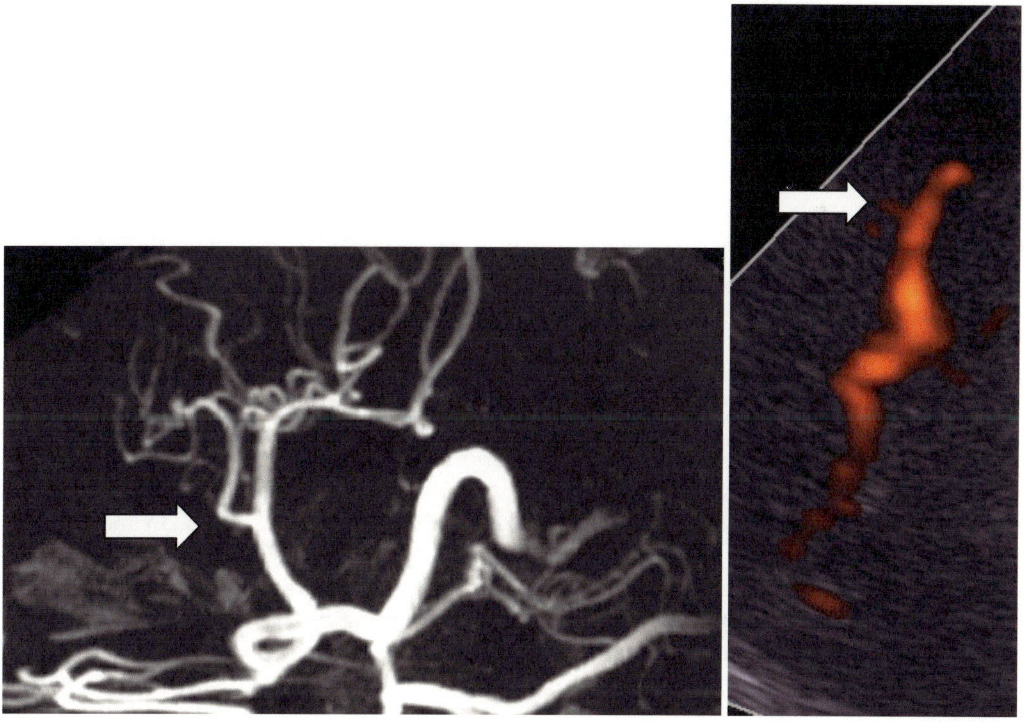

Fig. 8. In 8a, the top of the head is at the left of the image and the probe is placed at the top of the image. MRA (a) and TCCS (b) showing an ECB arising from the M1 segment at a right angle (c.f. arrows)

(blooming). Our study showed that TCCS can be used to obtain anatomical information on the M1 segment of the MCA. Nevertheless, the resolution of TCCS to detect MCA branches needs to be improved through technical developments.

Regardless of the technique used, it is quite possible for the main division branches to be taken for cortical branches and vice-versa (Tanriover, N. et al, 2003). In good conditions, TCCS enables the visualisation of the ECB despite their small diameter. The identification of these ECB using TCCS is also possible thanks to the application of anatomical criteria, in particular the almost 90° angle at which they branch from the M1 segment (Fig. 8).

Finally, it is also possible using TCCS to determine the site of the division as being before, at the level of, or distal to the genu.

To our knowledge, our study was the first to compare anatomical patterns as shown on MRA and TCCS images.

4. Pathological applications

The benefits of TCCS in detecting MCA stenosis or occlusion have been widely demonstrated (Kimura, K. et al, 1998; Baumgartner, R.W. et al, 1999; Tang, S.C. et al, 2005), particularly when contrast enhancement is used (Gerriets, T. et al, 2000; Ogata, T. et al, 2005). Similarly, as TCCS is a bedside tool that can be used easily and as required, it has become the test of choice for evaluating the recanalization of the M1 segment after thrombolysis (Gerriets, T. et al, 2000; Ogata, T. et al, 2005). These clinical applications of TCCS are based exclusively on an evaluation of flow velocities, particularly for the proximal part of the M1 segment. Yet with improvements in image quality, thanks to the recent advent of harmonic imaging and contrast enhancement (Burns, P.N., 1996), it is now possible to obtain precise morphological knowledge of various vascular lesions. Wherever the stenosis or occlusion in the M1 segment is located, it can now be identified and located more accurately with respect to the origin of the division of the branches of the M1 segment. It is also possible to specify the consequences of occlusion with regard to the ECB. These morphological data are essential in achieving a good understanding of the functional consequences of stenosis or occlusion.

Obviously, the same applies regarding the quality of recanalization of the M1 segment and the consequences of recanalization on its division branches, which can also be determined using morphological patterns. In addition, more precise localization of the blood clot can improve the capacity of low intensity ultrasound to accelerate thrombolysis (Alexandrov, A.V. et al, 2000; Molina, C.A. et al, 2004) or better guide the thrombectomy procedure. Hence, there is a need to pursue further TCCS studies with an increased focus on morphology. Moreover, the use of TCCS in pathological conditions and in the elderly population should now be easier. This would make it possible to implement clinical applications such as the localization of lesions and the time course of the morphological parameters of reperfusion, both of which may improve treatment strategies for stroke in the future.

5. References

Aaslid R, Markwalder TM, Nornes H: Noninvasive transcranial Doppler ultrasound recording of flow velocity in basal cerebral arteries. J Neurosurg 1982; 57: 769–774.

Alexandrov, AV, Demchuk AM, Felberg RA, et al: High rate of complete recanalization and dramatic clinical recovery during tPA infusion when continuously monitored with 2-MHz transcranial Doppler. Stroke 2000; 31: 610–614.

Baumgartner, RW, Mattle HP, Schroth G: Assessment of 6 50 and ! 50% intracranial sténoses by transcranial color-coded duplex sonography. Stroke 1999; 30: 87–92.

Bogdahn U, Becker G, Winkler J, Greiner K, Perez J, Meurers B: Transcranial color-coded real-time sonography in adults. Stroke 1990; 21: 1680–1688.

Burns P.N.: Harmonic imaging with ultrasound contrast agents. Clin Radiol 1996; 51(suppl 1):50-55.

Choi CG, Lee DH, Lee JH, Pyun HW, Kang DW, Kwon SU, Kim JK, Kim SJ, Suh DC (2007) Detection of intracranial atherosclerotic steno-occlusive disease with 3D time of flight magnetic resonance angiography with sensitivity encoding at 3T. AJNR Am J Neuroradiol 28:439-446.

Droste DW, Llull JB, Pezzoli C, Bogdahn U, Kaps M: Sonovue (BR1), a new long-acting echocontrast agent, improves transcranial color-coded duplex ultrasonic imaging. Cerebrovasc Dis 2002; 14: 27–32.

Duret H (1874) Recherches anatomiques sur la circulation de l'encéphale. Archives de Physiologie Normale et Pathologique 6:60-91.

Foix C, Lévy M (1927) Les ramollissements sylviens. Syndromes des lesions en foyer du territoire de l'artère sylvienne et de ses branches. Revue Neurologique 43:1-51.

Gerriets T, Postert T, Goertler M, et al: DIAS I: duplex-sonographic assessment of the cerebrovascular status in acute stroke: a useful tool for future stroke trials. Stroke 2000; 31: 2342–2345.

Gibo H, Carver CC, Rhoton AL, Lenkey C, Mitchell RJ (1981) Microsurgical anatomy of the middle cerebral artery. J neurosurg 54:151-169.

Griewing B, Schminke U, Motsch L, Brassel F, Kessler C: Transcranial duplex sonography of middle cerebral artery stenosis: a comparison of colour-coding techniques – frequency- or power-based Doppler and contrast enhancement. Neuroradiology 1998; 40: 490–495.

Herman L.H, Ostrowski A.Z, Gurdjian E.S (1963) Perforating branches of the middle cerebral artery; an anatomical study. Arch.Neurol (chic) 8:32-34.

Itoh T, Matsumoto M, Handa N, Maeda H, Hougaku H, Hashimoto H, Etani H, Tsukamoto Y, Kamada T: Rate of successful recording of blood flow signals in the middle cerebral artery using transcranial Doppler sonography. Stroke 1993; 24: 1192–1195.

Kimura K, Yasaka M, Wada K, Minematsu K, Yamaguchi T, Otsubo R: Diagnosis of middle cerebral artery stenosis by transcranial color-coded real-time sonography. AJNR Am J Neuroradiol 1998; 19: 1893–1896.

Krayenbuhl H.A, Yasargil M.G (1968) Cerebral angiography. Butterworth, London pp 58-60.

Martin PJ, Evans DH, Naylor AR: Measurement of blood flow velocity in the basal cerebral circulation: advantages of transcranial color-coded sonography over conventional transcranial Doppler. J Clin Ultrasound 1995; 23: 21–26.

Molina CA, Montaner J, Arenillas JF, Ribo M, Rubiera M, Alvarez-Sabin J: Differential pattern of tissue plasminogen activator-induced proximal middle artery recanalization among stroke subtypes. Stroke 2004; 35: 486–490.

Newton TH, Potts DG (1974) Radiology of the skull and brain. Angiography. The C.V Mosby Company, Saint-Louis.

Nomura T (1970) Atlas of cerebral angiography. Springer-Verlag, Tokyo.

Ogata T, Kimura K, Nakajima M, Naritomi H, Minematsu K: Diagnosis of middle cérébral artery occlusive lesions with contrastenhanced transcranial color-coded realtime sonography in acute stroke. Neuroradiology 2005; 47: 256–262.

Postert T, Meves S, Bornke C, Przuntek H, Buttner T: Power Doppler compared to color-coded duplex sonography in the assessment of the basal cerebral circulation. J Neuroimaging 1997; 7: 221–226.

Tang SC, Jeng JS, Yip PK, Lu CJ, Hwang BS, Lin WH, Liu HM: Transcranial color-coded sonography for the detection of middle cérébral artery stenosis. J Ultrasound Med 2005;24 :451-457.

Tanriover N, Kawashima M, Rhoton AL, Ulm AJ, Mericle RA (2003) Microsurgical anatomy of the early branches of the middle cerebral artery: morphometric analysis and classification with angiographic correlation. J neurosurg 98:1277-1290.

Umansky F, Juarez SM, Dujovny M et al. (1984) Microsurgical anatomy of the proximal segments of the middle cerebral artery. J Neurosurg 61:458-467.

Willinek W.A., Born M., Simon B., et al: Time-of-flight MR angiography: comparison of 3.0-T imaging and 1.5-T imaging - initial experience. Radiology 2003;229:913-920.

Yasargil MG (1984) Middle cerebral artery, Microneurosurgery (vol 1), Georg Thieme Verlag, Stuttgart pp 72-91.

Zunker P, Wilms H, Brossmann J, Georgiadis D, Weber S, Deuschl G: Echo contrast-enhanced transcranial ultrasound: frequency of use, diagnostic benefit, and validity of results compared with MRA. Stroke 2002; 33: 2600–2603.

14

Transcranial Doppler Sonography in Studies of Mental Effort

David A. Washburn, Natasha B. Schultz and Holly A. Phillips
Georgia State University
USA

1. Introduction

The history of experimental psychology—likely the history of every branch of science—is intimately and symbiotically connected with innovations in technologies and techniques for measurement. Although psychology's birth as a discipline was more about an idea (namely that mind and behavior can be studied objectively and empirically, for instance by observing how physical changes correspond to changes in experience and behavior) than about an apparatus, early advances in psychology as a science were facilitated, and in many cases catalyzed, by clever instrumentation. Often these innovations were simply novel applicants of existing technology to new scientific problems. For example, Wundt studied differences in reaction time to visual versus auditory information using a "pendulum apparatus for 'Complication' studies" (pictured in the online Museum of the History of Psychological Instrumentation at Monclair State University; *http://chss.montclair.edu/psychology/museum/x_073.htm*). This important apparatus was basically a modified metronome. The first tachistoscope for brief presentations of visual stimuli was an apparatus that resembled a guillotine (Turtle, 1997). Mueller's memory drum, which served for decades as the standard apparatus for studying memory for lists of items, was developed from a Ludwig-Baltzar kymograph, originally designed for the recording of blood pressure (Haupt, 2001). These and thousands of other devices found new useful life as research instruments in the study of behavior, and the scientific literature grew rapidly with findings reflecting each apparatus innovation.

The intersection of experimental psychology and biology, whether the offspring of that union is the field of physiological psychology or of cognitive neuroscience, illustrates this symbiotic relationship between science and technology. For example, cognitive neuroscience was established on the insights provided through the study of animal models and clinical populations, including individuals with brain damage that occurred as a result of injury, stroke, surgery, and so forth; however, the greatest gains (at least by quantitative measures, if not also by qualitative standards) in knowledge about brain-behavior relations have come in the years since the development of techniques for single-cell recording and neuroimaging of activity, structure and function. Electroencephalograhy (EEG), the event-related potential (ERP) paradigm, single-photon emission computed tomography (SPECT), magnetic resonance imaging (MRI), diffusion tensor imaging (DTI), transcranial magnetic stimulation (TMS), and transcranial Doppler (TCD) sonography are just a few of the technology-based neuroimaging techniques that are revolutionizing understanding of the physiological bases of psychological processes and their disorders.

Of course, instrumentation innovations do more than just opening doors for new questions to be investigated. They also constrain in some ways the answers that are obtained for those questions. Each new type of yardstick may provide an exciting novel method for measuring, but it also specifies the units of measurement, the types of things that can readily be measured, and the kinds of things that cannot. This is equally true of more sophisticated apparatus, including those used in neuroimaging. Each technique and tool provides some distinct advantages over alternate methods, but also carries specific limitations or disadvantages.

For example, the preeminent tool for contemporary neuroimaging, MRI, provides noninvasive high-resolution structural images of the brain or other organs. Carefully combined with behavioral testing to produce the functional MRI (fMRI) paradigm, this technology yields brain activity patterns that can be registered to the structural images, and compared against baseline activity patterns to provide insights into the functions associated with brain regions or networks.

But there are limitations to the fMRI procedure, including of course that it does not really provide information about the functional and causal information about the brain regions that are relatively active during particular cognitive operations. The data provided by fMRI can be highly informative, but they are correlational in nature. Only in concert with other types of data (e.g., clinical observations of patients with brain damage, experimental work with animal models) can we infer whether these correlations reveal brain networks that are necessary and sufficient for particular cognitive competencies. Another limitation of the fMRI paradigm is a sequela of the massive amount of data that are produced in a whole-brain scan: Sophisticated techniques are required to process the data such that they support valid inferences rather than statistical artifacts that suggest localizations from spurious, correlations, including those that Vul and collaborators called "voodoo correlations" (2009). Another limitation is cost. Although the hardware, software, and procedures for doing fMRI have improved in recent years, this neuroimaging strategy is still relatively expensive. It also remains difficult to conduct fMRI research with certain populations, as the procedure requires participants to remain motionless and to tolerate the ambient noises and enclosed spaces of the magnetic chamber. Many conditions, from metal implants to certain psychological disorders, are counterindicators of fMRI, disqualifying individuals from participation for research purposes. Thus, fMRI is a powerful neuroimaging tool that has a specific utility and value, but that also has specific limitations. This of course is true of *every* tool. That's why a plumber or carpenter needs a box of tools, rather than one general-purpose fix-all gadget.

In recent years, sonography has provided another instrument for the cognitive scientists' toolbox. Transcranial Doppler (TCD) sonography provides relatively inexpensive, noninvasive and painless, continuous measures of bloodflow velocity, as a proxy for neural activity, which serves as a measure of cognitive processing. TCD offers high temporal resolution—much higher, for example, than fMRI—but low spatial resolution. It is a wearable technology, and thus does not require participants to remain motionless during the test. Conditions like pacemaker implants, ferrous metal dental-work, tattoos, piercings, and claustrophobia that can disqualify a person from participating in an fMRI study do not affect the individual's suitability for TCD. On the other hand, it is difficult or impossible to obtain stable TCD signals from some participants, often for unknown reasons, and in every case for reasons that are not as obvious as tattoos or piercings or metallic implants. Thus, TCD studies and fMRI studies both have participant-inclusion issues, but one usually cannot predict in advance which participants will fail to produce stable TCD data. Also like fMRI, TCD produces correlational data (i.e., changes in cerebral blood flow velocity, CBFv, relative to baseline, that correspond to mental or behavioral activity).

Procedural details for TCD have been described elsewhere (e.g., Aaslid, 1987; McCartney, Thomas-Lukes, & Gomez, 1997; Ringelstein et al., 1990; Stroobant & Vingerhoets, 2000; Tripp & Warm, 2007). Generally, TCD requires the use one or more (typically two, for simultaneous bilateral recordings) 2-MHz ultrasound transducers to generate and receive sonic signals. The transducers are positioned against the head at the cranial windows, or locations where the bone in the skull is thin enough (or absent altogether in the case of foramina) to permit the ultrasonic signal to pass and to be focused on one of the three major cranial arteries. TCD can be used to measure CBFv through the anterior cerebral artery, the middle cerebral artery, or the posterior cerebral artery. For most studies, the middle cerebral artery is targeted with TCD, because of the large areas that are perfused by this artery within each hemisphere; thus, the transducers are typically positioned at the transtemporal windows, at the temples on either side of the forehead, lateral to each of the eyes. By adjusting the angle at which the transducer is aimed and the depth of the sonated signal, and by examining the direction in which blood is flowing, one can identify whether the ultrasonic signal is bouncing off blood cells in the medial cerebral artery or one of the other arteries. Once the desired artery is located and a strong and stable signal is obtained, the transducers are locked in place on a headband. Subsequently, the signal provides continuous measures of CBFv through each transducer, even with head and body movements.

Because the speed with which blood cells move through the arteries varies across the heartbeat, the signal recorded through the TCD transducer/receivers are typically averaged across the heartbeat to produce a mean CBFv value (Saver & Feldmann, 1993). Commercial TCD systems (such as the Nicolet Vascular/Viasys Healthcare Companion-III unit in our laboratory) compute these averages automatically, and also transform the Doppler sonography readings for visual display and digital storage. Task-related changes in mean CBFv values are compared to resting baseline measures. For example, one might record baseline values when participants are simply relaxing and staring at a blank wall.

Since Asslid and colleagues (1982) documented the use of TCD for recording cerebral bloodflow velocity (CBFv), the tool has been explored and tested in a wide range of studies. Clinically, the instrument is used as a diagnostic tool for examining the rate of blood flow through cerebral or other arteries, in connection with the study of stroke, coronary artery disease, and similar conditions. For the present review, we are primarily concerned with the use of TCD to measure changes in CBFv that correspond to mental activities. Increase in mental activity, as when a participant performs a cognitive operation or exerts mental effort, is associated with localized increases in neural firing. This neural activity demands additional blood flow to supply oxygen and to remove metabolic waste materials. Thus, changes in CBFv provide an index of the increase in cognition-related neural activity (e.g.,

Aaslid, 1987; Droste et al., 1989; Stroobant & Vingerhoets, 2000) in much the same way that bioelectrical activity registered by electroencephalography electrodes and radioisotope traces used in single-photon emission computed tomography (SPECT) indicate active brain regions associated with mental functions.

2. TCD for cognitive neuroscience

What value is there in TCD as an indirect measure of mental activity? That is, TCD does not directly measure cognitive activity. Even if cognitive psychology could provide a behavioral task that was a pure manipulation of a single cognitive process (which is impossible, as even the simplest tasks allow that multiple cognitive operations—perception, attention, memory, imagery, language, and the like—may be simultaneously operating, and not necessarily in service of the same outcomes), TCD still would not measure the cognitive operation itself. TCD does not even provide a direct measure of the neural activity that corresponds to the cognitive operations. Rather, TCD yield a measure of the speed of blood flow, which has been shown to be a function of neural activity somewhere in the perfusion zone, which has been shown to increase as mental activity increases. Further, TCD is spatially limited to the three broad, overlapping perfusion areas in each hemisphere that are served by the cerebral arteries. The skeptic might argue that examining the neurocognitive basis of behavior with TCD is like trying to measure the quality of an artist's work by recording patterns of carpet wear in the museum (although at least TCD has the temporal resolution advantage of rapid changes, which would be difficult to capture in the cynical analogy).

Notwithstanding these accurate criticisms, we contend that TCD does indeed have value for cognitive neuroscience, and will point to studies from the literature and from our laboratory that illustrate these benefits. As an overview, we suggest the following uses for TCD from the perspective of cognitive science:

a. Hemispheric differences: A wide range of methods have been used to study the differences between the left and right cerebral hemispheres. Although the popular conceptions of "left brain / right brain" (to borrow the title of Springer & Deutsch's excellent 2001 review of the literature) fail to do justice to the unity, interhemispheric communication and coordination, and plasticity of the brain, it is undeniable that the cerebral hemispheres differ reliably in structural and functional ways. The popular caricature of the left hemisphere as specializing in verbal, analytic, and sequential processing, with the right hemisphere as the home of visuospatial, holistic, parallel processing is at minimum over-simplified, and in many ways simply incorrect. Nevertheless, the localization to the left hemisphere of neural structures involved with language production and comprehension, at least for most right-handed participants, anchors the search for functional cerebral asymmetries that serve to enhance the cognitive competencies of animals (particularly humans) with large, highly encephalized, bilateral brains. The methods for examining these structural and functional asymmetries include all those subsumed under the label of neuroimaging (e.g., fMRI, EEG) as well as the clinical explorations of individuals with brain damage, split-brains (surgical severing of the corpus collosum, for example as an extreme treatment for epilepsy), and so forth. Additionally, a number of noninvasive behavioral paradigms have been used successfully to examine functional cerebral asymmetries, including divided visual-field paradigms and dichotic-listening paradigms which capitalize on the contralateral organization of perceptual-motor processing (e.g., the left hemisphere receives first input from the right side of visual space and from the right ear and controls motor function on the left side of the body, and vice versa). Attempts to measure functional cerebral asymmetries with psychophysiological measures such as tympanic-membrane temperature (e.g., Helton, 2010; Hopkins & Fowler, 1998) have also revealed interesting differences. TCD is arguably a more direct and more sensitive measure of task-related brain activity than is tempanic-membrane temperature, and in any case is a complementary measure in a field where converging evidence from behavioral, psychophysiological, and clinical data are important. Although there is certainly localization of cognitive functions without lateralization, hemispheric asymmetries in cognition do provide broad evidence about localization, which in turn may inform theoretical dissociations. For example, the theoretical dissociation between vigilance (sustained attention) and concentration (executive attention) as components of the construct "attention" has been supported with a variety of neuroimaging and cognitive paradigms (e.g., Posner & Rothbart, 2007)—including TCD, which indicates a right-hemisphere advantage for the control of vigilance (Warm, Matthews, & Parasuraman, 2009).

b. Individual and group differences: Even if TCD provided no information about localization, it provides a behaviorally relevant psychophysiological measure that shows task-related variability that needs to be explained. There are many examples of insights from psychophysical measures that complement, and in many cases that are more sensitive than, overt behavioral responses. Tiny movements of facial muscles, unobservable to the naked eye but recordable through electromyography reflect implicit attitudes about social-category membership (e.g., Vanman, Saltz, Nathan, & Warren, 2004). Variations in skin conductance reveal the contributions of affective states in judgment and decision making (e.g., Naqvi & Bechara, 2006). Occulomotor measures (eye gaze and pupil dilation) reflect the strategy and intensity of cognitive processing in reading and other operations (e.g., Just & Carpenter, 1995). Similarly, TCD provides value to cognitive neuroscience as another measure in which individuals and groups differ, and thus another potential predictor of the massive amount of unexplained variance that characterizes behavior. As will be discussed below, this measure is being used already in research on the cognitive differences between various groups, including females/males, children/adults, old/young, clinically diagnosed/control, and so forth.

c. Third, CBFv from TCD has value as a marker for mental effort. Vingerhoets & Luppens (2001) argued this point specifically (ironically in a study designed to show lateralization effects, which were largely absent in the results). Within a task, within a group, even within a participant, variations in workload or mental effort can alter performance and/or create error in measures of response latency, response accuracy, response topography, and so forth. Changes in CBFv may provide important insights into the intensity of mental activity, even in the absence of overt behavior to indicate stimulus processing. Many theorists have differentiated between two sources or types of cognitive control, in which some behaviors are determined automatically, reactively, through stimulus control or contention scheduling, whereas other behaviors are controlled, proactive, executively or willfully controlled (e.g., Banich, 2009; Braver, Paxton, Locke, & Barch, 2009; Cooper & Shallice, 2000; Hickey, van Zoest, & Theeuwes, 2010; Norman & Shallice, 1986; Schneider & Chein, 2003; Washburn & Taglialatela,

2006). Both automatic and controlled processing involves neural activity, of course, but by definition, automaticity is not cognitively demanding. Thus, one way of distinguish processing that is controlled, willful, and executive in nature (ultimately with the goal of understanding each of these terms in a way that does not require a homunculus) is to look for evidence of mental effort. The changes in CBFv measured by TCD promise to be one such measure. These data would complement other indicators of executive control versus contention scheduling (e.g., another criterion of automaticity is that it is fast, and so chronometric measures have been used to suggest when mental processing is controlled and proactive versus automatic and reactive).

3. Cognitive task-related changes in CBFv

As further evidence of the value of TCD for cognitive neuroscience, consider the studies that currently appear in the literature. Researchers have examined TCD-assessed changes in CBFv as a function of a wide range of cognitive activities. Table 1 shows how the number of PsycINFO-registered publications in which TCD was used has increased over the last three decades, suggesting that the paradigm is currently enjoying a surge in popularity (although it remains the case that most TCD publications are written by scholars in Europe). For comparison purposes, similar publication counts are provided for another relatively inexpensive new transcranial neuroimaging technique, transcranial magnetic stimulation (TMS). For TMS, an electromagnetic coil is used to stimulate neural firing, effectively creating a temporary functional "lesion" that disappears when the magnetic stimulation abates (Walsh & Pascual-Leone, 2005). Like TCD, TMS is noninvasive as the magnetic stimulation passes painlessly and harmlessly through bone and other tissue. Note that the rate of TMS publications has also increased dramatically in recent years; indeed, the rate of growth of cognitive neuroscience studies using TMS far exceeds those using TCD. Nevertheless, neither transcranial technique is being used and published at levels comparable to, or consistent with the growth characteristic of, MRI studies over this same period. (Of course, these publications referenced by PsycINFO reflect only a fraction of the total publications in which TCD, TMS, and MRI are used. For example, MEDLINE shows over 1,300 publications since 2007 using TCD. Some of these surely document CBFv effects of cognitive activity, just like the PsycINFO-referenced articles reviewed in the present chapter; however, it seems reasonable to suppose that most researchers who use TCD to study cognition would select a psychology-related outlet for the publication.)

	1981-1986	1987-1991	1992-1996	1997-2001	2002-2006	2007-2011
TCD	0	15	33	61	95	274
TMS	0	9	61	380	1074	2042
MRI	66	533	1511	3153	6822	16526

Table 1. PsycINFO publications for three neuroimaging methods, by 5-year periods

3.1 Hemispheric differences in CBFv

As Stroobant and Vingerhoets (2000) noted in their review, the primary question in most TCD studies is, "How do the cerebral hemispheres differ with respect to cognitive processing?" Given that the spatial resolution of TCD is limited to the perfusion areas of the cortical arteries being measured, it is difficult to do neuroimaging studies that require localization more specific than broad functional hemispheric asymmetries. (By measuring anterior versus posterior cerebral arteries, it is also possible to examine some general differences between lobes within each hemisphere, but the lateralization studies constitute the preponderance of the TCD literature.) Accordingly, Stroobant and Vingerhoets reviewed clear CBFv evidence for left-hemisphere specialization for processing language-related stimuli, and some less-consistent evidence from TCD studies of right-hemisphere advantages for visuospatial processing.

Lateralization studies since 1999 show similar patterns of results, but not without exceptions. For example, Kratch, Chen, and Hartje (2006) assessed functional cerebral asymmetries using TCD as well as a divided visual field paradigm. Although both measures showed lateralization effects for lexical-decision performance, the effects were not reliably correlated across paradigms. This task showed the predicted left-hemisphere advantage in the divided visual field procedure, but produced faster right-hemisphere than left-hemisphere CBFv. Similarly, Knetch and colleagues (2001) focused on participants with atypical, right-hemisphere specialization for language, as revealed by TCD, but did not find these participants to be deficient in linguistic performance on a variety of measures. Conversely, Szirmai and colleagues (2005) examined lateralization for verbal fluency and mental arithmetic tasks using both TCD and electroencephalography measures, and found significant correlations, at least for verbal fluency.

In our laboratory, we have also examined functional cerebral asymmetries in cognitive performance using a variety of paradigms, including TCD. In studies of individual differences in attention skills, we required participants to monitor a scene and to make rapid and accurate shoot/don't-shoot responses to target/nontarget stimuli (Schultz, Matthews, Warm & Washburn, 2009). The scene was projected on a wall so as to fill the visual field, and participants used a laser-modified handgun to respond to infrequent target images that appeared during a 36-minute vigil (see Figure 1). CBFv was bilaterally recorded throughout the vigil, and during a resting baseline period, to determine whether TCD measures would show vigilance decrements corresponding to the changes in task performance (response time, target detection hits and misses, marksmanship accuracy) as a function of time-on-task. As will be discussed below, systematic vigilance effects were observed. Of relevance to the present discussion, we also reported significant hemispheric differences for this task (albeit in the opposite direction from what was predicted). Parallel vigilance decrements were obtained for both cerebral hemispheres, but mean CBFv was consistently faster (relative to baseline) in the left hemisphere than in the right hemisphere, across the vigil.

In follow-up studies (e.g., Schultz, Phillips, & Washburn, 2010), we further investigated this cerebral asymmetry. The right-hemisphere advantage was unexpected, given the sustained-attention demands of this shoot/don't-shoot task. A speeded threat/nonthreat determination was required of participants every 3 seconds on average (interstimulus interval was randomized between 1 and 5 seconds), but only 25% of the stimuli required a "shoot" response. Given the long watchkeeping period and indeed the clear vigilance decrements that were observed across this period in response latency, decision accuracy (hits, misses, false alarms), and marksmanship accuracy, we expected to see evidence in the TCD data for a right-hemisphere specialization in vigilance. This prediction was based on findings that right frontal regions and right parietal cortex serve, along with the locus coeruleus, as a brain network for alertness or vigilance (Posner & Raichle, 1997; Warm et al., 2009). Our finding of elevated CBFv in the left hemisphere compared to the right hemisphere—an advantage that was stable across the vigil—was surprising.

The stability of the hemispheric difference in CBFv across the watchperiod provides one clue toward unpacking this curious result. In earlier TCD studies of vigilance (Helton et al, 2007; Hitchcock et al., 2003; Warm et al., 2009), the right-hemisphere advantage became evident as time-on-task increased. Early in the vigil, mean CBFv (relative to resting baseline) was comparable in the two hemispheres, but as the demands on sustaining attention increased over time, a cerebral asymmetry emerged reflecting activity in the right cerebral hemisphere. This consistent and intuitive finding is *not* what was observed in the TCD data of the Schultz and collaborators (2009) study. In our task, faster CBFv in the left hemisphere was observed even in the first quarter of the watchperiod. Indeed, in follow-up analyses we noted that the left-hemisphere advantage in CBFv is statistically significant within the very first minute of the task (Schultz, Phillips, & Washburn, 2010). This is presumably before vigilance would be required, or at least when the demands on sustained attention should be minimal. That this level of asymmetry was then stable throughout the vigil suggests that our left-hemisphere advantage for this task was not indicative of the lateralization of vigilance,

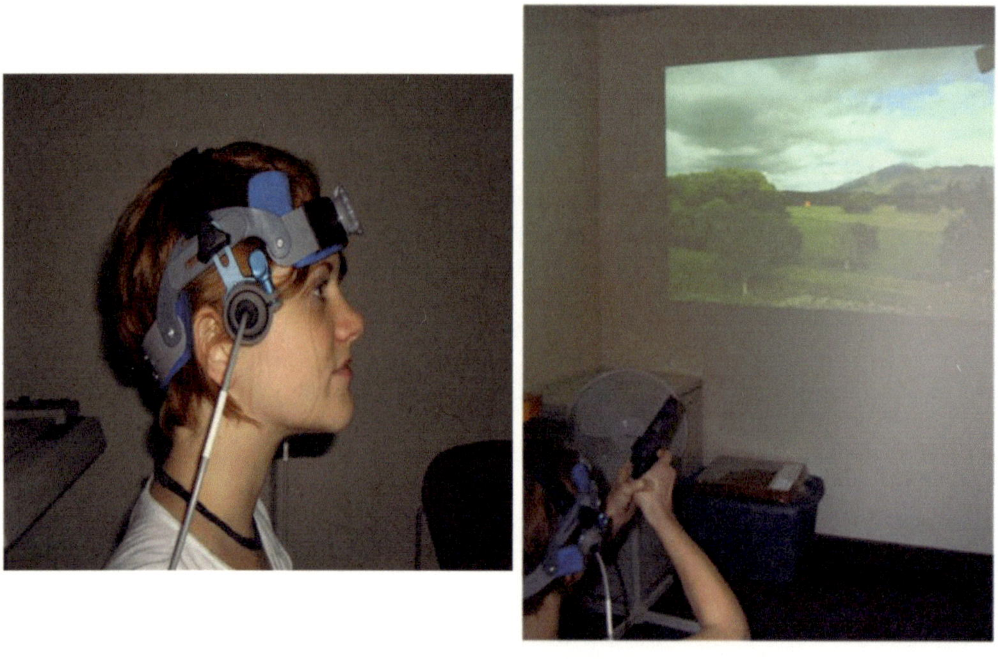

Fig. 1. Apparatus used in the Schultz et al. (2009) study. Left: The Transcranial Doppler Sonography transducers positioned at the right and left (not pictured) transtemporal window for recording changes in cerebral blood flow velocity through the middle cerebral artery of each hemisphere. The two 2-MHz transducers are connected to a Companion III TCD system (Nicolet/EME, Madison, WI), which uses Fast Fourier analysis to transform the signals and displays mean CBFv for each heartbeat-cycle envelope. Right: The participant uses a laser-modified handgun to respond to computer-generated stimuli projected on a wall. Shots were automatically detected and recorded (time, location) by LaserShot (Stafford, TX) hardware and software

but rather a lateralization of the shoot/don't-shoot judgments themselves that whelmed any right-hemisphere localization of sustained attention. In our study, the encoding and discrimination of threat/nonthreat images and the motor-preparation/aim/fire components of responding showed a left-hemisphere lateralization. With respect to this conclusion, it is important to note that all of our participants were right handed (as assessed by self-report); thus, it remains to be determined the proportion of this left-hemisphere advantage that is directly related to motor versus cognitive factors.

3.2 Group differences in CBFv

Stroobert and Vingerhoets (2000) reviewed the literature on cerebral hemodymanic effects of cognitive task performance. The tasks included in this review span a wide range, including simple motor tasks, linguistic tasks (e.g., reading, synonyms, syntax, word association, sentence completion, verbal fluency), visuospatial tasks (e.g., faces, designs, imagination, picture matching, cube comparison, mental rotation), numeric tasks (e.g., multiplication, dot estimation), and other tasks (e.g., music, sorting, vibratory stimulation, passive viewing). Their review summarized major themes of research and findings to that date. For example, they summarized TCD studies on the effects of gender, age, and handedness on CBFv and lateralization (i.e., hemispheric differences) in CBFv. They noted that blood flow velocity declines in older adults, as does lateralization. Where gender differences were reported, females produced higher CBFv. Handedness effects on lateralization were also reported, with consistent left-hemisphere advantages for the processing of linguistic stimuli among right-handed participants. The pattern of cerebral asymmetries in CBFv were less clear for left-handed participants (as is typically found using other paradigms as well).

Studies along these lines have continued in the years since the Stroobant and Vingerhoets (2000) review. For example, Bracco and colleagues (2011) used TCD with a memory task, and found that both males and females showed material-specific lateralization effects (e.g., memory for verbal material was lateralized to the left hemisphere, whereas memory for visuospatial material was right-hemisphere lateralized), although the lateralization of nonverbalizable material was attenuated with aging. Sorond and colleagues (2008) also found effects of aging on TCD values as participants performed word-stem completion and visual-search tasks. CBFv increase differentially in the anterior and posterior cerebral arteries for the elderly compared to the young-adult participants.

Although the Bracco et al. (2011) study reported no gender differences in CBFv, Walter, Roberts and Brownlow (2000) reported gender differences in CBFv (women faster than men) and lateralization patterns during performance of visuospatial tasks (mental rotation, visualizing). Similarly, Njemanze (2005) observed different hemispheric advantages for females and males solving the Raven's Progressive Matrices test, with females showing a left-hemisphere advantage and males showing a right-hemisphere effect. Schuepbach and colleagues (2009) used the Wisconson Card Sorting Test, and found linkages between the mental slowing that occurs during set-shifting and increases in CBFv, but only for females. Misteli and colleagues (2011) tested participants with a different executive functioning task (Trail-making) and found a similar gender difference in TCD data, with females showing a lateralization shift that was synchronized to a frequency peak in middle cerebral artery CBFv.

There have been many studies in which TCD was collected as part of comparisons between groups formed on the basis of clinical diagnoses. Cognitive testing has been complemented with TCD measures of CBFv to study the executive-function skills (Kral & Brown, 2004; Kral et al., 2003) and language functioning (Sanchez, Schatz, & Roberts, 2010) of children with sickle cell disease; to examine the executive-function deficits, particularly those involved in planning, associated with schizophrenia (Feldmann et al., 2006; Schuepback, Weber, Kawohl, & Hell, 2007); in the attention skills of participants with and without hypotension (Duschek & Schandry, 2004); in elderly adults with versus without depression (Tiemeier et al., 2002); to examine executive functioning in patients with Huntington's disease versus healthy controls (Deckel, Cohen, & Duckrow, 1998); and in the mental activity patterns of healthy individuals versus individuals recovering from stroke versus individuals who have shown no recovery from stroke (Bragoni et al., 2000). The results of these patterns are not as simple as "clinical conditions are associated with slower CBFv"—although that is what one sees for planning by individuals with schizophrenia compared to healthy controls (Feldmann et al., 2006), for depressed individuals compared to their nondepressed cohort (Tiemeier et al., 2002), and for individuals with Huntington's disease compared to healthy individuals (Deckel et al., 1998). Conversely, poorer cognitive performance by children with sickle cell disease is associated with abnormally high CBFv (Krall and colleagues, 2003, 2004; Sanchez et al., 2010). Another pattern of results is apparent in several studies, where CBFv is comparable between the comparison groups, but the clinical population shows less modulation or lateralization of blood flow, compared to healthy controls. This result was reported for individuals with schizophrenia (Schuepback et al., 2007) and for hypotensive compared to normotensive patients (Duschek & Schandry, 2004).

As was discussed above, one drawback to the TCD method is that there are participants for whom it is difficult or impossible to acquire CBFv readings from the middle cerebral artery on both sides of the brain. For many participants, bilateral measurement of this artery is easy to acquire, whereas even highly skilled experimenters are unable to sonate one or both arteries for other participants. We were interested in whether there are cognitive differences to correspond to these groups (i.e., participants from whom left+right hemisphere signals were obtained, compared to participants with left-hemisphere readings only, those with right-hemisphere readings, and those for whom neither hemisphere could be reliably sonated. Each of 540 undergraduate volunteers were tested on a shoot/don't-shoot task like the one described above (Schultz et al., 2009). For 47% of these volunteers, bilateral recording was possible. For 17% of the sample, only the right hemisphere could be sonated, whereas 5% of the participants contributed CBFv data only for the left hemisphere. The remaining 31% of the participants completed the shoot/don't-shoot task wearing the TCD apparatus, but a reliable signal for the cerebral artery of interest could not be located on either side of the brain.

We examined performance measures to determine whether these group differences were meaningful and diagnostic in any way. Table 2 summarizes shoot/don't-shoot performance for these four groups of participants. No differences were observed between the groups in decision accuracy (i.e., hit rate or false-alarm rate) or shot latency. For marksmanship error, there was a significant difference, which post doc analyses revealed to be the result of significantly ($p < .02$) poorer marksmanship by the group in which no TCD signal was obtained, compared to the other three groups. Participants for whom we were unable to locate a stable middle-cerebral-artery signal in either hemisphere produced shots about 15%

less accurate (further from the target) than the other participants. Perhaps this difference in marksmanship was a function, at least in part, of the relatively longer experimental sessions for these participants (i.e., the experimenters would try as long as possible to find a stable signal, and thus participants without a signal spent more time on average in the pre-task phase of the study than did the other volunteers). In any case, this difference seems fairly inconsequential in comparison to the more general finding: The subset of the sample for which good, bilateral recording was possible appears to be representative of the entire pool of volunteers, at least with respect to performance measures on this shoot/don't-shoot task. We see little reason to conclude that there is anything worrisome or diagnostic in this particular between-groups variable.

	Hit Rate	False-alarm Rate	Shot Latency	Marksmanship error
Both hemispheres	86%	1%	987 msec	2.79 cm
Left hemisphere only	83%	1%	1035 msec	2.56 cm
Right hemisphere only	86%	1%	994 msec	2.80 cm
Neither hemisphere	86%	1%	982 msec	3.20 cm

Table 2. Shoot/don't-shoot decision making, decision latency, and marksmanship accuracy as a function of groups formed on the basis of whether we were able to obtain stable TCD signals from the left and right cerebral hemispheres

One can also compare cognitive-task performance and CBFv measures between groups that are formed on the basis of performance on some criterial task or measure. Researchers who study working-memory capacity, for example, have been using this extreme-groups design strategy to reveal the cognitive and neural differences between individuals with high-span versus low-span memories (e.g., Chein, Moore & Conway, 2011; Kleider, Parrot, & King, 2010; Osaka et al., 2004; Unsworth & Engle, 2008)—although it appears that no one to date has compared CBFv of span-based groups using TCD. Duschek, Schuepbach and Schandry (2008) did however compare CBFv values derived from TCD between two groups that were formed on the basis of performance on a simple reaction-time task with an auditory attention cue. High-performance participants were characterized by greater increases in bilateral CBFv than low-performance participants—a difference that was significant even two seconds after the alerting tone (i.e., three seconds before presentation of the visual stimulus that required a response).

In our laboratory, we routinely test participants on a battery of attention-related tasks (the Assessment Software for Attention Profiles or ASAP battery), and subsequently form and compare groups on the basis of these attention profiles (e.g., Washburn, Smith & Taglialatela, 2005). The ASAP battery was constructed to include tasks that load on each component factor or dimension of attention (see Table 3). For example, previous factor analyses of the ASAP battery show that performance on incongruent Stroop trials clusters together with performance on a stop-signal inhibition task and response times on the "executive" component of the Attention Network Test (incongruent - congruent flanker stimuli; see Fan et al., 2005). Quartile splits were used to divide participants into groups, so that the top- and bottom-quartile-groups might be compared with respect to CBFv.

Factor or Dimension (with alternate names from the literature)	ASAP tasks (determined by prior factor analyses)	Left hemisphere mean CBFv, relative to resting baseline	Right hemisphere mean CBFv, relative to resting baseline	*p*
Attention focusing (executive attention, concentration)	Stroop, Stop-signal, ANT-executive	1.967 (0.28)	1.533 (0.22)	$p < .01$
Attention scanning (orienting, shifting, selection)	Cue task, Antisaccade task, Visual Search	-1.202 (0.77)	-1.032 (1.06)	$p > .10$
Attention sustaining (alerting, vigilance)	Continuous Performance Task, ANT-alerting	0.150 (0.78)	0.75 (0.67)	$p < .05$

Table 3. Mean CBFv values (expressed relative to resting baseline, such that positive numbers indicate that blood flow had increased compared to baseline, whereas negative numbers denote slower-than-baseline blood flow) and standard deviations by cerebral hemisphere and attention-factor

A similar extreme-groups strategy was used to analyze task performance described by Schultz et al. (2009), described above. Participants in the shoot/don't-shoot study were grouped according to quartiles, based on response latency and marksmanship accuracy. That is, we grouped the fastest shooters together in a group, using only those trials in which the stimulus was in fact a threat or "shoot" target, and the slowest shooters together in another group. Similarly, we grouped the most accurate shooters—again, not in terms of decision accuracy, as each of these responses was a "hit" in the sense of being a "shoot" response to a threat stimulus, but rather in terms of marksmanship accuracy, measured by the distance between the target and the location of the fired laser shot. Participants with least-accurate marksmanship were grouped together for comparison. Mean CBFv values were then computed from the middle cerebral artery of each hemisphere for each of these groups. Figure 2 summarizes the results of these analyses.

When the fastest-shooters were compared to the slowest-shooters group, a significant interaction was observed. The fastest shooters were characterized by a significant left-hemisphere advantage in CBFv. For the slowest-shooter group, CBFv was slightly but not significantly faster in the right hemisphere. This interaction was not seen in the extreme-groups analysis based on marksmanship accuracy, where both groups displayed left-lateralized CBFv for the task (as was seen for the overall analysis of all participants).

These same data also illustrate how TCD has been used to provide an individual-differences measure for psychometric studies of cognition. Recall the nature of the laboratory task discussed here: A participant is required to monitor a naturalistic scene and to make repeated threat/nonthreat (shoot/don't-shoot) judgments on the basis of stimulus appearance. The task was designed to mimic some of the elements of the real-life task performed by security officers, sentries, or police officers, or soldiers on a peacekeeping mission. These individuals must maintain vigilant attention across time, while they make

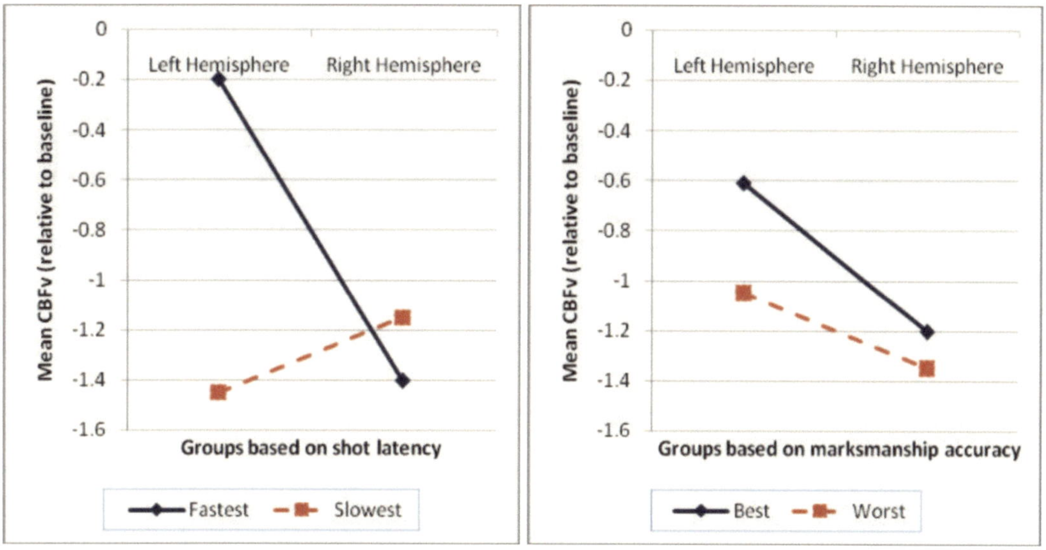

Fig. 2. Comparison of mean CBFv, relative to baseline, between performance-based groups in the shoot/don't-shoot task. Left: Groups formed on the basis of shot latency. Right: Groups formed on the basis of marksmanship accuracy

threat/nonthreat judgments about events around them. Threatening events are rare in most cases, but the life-or-death costs of making a poor decision (e.g., being too slow to shoot if there is a threat, or too quick to shoot at what turns out to be a nonthreat stimulus) are severe. Ideally, one would want a way of monitoring vigilance so that individuals faced with these critical decisions could be maximally attentive, or perhaps so interventions could be introduced at points when vigilance is flagging. This was the rationale behind the shoot/don't-shoot study designed by Schultz and colleagues (2009), who attempted to use measures available prior to a "shoot" response to predict the speed with which participants would respond to threat stimuli.

We found that response latency to a threat stimulus was significantly predicted by the participant's response time on the previous "shoot" trial, irrespective of how long it had been since that response ($R^2 = .098$, $p < 01$). By adding time-on-task to the regression equation, one could significantly increase the proportion of variance accounted for ($\Delta R^2 = .024$, $p < 01$). One could significantly augment this prediction further by adding a measure of CBFv in the left hemisphere. In fact, the prediction of shot latency was improved by CBFv values from the left hemisphere even if those values were selected as far back as 18 seconds before the threat image appeared on the screen ($\Delta R^2 = .015$, $p < 01$). Overall, we were able to account for 13% of the variance in shot latency by knowing how quickly the participant tends to shoot when the response is appropriate, how long the participant has been required to remain vigilant on the task, and how rapidly blood is flowing through the middle cerebral artery of the left hemisphere. Of course, 13% of explained variability means that 87% of the variability remains unexplained, and further investigation with additional predictors is required to make this statistically significant prediction more practical. For the present discussion however, the fact that CBFv measures reliably augment the prediction of task performance is sufficient to illustrate the ways that TCD has been, and can be, used in the study of individual differences.

The Matthews and colleagues, 2010, study discussed below also illustrates this use of TCD as a diagnostic tool. Further, Warm and colleagues (2009) reported that TCD measures may be useful as a selection tool for assigning personnel to vigilance duties. Reporting on the results of a study in their laboratory by Reinerman and collaborators (2006), these authors argue that CBFv changes during a battery of demanding tasks, combined with self-report measures of task engagement, significantly predicted subsequent vigilance performance. As was discussed above, these measures combined to account for 13% of the variance in subsequent vigilance performance.

3.3 TCD studies of attention and executive function

As summarized above and by Stroobant and Vingerhoets (2000), many researchers designing TCD studies over the last three decades have included explicitly verbal or visuospatial tasks, primarily to study lateralization effects (e.g., Dorst et al., 2008; Haag et al., 2010; Horton-Lambirth & Roberts, 1998; Lust, Geuze, Groothuis, and Bouma, 2010). A more recent development in the TCD literature is the increase in tasks designed to measure attention and closely related processes like inhibition, set-switching, planning, and maintaining/monitoring (i.e., the so-called "executive functions" or EF; see Banich, 2009; Barkley & Murphy, 2011; Latzman & Markon, 2010; Lyon & Krasnegor, 2005; Wiebe et al., 2011). Discussed already are recent studies in which popular attention and EF tasks like Wisconsin Card Sort, Trail-making, Stroop task, and Visual Search were used, albeit those discussions were focused on the group (e.g., gender) differences that were revealed in these tasks and in task-relevant changes in CBFv. Beyond this use of attention and EF tasks as potential measures on which differences may seen across genders, ages, diagnostic categories, and so forth, TCD may contribute to understanding of cognitive control and the ways that mental effort is allocated (or in the instances of cognitive disorders, is not allocated or controlled) to produce goal-appropriate performance.

One of the significant developments in the TCD field over the last decade is the emergence of a productive research team at the University of Cincinnati, anchored by Gerald Matthews, Joel Warm, and their collaborators. This research team studies cognition in applied settings, with particular attention to the relation between individual differences in cognitive and personality profiles and performance in human-machine (human factors) environments. For these scientists, with their backgrounds in research on topics like mental workload, stress states, and vigilance, TCD provided an ideal tool for continuous and noninvasive assay of cognitive activity. To quote the title of one of their publications (Warm, Parasuraman & Matthews, 2008), "vigilance requires hard mental work and is stressful" and it seemed reasonable to suppose that TCD would provide a way to As was discussed above, these researchers quickly established a literature on the cerebral hemodynamics of vigilance, documenting the decline of CBFv as a function of time-on-task that reflects the gradual shift from controlled toward automatic, less-attentive processing across the watchperiod (Helton et al., 2007; Schultz et al., 2009; Warm & Parasuraman, 2007; Warm et al., 2009). They also demonstrated that salient signals from the environment in the form of automation cuing of potential threats during the vigil can attenuate this decline in CBFv and mitigate the vigilance decrement (Hitchcock et al., 2003).

Matthews and colleagues (2010) used TCD as part of a battery of personality, psychophysiological, stress-state, and cognitive measures to predict vigilance performance of two groups of participants, each completing one of two vigilance tasks. As has been demonstrated consistently across many studies, CBFv declined across the watchperiod, and correlated with decrements in performance measures. Interestingly, CBFv was faster in the left hemisphere than the right hemisphere in this study, as had been reported by Schultz and collaborators (2009). Indeed, the pattern of performance from a sensory vigilance task in which participants monitored a display for 36 minutes and made judgments about a series of stimuli that depicted either "safe" or "threat" air-traffic situations. In contrast however, the decline in CFBv was more precipitous for the TCD data from the right hemisphere than from the left hemisphere for the vigilance task that required participants to retain and manipulate information in memory across the 36-minute test. For both vigilance tasks, CBFv was comparable in the blateral middle cerebral arteries at the outset of the vigil, but for the more cognitively demanding task the degree of lateralization was modulated across the vigil.

Matthews and colleagues (2010) used structural equation modeling to test a series of latent-factor models of effortful, sustained attention in tasks that require vigilance. The model that successfully fit the data included latent variables representing task engagement, derived from a self-report instrument administered during a pre-test baseline period and after the participants performed several cognitive tasks. The model also included CBFv, which appeared to index another resource-related energizing function, such as a psychophysiological proxy of mental effort. The addition of other predictors did not substantively improve the fit of this model, which accounted for 19% of the variance in performance on the the sensory (air-traffic control) vigilance task, and 18% of the variability in the cognitively demanding (working memory) vigilance task.

Of course, the hemodynamic correlates of cognitive control have been investigated by other researchers as well. In several studies, Duschek, Schuepbach, and colleagues provided elegant evidence for TCD as a tool for measuring the bilateral increases in CBFv as participants prepare and process task relevant information (Duschek, Schuepbach & Schandry, 2008; Schuepbach, Boeker, Duschek & Hell, 2007). In each study, the authors traced the time-course of CBFv changes, and linked those changes to pre-response cognitive processes such as preparatory attention and planning, respectively. Similarly, Schuepbach and collaborators (2004) examined the effects of set-maintenance and set-switching on CBFv in the anterior and middle cerebral arteries of each hemisphere, and found significant increases in peak CBFv in the anterior perfusion region. In In another study from this general research team, Duschek, Werner, Kapan, and Reyes del Paso (2008) used TCD and various other instruments to study psychophysiological changes during mental arithmetic, and attributed the observed left-hemisphere increase in CBFv to the cognitive effort required to perform the "cross sum" task (i.e., to add four single-digit numbers, and then to add the digits of the result). In our laboratory, we also used a mental arithmetic task as a distractor condition during a vigilance task, to show that the hemodynamic and behavioral patterns produced by inattention are discernable from the hemodynamic and performance patterns produced by distraction (i.e., of covertly switching attention to task-irrelevant processing; Washburn & Schultz, 2009).

4. Summary

Despite the limitations of the TCD paradigm, evidence is growing that it is a valuable tool in the study of brain-behavior relations that constitute cognitive competence. Many questions remain about the structural and functional differences between the cerebral hemispheres, and how those differences interact with grouping variables like gender, age, and diagnostic category; however, the present authors are most excited about the potential for using TCD to provide a measure of mental effort and cognitive control. Recent studies from scholars on both sides of the Atlantic Ocean illustrate the several ways that this noninvasive paradigm for the continuous, bilateral measurement of CBFv can inform our understanding of mental effort—providing in some instances converging evidence that can be integrated with behavioral observations (e.g., response latencies or accuracy levels), and in other cases a method for measuring the intensity of cognitive processing even in the absence of corresponding overt behavior.

5. Acknowledgments

The authors acknowledge the assistance of Gerald Matthews and Joel Warm in establishing our TCD laboratory, and the assistance of Jared Taglialagela, Frances James and R. Thompson Putney in some of the tasks reviewed here. This research and development, and preparation of this chapter were supported by grants and contracts from the National Institute of Child Health and Human Development (HD-060563), the United States Army Medical Research and Materiel Command (W81XWH-04-C-0002), and by Georgia State University. For more information, contact David A. Washburn, Department of Psychology, Georgia State University, Box 5010, Atlanta, GA 30302-5010, USA or dwashburn@gsu.edu.

6. References

Aaslid, R. (1987). Visually evoked dynamic blood flow response of the human cerebral circulation. *Stroke* 18: 771–775.

Aaslid, R., Markwalder, T. M., and Nornes, H. (1982). Noninvasive transcranial Doppler ultrasound recording of flow velocity in basal cerebral arteries. *Journal of Neurosurgery* 57: 769–774.

Banich, M. T. (2009). Executive Function: The Search for an Integrated Account. *Current Directions in Psychological Science (Wiley-Blackwell)*, 18(2), 89-94. doi:10.1111/j.1467-8721.2009.01615.x

Barkley, R. A., & Murphy, K. R. (2011). The Nature of Executive Function (EF) Deficits in Daily Life Activities in Adults with ADHD and Their Relationship to Performance on EF Tests. *Journal of Psychopathology & Behavioral Assessment*, 33(2), 137-158. doi:10.1007/s10862-011-9217-x

Bragoni, M. M., Caltagirone, C. C., Troisi, E. E., Matteis, M. M., Vernieri, F. F., & Silvestrini, M. M. (2000). Correlation of cerebral hemodynamic changes during mental activity and recovery after stroke. *Neurology*, 55(1), 35-40.

Braver, T. S., Paxton, J. L., Locke, H. S., & Barch, D. M. (2009). Flexible neural mechanisms of cognitive control within human prefrontal cortex. *Proceedings of the National Academy of Sciences of the United States of America*, 106(18), 7351-7356.

Chein, J. M., Moore, A. B., & Conway, A. A. (2011). Domain-general mechanisms of complex working memory span. *NeuroImage*, 54(1), 550-559. doi:10.1016/j.neuroimage.2010.07.067

Cooper, R., & Shallice, T. (2000). Contention Scheduling and the Control of Routine Activities. *Cognitive Neuropsychology*, 17(4), 297-338. doi:10.1080/026432900380427

Demarin, V., Kes, V., Morović, S., & Zavoreo, I. (2009). Evaluation of aging vs dementia by means of neurosonology. *Journal of the Neurological Sciences*, 283(1-2), 9-12. doi:10.1016/j.jns.2009.02.006

Deckel, A., Cohen, D., & Duckrow, R. (1998). Cerebral blood flow velocity decreases during cognitive stimulation in Huntington's disease. *Neurology*, 51(6), 1576-1583.

Dorst, J. J., Haag, A. A., Knake, S. S., Oertel, W. H., Hamer, H. M., & Rosenow, F. F. (2008). Functional transcranial Doppler sonography and a spatial orientation paradigm identify the non-dominant hemisphere. *Brain and Cognition*, 68(1), 53-58. doi:10.1016/j.bandc.2008.02.123

Droste, D. W., Harders, A. G., and Rastogi, E. (1989). Two transcranial Doppler studies on blood flow velocity in both middle cerebral arteries during rest and the performance of cognitive tasks. *Neuropsychologia* 27: 1221–1230.

Duschek, S., Hadjamu, M., & Schandry, R. (2007). Enhancement of cerebral blood flow and cognitive performance following pharmacological blood pressure elevation in chronic hypotension. *Psychophysiology*, 44(1), 145-153. doi:10.1111/j.1469-8986.2006.00472.x

Duschek, S., & Schandry, R. (2004). Cognitive performance and cerebral blood flow in essential hypotension. *Psychophysiology*, 41(6), 905-913. doi:10.1111/j.1469-8986.2004.00249.x

Duschek, S., Werner, N., Kapan, N., & Reyes de Paso, G. A. (2008). Patterns of cerebral blood flow and systemic hemodynamics during arithmetic processing. *Journal of Psychophysiology*, 22(2), 81-90. doi:10.1027/0269-8803.22.2.81

Fan, J., McCandliss, B. D., Fossella, J., Flombaum, J. I., & Posner, M. I. (2005). The activation of attentional networks. *NeuroImage*, 26(2), 471-479. doi:10.1016/j.neuroimage.2005.02.004

Feldmann, D., Schuepbach, D., von Rickenbach, B., Theodoridou, A., & Hell, D. (2006). Association between two distinct executive tasks in schizophrenia: A functional transcranial Doppler sonography study. *BMC Psychiatry*, 6doi:10.1186/1471-244X-6-25

Haag, A., Moeller, N., Knake, S., Hermsen, A., Oertel, W. H., Rosenow, F., & Hamer, H. M. (2010). Language lateralization in children using functional transcranial Doppler sonography. *Developmental Medicine & Child Neurology*, 52(4), 331-336. doi:10.1111/j.1469-8749.2009.03362.x

Haupt, E. J. (2001). Laboratories for experimental psychology: Göttingen's ascendancy over Leipzig in the 1890s. In R. W. Rieber, D. K. Robinson, R. W. Rieber, D. K. Robinson (Eds.) , *Wilhelm Wundt in History: The Making of a Scientific Psychology* (pp. 205-250). New York, NY US: Kluwer Academic/Plenum Publishers.

Helton, W. S. (2010). The relationship between lateral differences in tympanic membrane temperature and behavioral impulsivity. *Brain and Cognition*, 74(2), 75-78. doi:10.1016/j.bandc.2010.06.008

Helton, W. S., Hollander, T. D., Warm, J. S., Tripp, L. D., Parsons, K., Matthews, G., Dember, W. N., Parasuraman, R., & Hancock, P. A. (2007). The abbreviated vigilance task and cerebral hemodynamics. *Journal of Clinical & Experimental Neuropsychology*, 29(5), 545-552. doi:10.1080/13803390600814757

Hickey, C., van Zoest, W., & Theeuwes, J. (2010). The time course of exogenous and endogenous control of covert attention. *Experimental Brain Research*, 201(4), 789-796. doi:10.1007/s00221-009-2094-9

Hitchcock, E. M., Warm, J. S., Matthews, G., Dember, W. N., Shear, P. K., Tripp, L. D., Mayleben, D. W., & Parasuraman, R. (2003). Automation cueing modulates cerebral blood flow and vigilance in a simulated air traffic control task. *Theoretical Issues in Ergonomics Science*, 4(1-2), 89-112. doi:10.1080/14639220210159726

Hopkins, W. D., & Fowler, L. A. (1998). Lateralized changes in tympanic membrane temperature in relation to different cognitive tasks in chimpanzees (Pan troglodytes). *Behavioral Neuroscience*, 112(1), 83-88. doi:10.1037/0735-7044.112.1.83

Horton-Lambirth, A., & Roberts, A. E. (1998). Cerebral blood flow velocities modulate during cognitive tasks using vision and vision-like requirements: A TCD study. *Psychobiology*, 26(3), 183-189.

Just, M., & Carpenter, P. A. (1995). The intensity dimension of thought: Pupillometric indices of sentence processing. In J. M. Henderson, M. Singer, F. Ferreira, J. M. Henderson, M. Singer, F. Ferreira (Eds.), *Reading and language processing* (pp. 182-211). Hillsdale, NJ England: Lawrence Erlbaum Associates, Inc.

Kleider, H. M., Parrott, D. J., & King, T. Z. (2010). Shooting behaviour: How working memory and negative emotionality influence police officer shoot decisions. *Applied Cognitive Psychology*, 24(5), 707-717. doi:10.1002/acp.1580

Knecht, S., Dräger, B. B., Flöel, A. A., Lohmann, H. H., Breitenstein, C. C., Henningsen, H. H., & Ringelstein, E. B. (2001). Behavioural relevance of atypical language lateralization in healthy subjects. *Brain: A Journal of Neurology*, 124(8), 1657-1665. doi:10.1093/brain/124.8.1657

Kral, M. C., & Brown, R. T. (2004). Transcranial Doppler ultrasonography and executive dysfunction in children with sickle cell disease. *Journal of Pediatric Psychology*, 29(3), 185-195. doi:10.1093/jpepsy/jsh020

Kral, M., Brown, R., Nietert, P., Abboud, M., Jackson, S., & Hynd, G. (2003). Transcranial Doppler ultrasonography and neurocognitive functioning in children with sickle cell disease. *Pediatrics*, 112(2), 324-331.

Latzman, R. D., & Markon, K. E. (2010). The Factor Structure and Age-Related Factorial Invariance of the Delis-Kaplan Executive Function System (D-KEFS). *Assessment*, 17(2), 172-184. doi:10.1177/1073191109356254

Lust, J. M., Geuze, R. H., Groothuis, A. G., & Bouma, A. A. (2010). Functional cerebral lateralization and dual-task efficiency—testing the function of human brain lateralization using ftcd. *Behavioural Brain Research*, doi:10.1016/j.bbr.2010.10.029

Lyon, G. R., & Krasnegor, N. A. (Eds.) 2005. *Attention, Memory, and Executive Function*. Baltimore, MD: Paul H. Brookes Publishing Company.

Matthews, G., Warm, J., Reinerman-Jones, L., Langheim, L., Washburn, D., & Tripp, L. (2010). Task engagement, cerebral blood flow velocity, and diagnostic monitoring for sustained attention. *Journal of Experimental Psychology: Applied*, 16, 187-203

McCartney, J. P., Thomas-Lukes, K. M., and Gomez, C. R. (1997). *Handbook of Transcranial Doppler*. New York, NY:Springer-Verlag.

Misteli, M., Duschek, S., Richter, A., Grimm, S., Rezk, M., Kraehenmann, R., & ... Schuepbach, D. (2011). Gender characteristics of cerebral hemodynamics during complex cognitive functioning. *Brain and Cognition*, 76(1), 123-130. doi:10.1016/j.bandc.2011.02.009

Naqvi, N. H., & Bechara, A. (2006). Skin Conductance: A Psychophysiological Approach to the Study of Decision Making. In C. Senior, T. Russell, M. S. Gazzaniga, C. Senior, T. Russell, M. S. Gazzaniga (Eds.) , *Methods in mind* (pp. 103-122). Cambridge, MA US: MIT Press.

Njemanze, P. C. (2006). Cerebral lateralisation for facial processing: Gender-related cognitive styles determined using Fourier analysis of mean cerebral blood flow velocity in the middle cerebral arteries. *Laterality: Asymmetries of Body, Brain and Cognition*, 12(1), 31-49. doi:10.1080/13576500600886796

Norman, D.A., & Shallice, T. (1986). Attention to action: Willed and automatic control of behaviour. In R. Davidson, G. Schwartz, & D. Shapiro, (Eds.), *Consciousness and self regulation: Advances in research and theory*, Vol. 4 (pp. 1–18). New York: Plenum.

Osaka, M., Osaka, N., Kondo, H., Morishita, M., Fukuyama, H., Aso, T., & Shibasaki, H. (2003). The neural basis of individual differences in working memory capacity: an fMRI study. *NeuroImage*, 18(3), 789. doi:10.1016/S1053-8119(02)00032-0

Posner, M. I., & Raichle, M. E. (1997). *Images of Mind*. New York, NY: W. H. Freeman

Posner, M. I., & Rothbart, M. K. (2007). Research on Attention Networks as a Model for the Integration of Psychological Science. *Annual Review of Psychology*, 581-23. doi:10.1146/annurev.psych.58.110405.085516

Reinerman, L. E., Matthews, G.,Warm, J. S., Langheim, L. K., Parsons, K., Proctor, C. A., et al. (2006). Cerebral blood flow velocity and task engagement as predictors of vigilance performance. *Proceedings of the Human Factors and Ergonomics Society*, 50, 1254–1258.

Ringelstein, E. B., Kahlscheuer, B., Niggemeyer, E., and Otis, S. M. (1990). Transcranial Doppler sonography: Anatomical landmarks and normal velocity values. *Ultrasound in Medicine and Biology* 16, 745–761.

Risberg, J. (1986). Regional cerebral blood flow in neuropsychology. *Neuropsychologia* 24: 135–140.

Sanchez, C. E., Schatz, J., & Roberts, C. W. (2010). Cerebral blood flow velocity and language functioning in pediatric sickle cell disease. *Journal of the International Neuropsychological Society*, 16(2), 326-334. doi:10.1017/S1355617709991366

Saver, J. L., and Feldmann, E. (1993). Basic transcranial Doppler examination: Technique and anatomy. In V. L. Babikian and L. R. Wechsler (Eds.), *Transcranial Doppler Ultrasonography* (pp. 11-28). St. Louis, MO: Moseby.

Schneider, W., & Chein, J. M. (2003). Controlled & automatic processing: behavior, theory, and biological mechanisms. *Cognitive Science*, 27(3), 525. doi:10.1016/S0364-0213(03)00011-9

Schuepbach, D., Bader, J., Hell, D., & Baumgartner, R. W. (2004). Cerebral hemodynamics and processing speed during category learning. *NeuroReport: For Rapid Communication of Neuroscience Research*, 15(7), 1195-1198. doi:10.1097/00001756-200405190-00023

Schuepbach D, Boeker H, Duschek S, Hell D. (2007) Rapid cerebral hemodynamic modulation during mental planning and movement execution: evidence of time-locked relationship with complex behavior. *Clinical Neurophysiology*, 118, 2254–62.

Schuepbach, D., Huizinga, M., Duschek, S., Grimm, S., Boeker, H., & Hell, D. (2009). Rapid cerebral hemodynamic modulation during set shifting: Evidence of time-locked associations with cognitive control in females. *Brain and Cognition*, 71(3), 313-319. doi:10.1016/j.bandc.2009.07.006

Schuepbach, D., Merlo, M. G., Goenner, F. F., Staikov, I. I., Mattle, H. P., Dierks, T. T., & Brenner, H. D. (2002). Cerebral hemodynamic response induced by the Tower of Hanoi puzzle and the Wisconsin Card Sorting test. *Neuropsychologia*, 40(1), 39-53. doi:10.1016/S0028-3932(01)00074-4

Schuepbach, D., Weber, S., Kawohl, W., & Hell, D. (2007). Impaired rapid modulation of cerebral hemodynamics during a planning task in schizophrenia. *Clinical Neurophysiology*, 118(7), 1449-1459. doi:10.1016/j.clinph.2007.03.001

Schultz, N. B., Phillips, H. A., & Washburn, D. A. (2010). Lateral asymmetries in cerebral bloodflow velocity related to attention-task performance. Poster presented at the annual meeting of the Psychonomic Society (manuscript in preparation).

Schultz, N. B., Matthews, G., Warm, J. S., & Washburn, D. A. (2009). A transcranial Doppler sonography study of shoot/don't-shoot responding. *Behavior Research Methods*, 41(3), 593-597. doi:10.3758/BRM.41.3.593

Sorond, F. A., Schnyer, D. M., Serrador, J. M., Milberg, W. P., & Lipsitz, L. A. (2008). Cerebral blood flow regulation during cognitive tasks: Effects of healthy aging. *Cortex: A Journal Devoted to the Study of the Nervous System and Behavior*, 44(2), 179-184. doi:10.1016/j.cortex.2006.01.003

Springer, S. P., & Deutsch, G. (2001). *Left Brain, Right Brain: Perspectives from Cognitive Neuroscience* (5th edition). New York: W. H. Freeman and Company.

Stroobant, N., & Vingerhoets, G. (2000). Transcranial doppler ultrasonography monitoring of cerebral hemodynamics during performance of cognitive tasks: A review. *Neuropsychology Review*, 10(4), 213-231. doi:10.1023/A:1026412811036

Szirmai I, Amrein I, Pálvőgyi L, Debreczeni R, Kamondi A. (2005). Correlation between blood flow velocity in the middle cerebral artery and EEG during cognitive effort. *Cognitive Brain Research*, 24, 33–40.

Tiemeier, H. H., Bakker, S. M., Hofman, A. A., Koudstaal, P. J., & Breteler, M. B. (2002). Cerebral haemodynamics and depression in the elderly. *Journal of Neurology, Neurosurgery & Psychiatry*, 73(1), 34-39. doi:10.1136/jnnp.73.1.34

Tripp, L. D., & Warm, J. S. (2007). Transcranial doppler sonography. In R. Parasuraman, M. Rizzo, R. Parasuraman, M. Rizzo (Eds.), *Neuroergonomics: The brain at work* (pp. 82-94). New York, NY US: Oxford University Press.

Turtle, A. M. (1997). Tachistoscope. In R. Bund & D. Warner (Eds). *Instruments of Science: A Historical Encyclopedia* (pp. 595-596). New York: NY US: Garland Publishing Inc.

Unsworth, N., & Engle, R. W. (2008). Speed and Accuracy of Accessing Information in Working Memory: An Individual Differences Investigation of Focus Switching. *Journal of Experimental Psychology. Learning, Memory & Cognition*, 34(3), 616-630. doi:10.1037/028-7393.34.3.616

Vanman, E. J., Saltz, J. L., Nathan, L. R., & Warren, J. A. (2004). Racial discrimination by low-prejudiced Whites facial movements as implicit measures of attitudes related to behavior. *Psychological Science*, 15(11), 711-714. doi:10.1111/j.0956-7976.2004.00746.x

Vingerhoets, G., & Luppens, E. (2001). Cerebral blood flow velocity changes during dichotic listening with directed or divided attention: A transcranial Doppler ultrasonography study. *Neuropsychologia*, 39(10), 1105-1111. doi:10.1016/S0028-3932(01)00030-6

Vul, E., Harris, C., Winkielman, P., & Pashler, H. (2009). Puzzlingly high correlations in fMRI studies of emotion, personality, and social cognition. *Perspectives on Psychological Science*, 4(3), 274-290.

Walsh, V., & Pascual-Leone, A. (2006). *Transcranial Magnetic Stimulation: A Neurochronometrics of Mind.* Cambridge, MA: MIT Press.

Walter, K. D., Roberts, A. E., & Brownlow, S. S. (2000). Spatial perception and mental rotation produce gender differences in cerebral hemovelocity: A TCD study. *Journal of Psychophysiology*, 14(1), 37-45. doi:10.1027//0269-8803.14.1.37

Warm, J. S., Matthews, G., & Parasuraman, R. (2009). Cerebral hemodynamics and vigilance performance. *Military Psychology*, 21(Suppl 1), S75 S100. doi:10.1080/08995600802554706

Warm, J. S., & Parasuraman, R. (2007). Cerebral hemodynamics and vigilance. In R. Parasuraman & M. Rizzo (Eds.), *Neuroergonomics: The brain at work* (pp. 146-158). New York: Oxford University Press.

Warm, J. S., Parasuraman, R., & Matthews, G. (2008). Vigilance Requires Hard Mental Work and Is Stressful. (Cover story). *Human Factors*, 50(3), 433-441. doi:10.1518/001872008X312152

Washburn, D. A., & Schultz, N. B. (2008, November). Inattention vs. task-irrelevant attention in the vigilance decrement. Paper presented at the annual meeting of the Psychonomic Society, Chicago, IL. Manuscript in preparation.

Washburn, D. A., Smith, J., & Taglialatela, L. A. (2005). Individual Differences in Metacognitive Responsiveness: Cognitive and Personality Correlates. *Journal of General Psychology*, 132(4), 446-461

Washburn, D. A., & Taglialatela, L. A. (2006). Attention as it is manifest across species. In T. R. Zentall & E. Wasserman (Eds.), *Comparative Cognition: Experimental Explorations of Animal Intelligence* (pp. 127-142), New York: Oxford University Press.

Wiebe, S. A., Sheffield, T., Nelson, J., Clark, C. C., Chevalier, N., & Espy, K. (2011). The structure of executive function in 3-year-olds. *Journal of Experimental Child Psychology*, 108(3), 436-452. doi:10.1016/j.jecp.2010.08.008

15

Future Uses of Three/Four Dimensional Power Doppler Signal in Fetal Medicine

Juan Carlos Bello-Munoz[1], Mauricio Ayala[2],
Elena Carreras[1], Paula Oliveros[1], Nazareth Campo[1],
Alexandra Casasbuenas[1], Silvia Arévalo[1] and Lluis Cabero[1]
[1]*Department of Obstetrics, Vall d'Hebron University Hospital;*
Universitat Autónoma de Barcelona; Catalonia
[2]*Department of Applied Physics and Mathematics;*
Universitat Autónoma de Barcelona; Catalonia
Spain

1. Introduction

Three-dimensional Ultrasound (3DUS) has grown quickly and constantly over the last fifteen years. However, some of its best clinical uses remain to be defined. The three-dimensional Power Doppler (PD) is based on the ability to register the signal amplitude of the ultrasound wave, which allows us to depict most moving particles in a given Region of Interest (ROI). It is also based on the three-dimensional US principles, that permit the collection of signals from such particles in a given Volume of Interest (VOI) The inclusion of a time sequencing protocol or a Space-Time Image correlation (STIC) algorithm, developed and made available to last generation US machines, adds the additional possibility of following the signal evolution during a pre-established lap. At first, this promising tool was used to evaluate vascularisation and perfusion in a series of foetal organs, finding neither adequate accuracy nor repeatability. Nowadays, its use in Foetal Medicine is restricted to certain foetal conditions, although new research is on-going and further uses for this technology are being unveiled.

As is it largely understood (Burns 1992), there are compelling scientific and medical reasons to seek measuring the volumetric flow rate, which means to estimate the volume of flow delivered per minute to a tissue bed. No doubt, the success in delivering oxygen and nutrients to the tissues depends, mainly, on the amount of blood delivered to such tissues per unit of time. At the beginning of the Doppler ultrasound era, a number of attempts to achieve this calculation were done (Gill 1979; Eik-Nes et al. 1982; Sauders et al. 1980). The standard method for estimating volume flow using sonography consists on multiplying the mean spatial velocity by the luminal cross-sectional area. However, it is well known that this technique has many problems; these include the inherent variability of vessel geometry, inaccurate assumptions about flow profile, B-dimensional sampling, and other important technical limitations derived from the way pulsed and spectral Doppler signals are registered, not to mention an unsustainable amount of human interaction in the final estimation (J M Rubin 1999). All of the abovementioned reasons caused those efforts to fail and led this pretension to be forsaken for two decades.

Then, the experimental analysis of the Doppler Effect was described – taking into account the amplitude of the wave and tracking the acoustic speckle pattern produced by the echoes from moving blood (J M Rubin et al. 1994; Forsberg et al. 1995; Harrington et al. 1996; J M Rubin 1999). From those initial approaches, the concept of Fractional Moving Blood Volume (FMBV) (J M Rubin et al. 1997) was developed, which was mainly a mathematical normalization process of the colour pattern obtained from the power Doppler signal acquisition (Tomas Jansson et al. 2003; A. Welsh 2004). Preliminary publications established a direct relationship between the data from FMBV acquired by registering the power Doppler signal in a given Region of Interest (ROI) and actual perfusion of the tissue as measured by invasive methods in animal models (E Hernandez-Andrade, T Jansson, et al. 2004; E Hernandez-Andrade, Thuring-Jönsson, et al. 2004). It has been recently described how, under certain foetal conditions such as foetal growth restriction, some perfusion patterns are objectively altered and significantly differ from "normal" patterns established by the authors (E Hernandez-Andrade et al. 2008; Rogelio Cruz-Martinez et al. 2009; R Cruz-Martinez et al. 2011).

Nonetheless, there are still enormous gaps between the information obtained by FMBV and the actual estimations of, either, flow or perfusion (A. Welsh 2004; Lai et al. 2010). There are some boundaries which will limit insurmountably the utility of this technique, such as the low repeatability when comparing one patient with the same in a better acquisition setting - or one patient with difficulties for exploration like obese or anxious mothers to a normal one. Additionally, it will be impossible to relate such magnitudes with flow whenever there is no time frame considered in the image quantification process (A. W. Welsh et al. 2005).

No additional experience in this technique has been published and very likely it will not in the future. The next logical step would be to evaluate the possibilities of three dimensional ultrasound and power Doppler as an alternative approach to this phenomenon.

2. Three-dimensional power Doppler signal and the vascular indexes

Three-dimensional power Doppler (PD) became available for medical purposes towards the end of the last century (Fenster, Lee, et al. 1998; Guo, Durand, et al. 1998). It exhibited some advantages, considering the higher sensitivity of the PD for detecting, and therefore depicting, moving particles. Its first clinical application was designed to evaluate vascularisation in compromised regions, trying to elucidate whether there was an obstruction or not in a given vessel (Guo & Fenster 1996). Considering its potential for depicting vascular structure accurately, it was employed as a tool for measuring potentially angiogenic structures as tumours (Bendick et al. 1998; Kupesic & Kurjak 2000). Also its potential for depicting vascular architecture and potential anomalies has been considered as promising (Fig. 1) (Heling, Chaoui, et al. 2000; Chaoui & Kalache 2001)

Nevertheless, the information given by this technique was rather limited, considering there was no quantification of the signal and no objective measurements would be done. Then, a mathematical algorithm was developed, firstly used in gynaecology (J M Rubin 1999; Pairleitner et al. 1999); based on the possibility of a direct correlation between PD signal

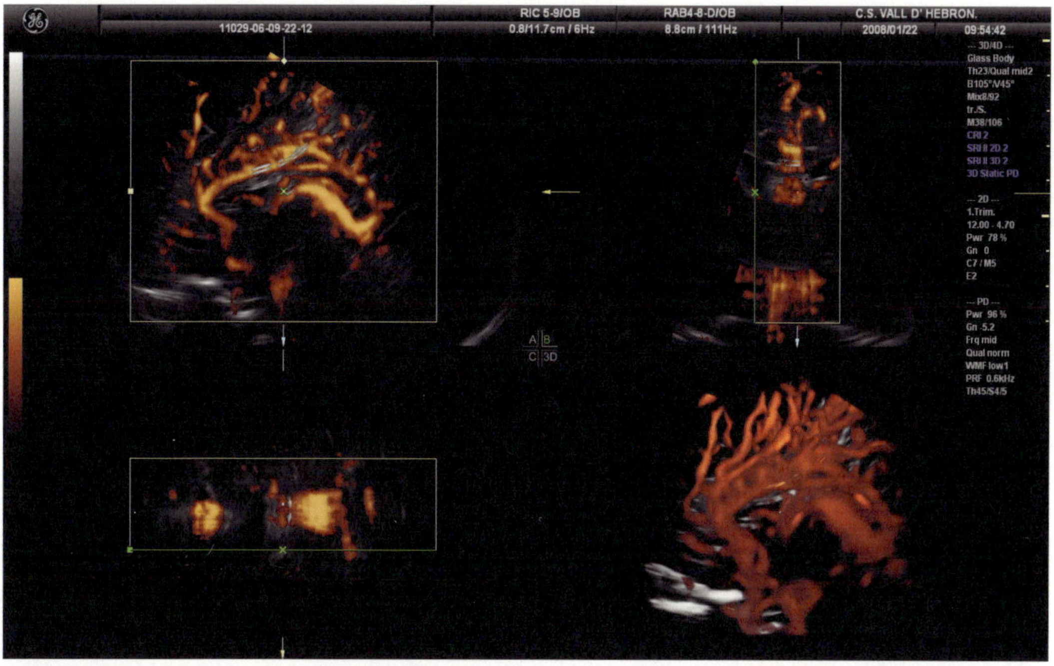

Fig. 1. Three dimensional PD angio mode rendering of intracranial blood vascularisation in a term fetus

intensity and, somehow, the velocity of the particles and the possible quantification of moving particles in a Volume of Interest (VOI) over the amount of grayscale, B-mode, particles in the same VOI. Three indexes were developed, which could indirectly give a mathematical expression of vascularisation and flow:

*Vascularization index (VI) = color voxels/(total voxels − background voxels)

$$VI = \frac{\sum_{c=1}^{100} hc(c)}{\sum_{g=1}^{100} hg(g) + \sum_{c=1}^{100} hc(c)} \tag{1}$$

Where
g= gray-scale value in the US image, normalized to 0-100: lowest intensity= 1; highest = 100
c= color value in the US image from power Doppler signal representation. Normalized to 0-100: lowest intensity= 1; highest = 100
hg(x) = frequency of gray-value x in US image
hc(x) = frequency of color value x in US image
*Flow index (FI) = weighted color voxels/color voxels

$$FI = \frac{\sum_{c=1}^{100} c \cdot hc(c)}{\sum_{c=1}^{100} hc(c)} \tag{2}$$

*Vascularization-flow index 1 (VFI) = weighted color voxels/(total voxels - background voxels)

$$VFI = \frac{\sum_{c=1}^{100} c \cdot hc(c)}{\sum_{g=1}^{100} hg(g) + \sum_{c=1}^{100} hc(c)} \tag{3}$$

Based on the above mentioned indexes, a number of research communications have been produced, evaluating the vascularity of benign versus malign ovarian masses (Kurjak et al. 1998; Juan Luis Alcázar & Jurado 2011) and prostatic tumours (Moskalik et al. 2001). Regarding the feto-placental unit, several attempts to correlate those indexes with regional perfusion of foetal brain (Hayashi et al. 1998; Nardozza et al. 2009), liver (C.-H. Chang et al. 2003), and lungs in normal (Dubiel et al. 2005) as well as pathologic *in-utero* conditions (Ruano et al. 2006). However, the clinical efficacy of this method remains unsupported by the evidence. No clinical findings can be drawn from those values so far. (Fig. 2)

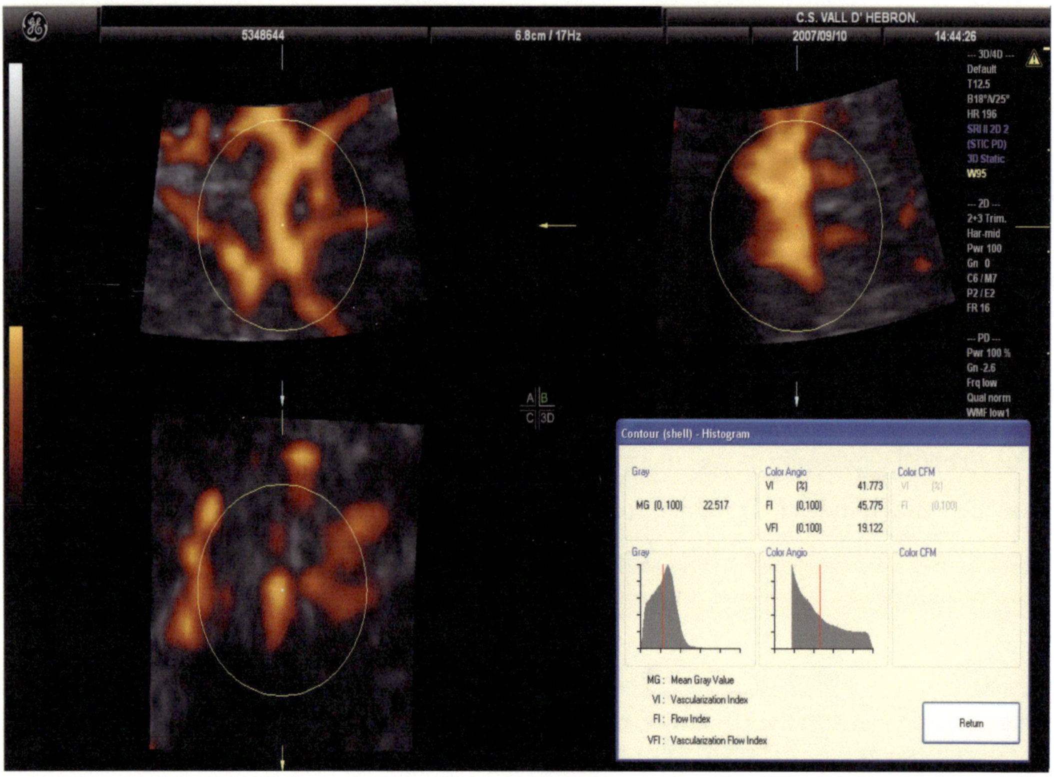

Fig. 2. Three dimensional PD angio mode rendering of intracranial blood vascularisation in a mid-trimester foetus with suspected brain sparing. In the right lower corner it is possible to visualize the histogram with the indexes obtained from the spherical shape -Volume of Interest

A promising field, still open to research, is the analysis of placental vasculature and its potential relationship to placental dysfunction (N. W. Jones et al. 2011). Some authors have found a positive correlation between low vascularisation indexes in early pregnancy and Fetal Growth Restriction (FGR) (Bozkurt, Başgül Yigiter, et al. 2010; Dar et al. 2010; Guimarães Filho et al. 2011; Morel et al. 2010; Negrini et al. 2011; A. O. Odibo et al. 2011;

Pomorski et al. 2011; Rizzo et al. 2009). It seems that the evaluation of first trimester placental vascularisation correlates, somehow, with a compromised placentation and therefore could predict some adverse perinatal outcomes of placental origin. Besides, the technique exhibits fairly good repeatability and accuracy (Tuuli et al. 2010; Martins & N J Raine-Fenning 2010; Yigiter et al. 2011).

The challenges for the future involve overcoming some of the technical problems that the three dimensional PD is plagued with and also to establish an adequate normalisation protocol, which it is currently lacking. (Fig. 3)

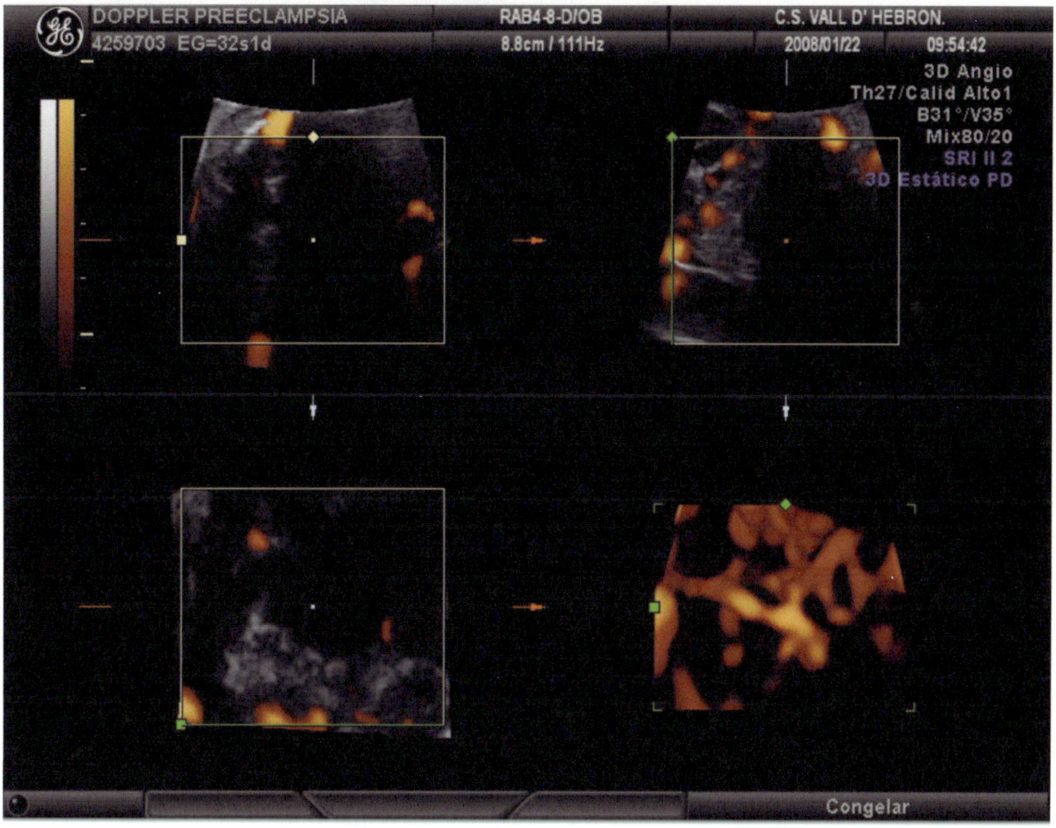

Fig. 3. Three dimensional angio mode rendering of placental vascularisation in a pre-eclampsia patient. Quantification of vascular branches suggests a lower flow in the corial plate when compared to volumes taken at the same gestational age from normal gestations

Another recently attempted and straightforward approach is to use 3D PD for the evaluation of progressive foetal conditions such as foetal goitrous hypothyroidism (Marín et al. 2010): In a given patient, under well-controlled conditions, it should be possible to evaluate the progression of either, an inflammatory response or the success of the treatment, which was thyroid hormone supplementation in that case. (Fig. 4).

Despite being rather promising, the 3D PD still has important limitations, some related to the power Doppler signal itself and some derived from acoustic impedance and mechanical interference. Some of these aspects are going to be discussed further in the next section.

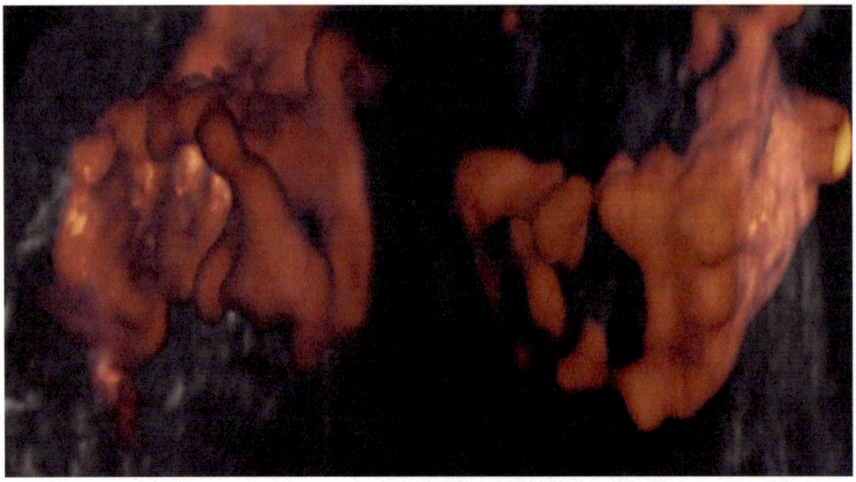

Fig. 4. Three dimensional PD angio mode rendered image of Thyroid gland of the same human foetus, before (left side) and after four weeks of intra-amniotic thyroid hormone supplementation (right side). Actual volume of the gland changed according to foetal growth, but vascularisation decreased markedly after treatment

2.1 The signal normalization problem and its consequences

To normalize the 3D PD signal, it is necessary to take into account three paramount boundaries:

- The signal can be altered by tissue impedance, which means that a low velocity flow in a deep vessel will produce completely different PD patterns depending on the mother's abdominal wall thickness, the amount of amniotic fluid and the position of the foetus (Schulten-Wijman et al. 2011).
- The settings of the machine can sensibly modify the amount of signal registered by the processor, and therefore, the amount of colour voxels inside the VOI: the algorithms for refining the B-mode signal, like the speckle reduction or the cross beam reduction post-process algorithms, mask the signal processed and "erase" a significant amount of moving particles. (N J Raine-Fenning, Nordin, Ramnarine, Campbell, Clewes, Perkins & Johnson 2008b)
- The post-processing software provided by the developers of the Volume Measurement software: 4DView and virtual organ computer-aided analysis (VOCAL®) by General Electric Medical division. Q-lab® by Philips Medical Division, as well as Sonoview® and Histogram by Samsung-Medison Co show no correlation in their measurements. Therefore, the same structure, under similar circumstances, draw off different results once measurement of the VOI is performed. (J L Alcázar 2008)

2.1.1 The biases behind the algorithm

Based on previous observations, we conducted a preliminary study, on five healthy foetuses on their 20th week of gestation, comparing the values obtained in the same foetus with different machines and adjusting settings as main gain in 600 Hz, medium wall filter in 60 Hz, cross beam reduction off and persistence of colour signal in 0. In all of them the structure was the Willis' polygon at the cranial base. Figure 5 shows the images obtained from the machines and the histograms.

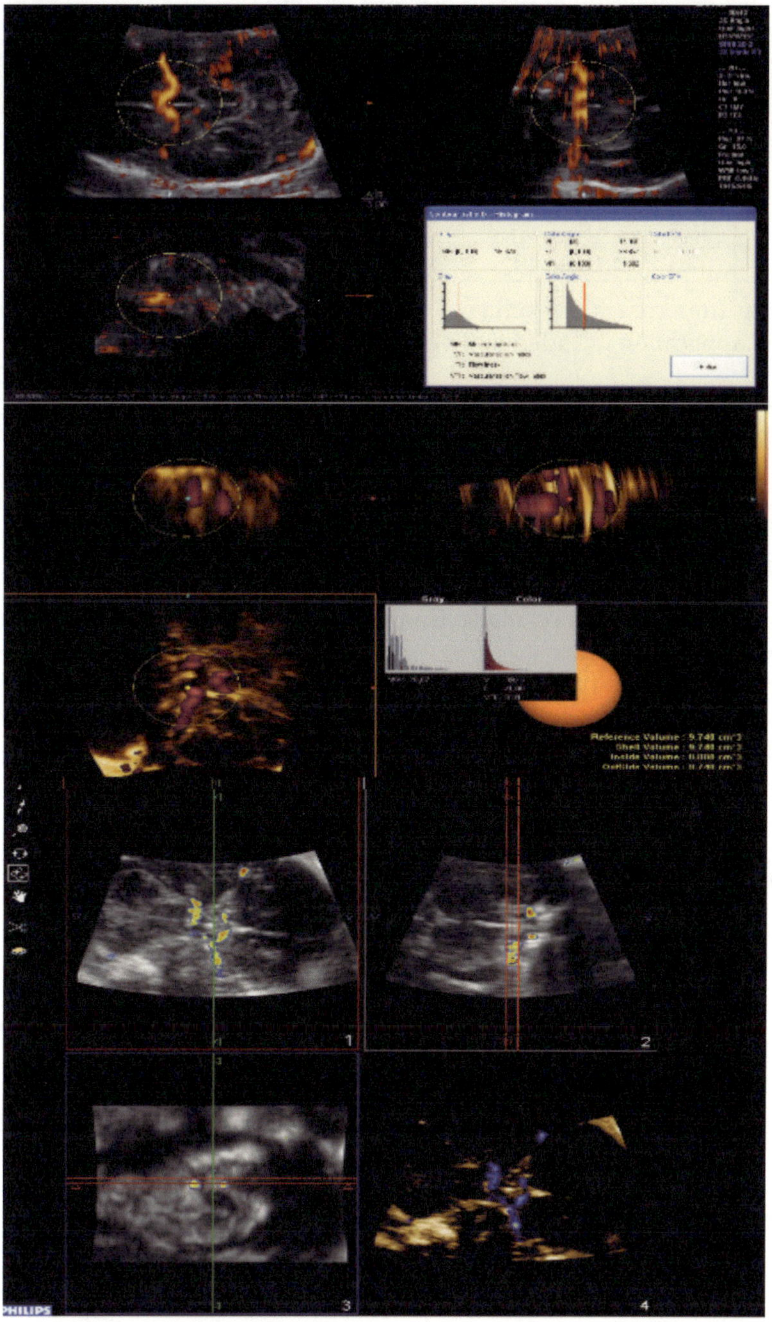

Fig. 5. Images obtained from a single foetus in cephalic presentation, from three different machines: General Electric Voluson E8 (Upper); Medison Accuvix V20 Prestige (Middle); Philips iU22 (Lower)

The results, summarized in the table 1, show how different the measurements are, depending on the brand. They also show how they differ among themselves, despite the same gestational age and similar maternal characteristics.

Foetus	GE Voluson E8			Philips iU22			Medison Accuvix V20		
	VI	FI	VFI	VI	FI	VFI	VI	FI	VFI
1	44.9	46.1	20.7	32.3	25..1	33.5	48.6	16.9	5.5
2	14.1	39.8	5.6	16.6	28.3	9.5	39.4	21.1	8.3
3	23.6	51.1	17.3	36.2	17.3	19.5	42.5	28.1	4.7
4	36.3	38.9	21.3	27.3	32.8	11.1	25.8	40.3	19.2
5	37.3	44.0	9.5	48.1	27.3	13.1	35.8	39.9	6.9

Table 1. Results from comparing similar VOI in three different machines, with the PD quantification application included in their software

In conclusion, normalizing the data from the 3D PD signal is currently not possible and reference ranges to discriminate normality from pathologic conditions are not available. Therefore, no feasibility for these indexes in obstetric clinical practice can be foreseen in the short term.

2.2 The regional normalization solution

Given that no decisions can be made from direct measurement of the abovementioned indexes, a possible approach could be to use two Regions of Interest (ROI) inside the same volume. The more reliable possibility after *in-vitro* testing was the VFI (N J Raine-Fenning, Nordin, Ramnarine, Campbell, Clewes, Perkins & Johnson 2008a). And the easier and more repeatable formula was a simple VFI index

$$VFI_1 / VFI_2 \tag{5}$$

2.2.1 The ductus venosus shunting as an example

In physiological conditions, few regions of foetal circulation can offer enough regional differences to be considered clinically relevant. But the most important of these is, no doubt, the physiological shunt in the ductus venosus which is not only a reliable indicator of preload, but also a sensitive mechanism of circulatory re-distribution in adverse circulatory conditions such as placental insufficiency (M Bellotti et al. 2000; Kiserud 2001).

The original description of Ductus Venosus Shunting (DVS) measurement was published by Belloti (Maria Bellotti et al. 2004), and was, simplifying, an index of estimated flow through Ductus Venosus (DV) over the one through Umbilical Vein (UV)

The classical way for estimating the flow through the UV is

$$Q_{UV} = 0.5 \times (V_{\max})_{UV} \times \pi \times (D_{UV}^2 / 4) \tag{6}$$

Where Vmax relates to the Umbilical Vein maximum velocity as measured by pulsed Doppler. 0,5 is a normalization constant related to foetal blood viscosity and DUV is the mean diameter of the umbilical vein in its abdominal portion.

Also, the calculation of DV flow, made by Belloti et al, is;

$$Q_{DV} = \left(-0.03 \times DR^2 + 0.189 \times DR + 0.43\right) \times (V_{\max})_{UV} \times \pi \times (D_{UV}^2 / 4) \tag{7}$$

Where Vmax DV is the maximum systolic velocity in the Ductus Venosus. DR respresents the ratio between the inlet (smaller) and the outlet (larger) of the ductus venosus, represented as part of a paraboloid equation

Therefore, the DVS could be expressed as

$$\left(Q_{DV} / Q_{UV}\right) \cdot \cdot 100 \tag{8}$$

A description of the ideal technique for measuring blood flow in both UV and DV has been published (Tchirikov et al. 2006). For UV blood volume flow measurement, a straight segment of the intra-abdominal part of the UV upstream of any hepatic branches should be selected, with the Doppler gate positioned so as to completely cover the vessel's diameter. The UV flow volume can also be measured in the umbilical cord. Authors suggest measuring blood flow volume following the 'maximum principle', which aims to determine the maximum diameter of the vessel, the maximum intensity weighted mean velocity (or time-averaged mean velocity, TAV) at the maximum vessel length in a straight longitudinal section. The inner vessel diameter is determined to the nearest tenth of a millimeter by placing the calipers at right angles to the vessel axis on a frozen B-mode image (without color). This is followed by the TAV measurement at the same vessel portion with a small insonation angle of insonation (less than 30°). The blood volume flow rate is calculated from diameter (D) and TAV as flow rate = TAV × π × $(D/2)^2$ mL/min. Regarding the DV, The inner diameter of the DV should be measured by insonating perpendicularly to the vessel wall at the isthmus. In order to reduce random error, the procedure must be repeated four or more times and the calculated mean diameter entered into the statistics (Kiserud et al. 2006). Doppler evaluations must be carried out in the absence of fetal breathing and body movements.

As it should become evident, the skills needed for achieving such measurements are prohibitively high; the time needed for every exploration is too long for a usual clinical exploration and the medical scope of this practice is quite reduced. Our proposal to address this issue is a far simpler, faster and repeatable approach, by using 3D PD. (Bello-Muñoz et al. 2009)

By taking a single volume of the foetal abdomen in Angio 3D PD mode, it was possible to measure the UV VFI by calculating it into a 1 cc sphere. After navigating through the volume, same measurement (DV VFI) was done in the DV, employing the same 1 cc sphere (Figure 6 summarizes both measurements)

Our study compared 162 volumes from normal foetuses and 36 from Foetal Growth Restriction (FGR) cases. In all of them we measured the DVS as described classically by Belloti et al (M Bellotti et al. 2007), and collected a volume of the foetal abdomen with 3D PD angio mode signal, always adjusting the same settings in the machine (General Electric Voluson E 8 GE Medical Systems Milwaukee USA) with a 3D RNA5-9-D Volume Convex Array Transducer Probe.

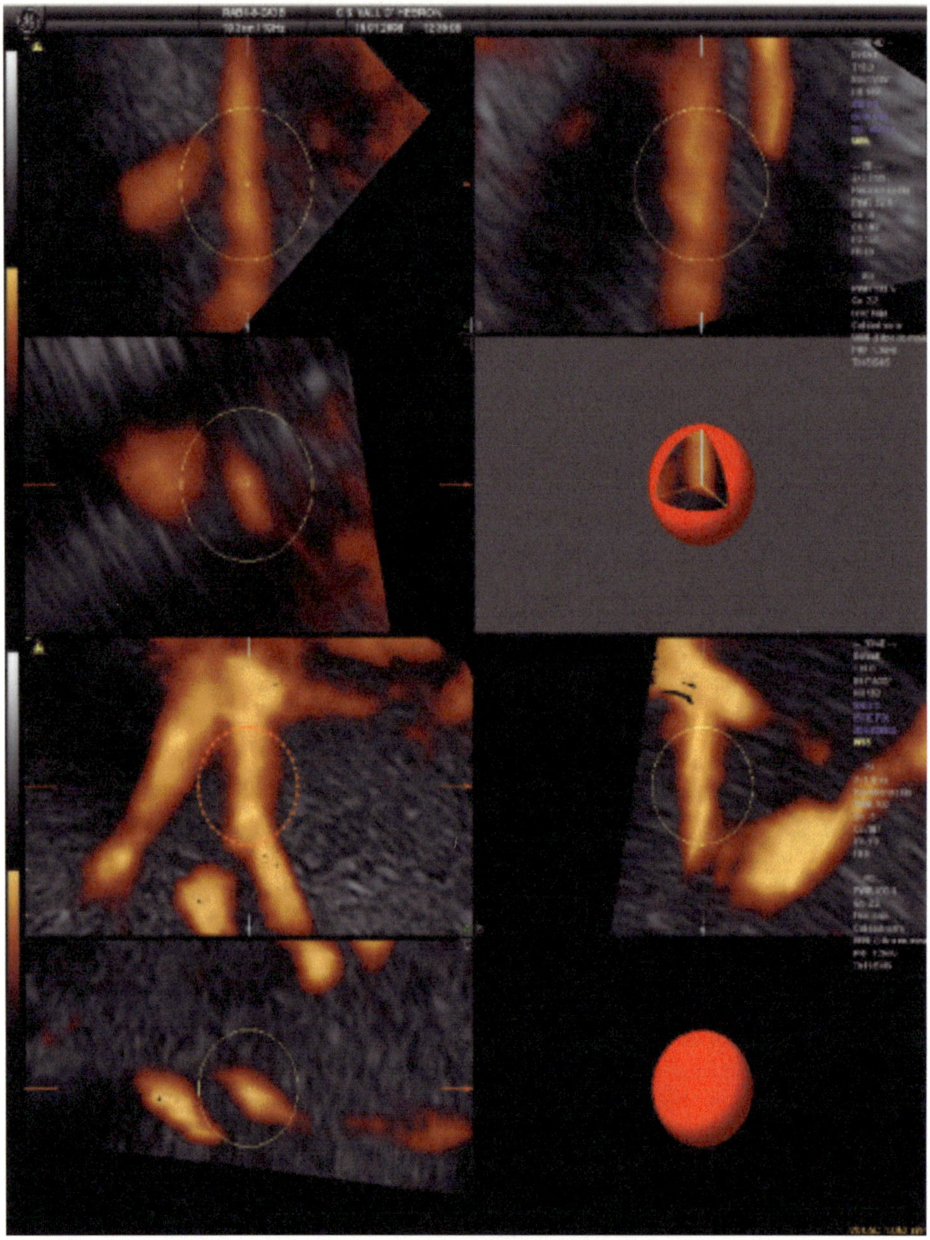

Fig. 6. VFI measurement in abdominal umbilical vein (upper) and in ductus venosus (lower). As the size of the sphere is exactly the same, the VOI remains unchanged

The calculation of the DV/UV VFI ratio was as simple as:

$$DV \cdot VFI \, / \, UV \cdot VFI. \cdot \cdot 100 \tag{9}$$

We found a significant positive correlation between DVS measured as described by Belloti et al and DVS measured as a ratio of DV/UV VFI (Figure 7)

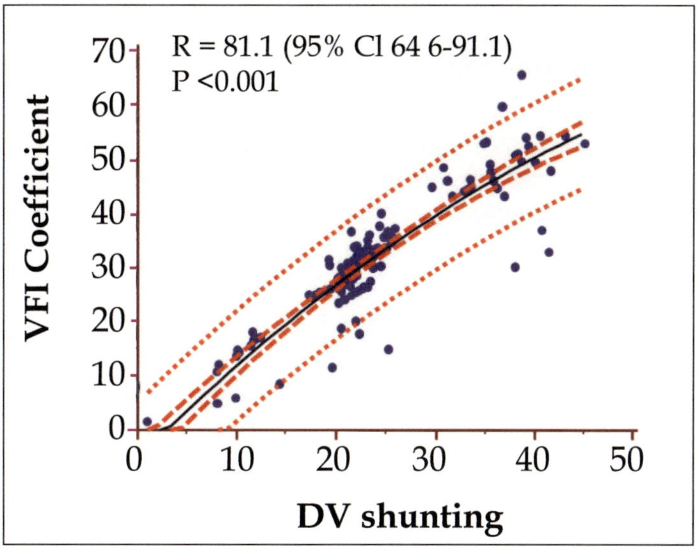

Fig. 7. Lineal regression plot comparing the DVS measured as classically described and the DV/UV VFI ratio r value = 0.81; P<0.001

Reference ranks equation $y = 0{,}6766 + 1{,}6542\ x + -0{,}007813\ x^2$

Also, as previously described, we found a significant difference in DV/UV VFI ratio between normal and FGR foetuses. Comparing results in growth restricted foetuses showed difference as plotted by gestational age mean (SD):39 (11,5) and 53(16,8) (p = 0,03). (Figure 8)

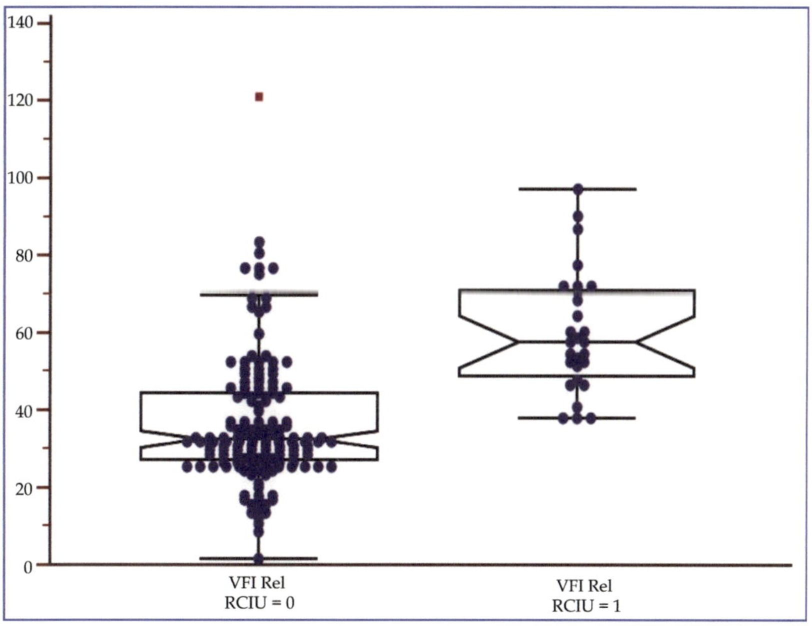

Fig. 8. Box Whisker plot of DV/UV VFI ratio comparing normal (left) to IUGR foetuses (right)

3. Four-dimensional power Doppler signal and the estimation of flow

3.1 The addition of a time sequence

Since the solution provided is already limited and only allows to estimate some regional changes in vascularity, applicable perhaps to the abovementioned DVS and to placenta (Odeh et al. 2011), but is still far away from depicting the flow phenomenon; it is necessary to move forward, towards two recently opened gates:

First is the integration of Power Doppler signal derived velocities profile, whose most reliable approach is the Surface Integration of Velocity Vectors, (Sun et al. 1995; J M Rubin et al. 2001; Berg et al. 2000) a clarifying concept which was developed for Color Dopler signal analysis, but has the handicap of the angle effect (Pemberton et al. 2005; Li et al. 2005), reason why it was left aside. Until the algorithms for calculating velocity of particles from power Doppler signals were developed (M. G. Jones et al. 2003; Kripfgans et al. 2006; Petersch & Hönigmann 2007)

Surface integration of velocity vectors is based on Gauss' theorem, which relates the divergence of the quantity (*v*) in an enclosed volume (*V*) to the flux through the surface (*S*) covering (*V*). In other words, a surface integral of *v* over the enclosing boundary *S* will yield the volume flow *Q*:

$$Q = \int_S \vec{v} \cdot \overrightarrow{dA} \,. \tag{10}$$

The easiest way to implement SIVV is to choose a surface that is locally perpendicular to each Doppler beam. For this case, the right side dot product in Equation 1 will be replaced by a regular multiplication of the Doppler velocity and the size of the surface element. In other words, this surface has a constant depth geometry with respect to the Doppler beams. (Kripfgans et al. 2006)

The most general scanning geometry is the surface of a torus because the center of rotation for the axial-lateral and axial-elevational beams can differ). Volume flow can be computed by integrating all Doppler acquisitions on the defined surface, as expressed by Kripfgans et al:

$$Q = \sum_{i \in S} v_i a_i \tag{11}$$

Where, *Q* is the total flux through the surface *S*, which equals volume flow; *vi* is the local Doppler velocity; *ai* is the associated cross-sectional area on *S* for this voxel, and · is the dot product between the local velocity vector and the local surface normal. In this case, the detected velocity is parallel to the surface normal.

In Kripfgans et al experiment, for the depicted type of tube-to-transducer orientation, the left-/right-most Doppler beam has the smallest/largest Doppler angle, respectively. This causes the velocity maximum to shift toward the left. However, warping of velocity values does not affect the measured SIVV value. Inherent compensation of this warping is due to nonuniform distribution of surface elements over the tube cross section.

A very important matter, mainly derived from biophysical characteristics of blood is the Rouleaoux' effect (J M Rubin et al. 1997; A. W. Welsh et al. 2005; N J Raine-Fenning, Nordin,

Ramnarine, B. K. Campbell, Clewes, Perkins & Johnson 2008a). The local Doppler power is largest inside the vessel and smallest outside because of the effect of partial volume averaging and the Doppler wall filter effect, which gives the pixels inside the vessel a higher power. All Doppler data is wall filter processed internally in the scanner by the smallest setting possible on the machine. Therefore, it is mandatory to minimize filtering for the selected Doppler frequency range.

Authors define a solution for surface integration of velocity vectors, which was weighted on the basis of the Doppler power in the respective voxels. A velocity masking algorithm which was generated, using the Doppler power value pT to weight the velocity values of the integration surface.

Therefore, the modified SIVV method that was used by the authors was

$$Q = \sum_{i \in S} (v_i \cdot a_i) p_i \,. \qquad (12)$$

Where, *pi* is a scaling factor based on the local Doppler power. Power weighting factors *pi* were set to 1 for all Doppler powers larger then *pT*. Values between 0 and *pT* were scaled between 0 and 1 on the basis of their Doppler power value. The justification for the selection/scaling process is that voxels near the wall, which partially contain flow and soft tissue, will show lower than- maximum Doppler power. Fractional power is therefore weighted by fractional scaling factors. So far, the threshold *pTwas* set empirically by developers. However, it was set constant for all measurements, and it could be shown that the *pT* contour fills the lumen. User-selected Doppler gain was adjusted as needed to compensate for signal reduction due to large angles between flow and Doppler beams.

The next addition to the conceptual framework was the estimation of pulsatile conditions by Richards and Kripfgans (Richards et al. 2009), by adding to the model the potential signal fluctuations derived from the wall movements and the local velocity profile changes derived from particles acceleration. As a first issue, authors defined the possibility of collecting not one, but *N* number of velocity profiles according to the local variations in time and position. Such local velocities were expressed as:

$$\widehat{v_i} = E\left(v_i\left(X_i\right)\right) = \frac{\sum_{j=1}^{N} v\left(X_i, t_j\right)}{N} \,, \qquad (13)$$

Where $E(vi(Xi))$ is the expected value of the local velocity estimates. $v(Xi,tj)$ are the local velocity estimates that are measured at randomly selected time increments defined by tj as follows:

$$t_{j+1} = t_j + t_s + t_r \,, \qquad (14)$$

Authors defined an experiment to obtain the average volume flow in the presence of pulsatility: 50 random time points distributed across the equivalent of a cardiac cycle were collected and averaged at each location. Power Doppler data were then used to correct for partial volume effects as described in the previous paragraph. Then, using seven previously defined surfaces for flow estimate, the equation for the modified SIVV method, became:

$$Q = \frac{1}{M} \sum_{i \in S_M} s_i \bullet w_i \bullet \widehat{v_i} \,, \tag{15}$$

where M is the number of integration surfaces and the surface of integration *(S)* has been modified to include the M surfaces *(SM)*.

In our opinion, Richards & Kripfgans' works have achieved a breakthrough in this matter, and the experiment we have developed is nothing but a logical consequence of their postulations.

Before describing the experiment, next consequent step was to add a regular time frame to the algorithm. Fortunately, the tool for getting the initial data was already developed and seated on the machine: The Spatio Temporal Image Correlation (STIC) is an automated volume acquisition in which the array inside the transducer housing performs a slow, single sweep, recording one single 3D data set. This volume consists of a high number of 2D frames, one behind the other. Due to the small region of interest required to image the foetal heart, the B-mode frame rate during the acquisition of the volume scan is very high, in the range of 150 frames/s. Assuming a volume acquisition time of 10 s and sweeping over an area of 25° (both parameters can be adjusted), there are 1500 B-mode images in the volume memory. During this acquisition time the fetal heart beats 20–25 times, which means there are 20–25 images showing a systolic peak contained within these 1500 B-mode frames (DeVore et al. 2003; Chaoui & Heling 2005). Concerning this application, further studies have shown how, the mere analysis of intra-ventricular stroke volume in left and right heart gave information reliable enough for calculating the cardiac output in foetuses from 16 to 32 weeks (Molina, Faro, Sotiriadis, Dagklis & Nicolaides 2008a).

Basis of volume calculation in VOCAL are performed by integration of polygon areas marked in parallel planes. The method used for the integration of the polygon areas is given by the formula

$$Vol - \frac{\pi}{N} \cdot \left[\sum_{i=1}^{2 \cdot N} TA_i \cdot ds_i \right] \tag{16}$$

Where N = number of marked polygon areas Ai = polygon area in plane i di,j = distance between plane i and plane j the sort order of planes 1,..., N is given by d1,2 £ d1,3 £... £ d1,N. (Sohn 1993; Robb et al. 1997).

And the basis for stroke volume calculation and cardiac output calculation were (Molina, Faro, Sotiriadis, Dagklis & Nicolaides 2008b):

$$CO = \lim_{n \to \infty} \left(1 + \frac{1}{n}\right)^n \cdot Vs \;\vdots - \vdots\; \lim_{n \to \infty} \left(1 + \frac{1}{n}\right)^n \cdot VD \tag{17}$$

Where CO = Cardiac Output, VS is Systolic Volume and VD is Diastolic Volume.

The abovementioned approach provides some additional information on cardiac output and has proven to be repeatable and more accurate than previous methods (Messing et al. 2007; Hamill et al. 2011; Simioni et al. 2011). Notwithstanding, it still has a substantial amount of human interaction, and is rather time-consuming as for being used in an actual clinical setting.

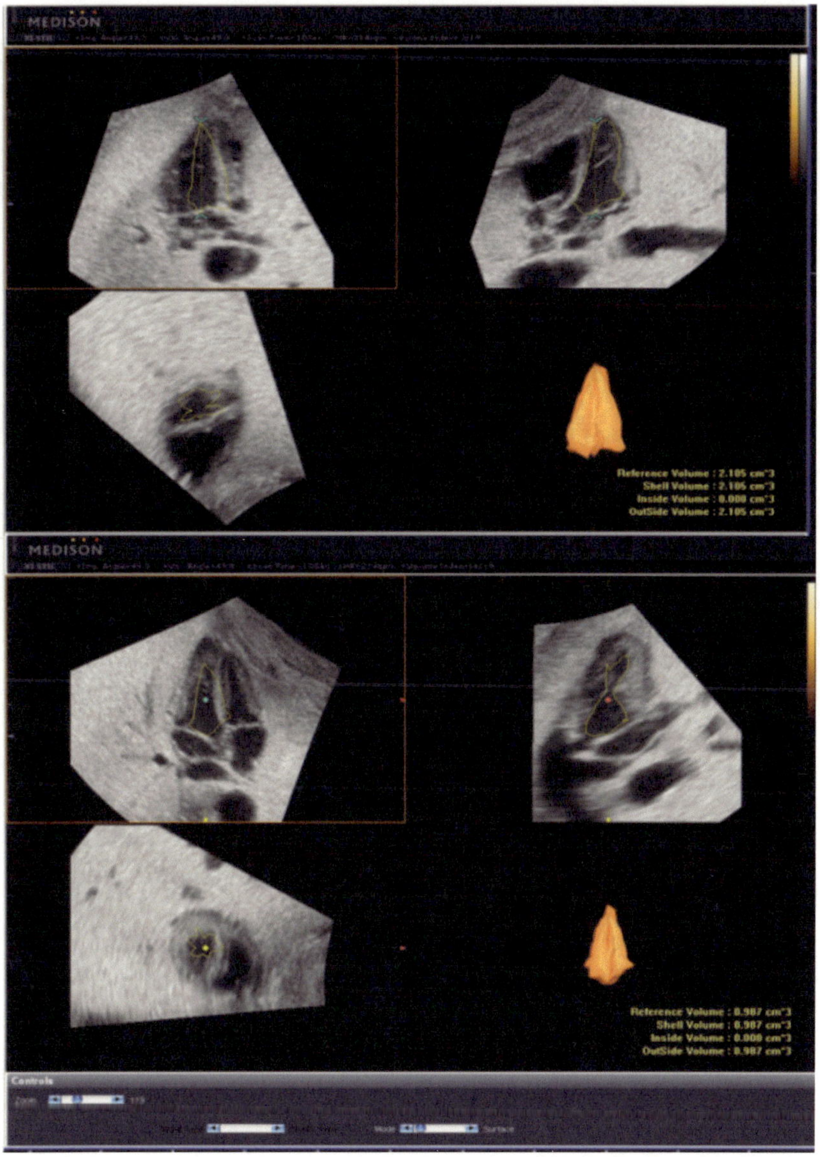

Fig. 9. Reproduction of STIC and VOCAL model for left ventricle output calculation in a term ovine foetus, taken by the authors during their experiment (Bello-Muñoz et al. 2010); as proposed by Molina et al.

3.1.1 The cardiac output model

Based on previous studies and encouraged by the works of Richards & Kripfgans, we decided to develop an algorithm of flow calculation, based on surface integration of velocity vectors and time frame sequences from STIC volumes. Volume datasets as obtained by the ultrasound machine Medison Accuvix V-20 prestige with a Medison 3D4-8ET 3D volumetric probe (Samsung Medical Co, Hoofddorp, Nz).

A total of eight foetuses from near term pregnant sheep (125-140 days) were exteriorized through a cesarean section and a modified central catheter inserted via umbilical cord and under direct echographic vision. An arterial line was also inserted in one of the umbilical arteries. Both transducers from the catheters were connected to a PICCO monitor for invasive testing (PULSION Medical Inc. Irving TX, USA). Continuous measurement of combined cardiac output was the registered as long as the experiment was carried out, meanwhile one of the authors (JB-M), recorded several volume datasets synchronizing the register of the data set with data obtained by monitorization. Analysis of all the data was made offline.

A complete spreadsheet of physiologic registers from the experimental subject was recorded for comparison and external validation of calculations. All images were processed by using the Mathematica® software (Wolfram Research Europe Ltd., Oxfordshire, UK). All data from VOI analysis was addded to the calculation spreadsheet and a polinomial regression fit model was designed

The mathematical background of this study was based on flow calculation:

$$Q = \sum_{i \in S} (v_i \cdot a_i) p_i \; . \tag{12}$$

And the concept of vector velocity profile described above. But with the addition of a time frame provided by the STIC algorithm, which means a continuous sum of velocity profiles, giving us a new profile of the area, represented as:

$$(1+A)^n = 1 + \frac{Ax}{1!} + \frac{A(n-1)x^2}{2!} + \cdots \tag{18}$$

And to the velocity profile, expressed also as

$$\sum vi(t1) + vi(t2) \ldots \ldots vi()tn \tag{19}$$

Where N is the entire amount of frames included in a cardiac cycle.

Once collected the sequences, information of velocity vector profile (VVP) form the VOI was collected in a series of frames, from the starting of the cardiac cycle (early start of diastole), denominated as t_0 until the end of same cycle (end of systole) hence called t_n. Information of VVP was then modified according to area variation in every frame. Therefore, the mathematical expression of this phenomenon could be expressed as a matrix of data:

$$\sum_{t=1}^{N} Qn = \big((A1.vi1)t1 \vdots (A2.vi2)t1 \vdots \cdots \vdots (Ax.vix)t1 \vdots (A1.vi1)t2 \vdots (A2.vi2)t2 \vdots \cdots \vdots \\ (Ax.vix)t2 \vdots (A1.vi1)tn \vdots (A2.vi2)tn \vdots \cdots \vdots (Ax.vix)tn\big) \tag{20}$$

Where A_x is an estimated area obtained by adding all the regional areas in the VOI and vi_x is the velocity vector profile in each sub-area, according to, previously described, sectorial variations in velocity. And t is the timeline described above.

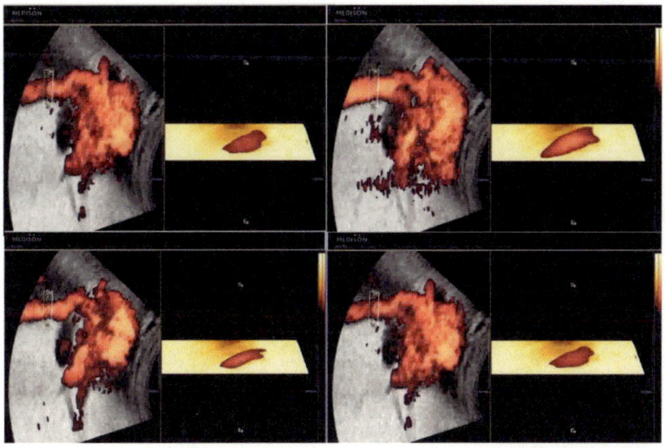

Fig. 10. Screen snapshot of descending aorta plane with selected volume of evaluation. Right side of the image is the VOI containing the $v_1 \ldots v_n$ information. A set of voxels like this one was added to the matrix, since t_1 till t_n where n=end of the cardiac cycle. (Actual experiment added measurements from the aortic isthmus, this image is for illustrative purposes)

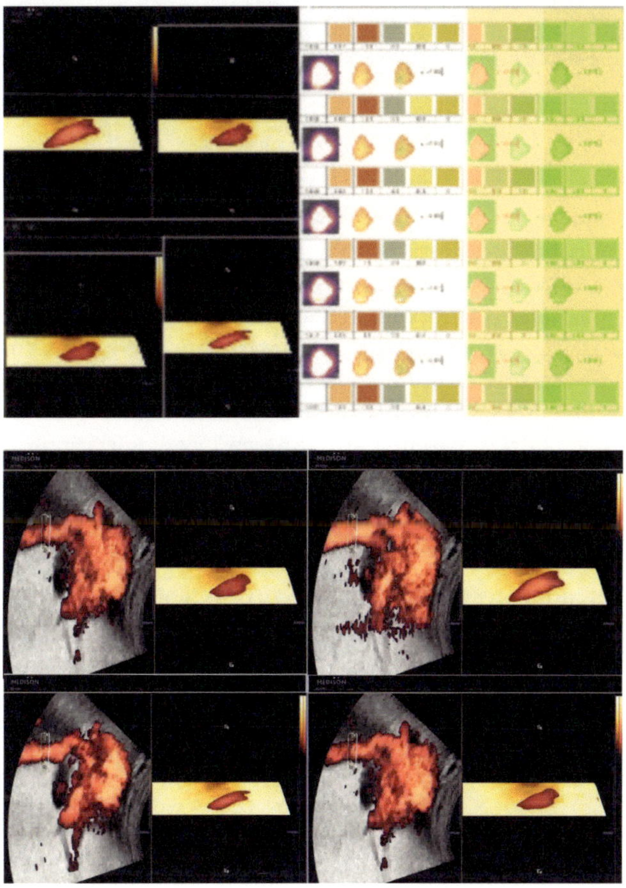

Fig. 11. Colour deconvolution algorithm as delivered by the Mathematica software ®

Regression analysis showed a strong correlation between actual measurement of Combined cardiac Output as obtained by invasive methods and the estimated flow 4D PD dataset as calculated by the authors. The reference polynomial equation and plot is showed in Figure 11

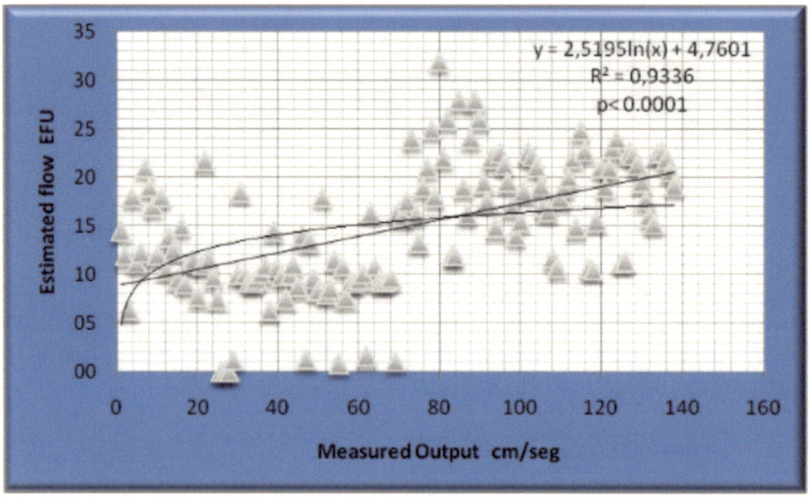

Fig. 12. Polinomial regression plot

4. Conclusion

Three dimensional power Doppler (3D PD), in its current state has no correlation with actual flow measurements, since there is no way of involving the time as a magnitude. Four dimensional power Doppler, by adding the surface integration of velocity vectors from power Doppler signal, and the Spatio Time Image correlation (STIC) might improve significantly its potential. An important amount of additional research on this field is mandatory in order to grant its utility in clinical conditions. But 4D PD could be, in the near future, the most reliable tool for non invasive assessment of physiological intrauterine magnitudes, as Cardiac Output, vascular shunting and flow variations, in normal as well as in pathological conditions

5. Acknowledgment

The authors wish to thank Drs Marielle Estevez and Carla Fonseca from the animal house of the Institut de Recerca de l'Hospital Universitari Vall d'Hebron for their invaluable help in animal care and preparation. They also wish to express their gratitude to Dr Jose Lluis Peiró for his surgical intervention on the mother sheep and the instrumentation of foetuses as well as for his generous teaching and support.

6. References

Alcázar, J L, 2008. Three-dimensional power Doppler derived vascular indices: what are we measuring and how are we doing it? Ultrasound in Obstetrics & Gynecology: The

Official Journal of the International Society of Ultrasound in Obstetrics and Gynecology, 32(4), págs.485-487.

Alcázar, Juan Luis & Jurado, M., 2011. Three-dimensional ultrasound for assessing women with gynecological cancer: a systematic review. Gynecologic Oncology, 120(3), págs.340-346.

Bello-Muñoz, J. et al., 2009. OP23.05: A three-dimensional power Doppler algorithm for ductus venosus shunting evaluation in normal and growth restricted fetuses. Ultrasound in Obstetrics & Gynecology, 34(S1), págs.136-137.

Bellotti, M, Pennati, G. & Ferrazzi, E., 2007. Re: ductus venosus shunting in growth-restricted fetuses and the effect of umbilical circulatory compromise. Ultrasound in Obstetrics & Gynecology: The Official Journal of the International Society of Ultrasound in Obstetrics and Gynecology, 29(1), págs.100-101; author reply 101-102.

Bellotti, M et al., 2000. Role of ductus venosus in distribution of umbilical blood flow in human fetuses during second half of pregnancy. American Journal of Physiology. Heart and Circulatory Physiology, 279(3), págs.H1256-1263.

Bellotti, Maria et al., 2004. Simultaneous measurements of umbilical venous, fetal hepatic, and ductus venosus blood flow in growth-restricted human fetuses. American Journal of Obstetrics and Gynecology, 190(5), págs.1347-1358.

Bendick, P.J. et al., 1998. Three-dimensional vascular imaging using Doppler ultrasound. American Journal of Surgery, 176(2), págs.183-187.

Berg, S. et al., 2000. Volumetric blood flow measurement with the use of dynamic 3-dimensional ultrasound color flow imaging. Journal of the American Society of Echocardiography: Official Publication of the American Society of Echocardiography, 13(5), págs.393-402.

Bozkurt, N., Başgül Yigiter, A., et al., 2010. Correlations of fetal-maternal outcomes and first trimester 3-D placental volume/3-D power Doppler calculations. Clinical and Experimental Obstetrics & Gynecology, 37(1), págs.26-28.

Burns, P.N., 1992. Measuring volume flow with Doppler ultrasound-an old nut. Ultrasound in Obstetrics & Gynecology: The Official Journal of the International Society of Ultrasound in Obstetrics and Gynecology, 2(4), págs.238-241.

Cruz-Martinez, R et al., 2011. Normal reference ranges of fetal regional cerebral blood perfusion as measured by fractional moving blood volume. Ultrasound in Obstetrics & Gynecology: The Official Journal of the International Society of Ultrasound in Obstetrics and Gynecology, 37(2), págs.196-201.

Cruz-Martinez, Rogelio et al., 2009. Cerebral blood perfusion and neurobehavioral performance in full-term small-for-gestational-age fetuses. American Journal of Obstetrics and Gynecology, 201(5), págs.474.e1-7.

Chang, C.-H. et al., 2003. Assessment of normal fetal liver blood flow using quantitative three-dimensional power Doppler ultrasound. Ultrasound in Medicine & Biology, 29(7), págs.943-949.

Chaoui, R. & Heling, K.S., 2005. New developments in fetal heart scanning: three- and four-dimensional fetal echocardiography. Seminars in Fetal & Neonatal Medicine, 10(6), págs.567-577.

Chaoui, R. & Kalache, K.D., 2001. Three-dimensional power Doppler ultrasound of the fetal great vessels. Ultrasound in Obstetrics & Gynecology: The Official Journal of the

International Society of Ultrasound in Obstetrics and Gynecology, 17(5), págs.455-456.

Dar, P. et al., 2010. First-trimester 3-dimensional power Doppler of the uteroplacental circulation space: a potential screening method for preeclampsia. American Journal of Obstetrics and Gynecology, 203(3), págs.238.e1-7.

DeVore, G.R. et al., 2003. Spatio-temporal image correlation (STIC): new technology for evaluation of the fetal heart. Ultrasound in Obstetrics & Gynecology: The Official Journal of the International Society of Ultrasound in Obstetrics and Gynecology, 22(4), págs.380-387.

Dubiel, M. et al., 2005. Computer analysis of three-dimensional power angiography images of foetal cerebral, lung and placental circulation in normal and high-risk pregnancy. Ultrasound in Medicine & Biology, 31(3), págs.321-327.

Eik-Nes, S.H. et al., 1982. Ultrasonic measurement of human fetal blood flow. Journal of Biomedical Engineering, 4(1), págs.28-36.

Fenster, A., Lee, D., et al., 1998. Three-dimensional ultrasound imaging of the vasculature. Ultrasonics, 36(1-5), págs.629-633.

Forsberg, F. et al., 1995. Volume flow estimation using time domain correlation and ultrasonic flowmetry. Ultrasound in Medicine & Biology, 21(8), págs.1037-1045.

Gill, R.W., 1979. Pulsed Doppler with B-mode imaging for quantitative blood flow measurement. Ultrasound in Medicine & Biology, 5(3), págs.223-235.

Guimarães Filho, H.A. et al., 2011. Reproducibility of three-dimensional power Doppler placental vascular indices in pregnancies between 26 and 35 weeks. Archives of Gynecology and Obstetrics, 283(2), págs.213-217.

Guo, Z. & Fenster, A., 1996. Three-dimensional power Doppler imaging: a phantom study to quantify vessel stenosis. Ultrasound in Medicine & Biology, 22(8), págs.1059-1069.

Guo, Z., Durand, L.G., et al., 1998. In vitro evaluation of multiple arterial stenoses using three-dimensional power Doppler angiography. Journal of Vascular Surgery: Official Publication, the Society for Vascular Surgery [and] International Society for Cardiovascular Surgery, North American Chapter, 27(4), págs.681-688.

Harrington, K., Deane, C. & Campbell, S., 1996. Measurement of volume flow with time domain and M-mode imaging: in vitro and in vivo validation studies. Journal of Ultrasound in Medicine: Official Journal of the American Institute of Ultrasound in Medicine, 15(10), págs.715-720.

Hayashi, T. et al., 1998. Three-dimensional reconstruction of the power flow Doppler imaging of intracranial vascular structures in the neonate. Journal of Neuroimaging: Official Journal of the American Society of Neuroimaging, 8(2), págs.94-96.

Heling, K.S., Chaoui, R. & Bollmann, R., 2000. Prenatal depiction of the angioarchitecture of an aneurysm of the vein of Galen with three-dimensional color power angiography. Ultrasound in Obstetrics & Gynecology: The Official Journal of the International Society of Ultrasound in Obstetrics and Gynecology, 15(4), pág.345.

Hernandez-Andrade, E et al., 2008. Changes in regional fetal cerebral blood flow perfusion in relation to hemodynamic deterioration in severely growth-restricted fetuses. Ultrasound in Obstetrics & Gynecology: The Official Journal of the International Society of Ultrasound in Obstetrics and Gynecology, 32(1), págs.71-76.

Hernandez-Andrade, E, Jansson, T, et al., 2004. Validation of fractional moving blood volume measurement with power Doppler ultrasound in an experimental sheep model. Ultrasound in Obstetrics & Gynecology: The Official Journal of the International Society of Ultrasound in Obstetrics and Gynecology, 23(4), págs.363-368.

Hernandez-Andrade, E, Thuring-Jönsson, A., et al., 2004. Fractional moving blood volume estimation in the fetal lung using power Doppler ultrasound: a reproducibility study. Ultrasound in Obstetrics & Gynecology: The Official Journal of the International Society of Ultrasound in Obstetrics and Gynecology, 23(4), págs.369-373.

Jansson, Tomas et al., 2003. Estimation of fractional moving blood volume in fetal lung using Power Doppler ultrasound, methodological aspects. Ultrasound in Medicine & Biology, 29(11), págs.1551-1559.

Jones, M.G., Shipley, J.A. & Robinson, T.M., 2003. Visualisation of 4-D colour and power Doppler data. Ultrasound in Medicine & Biology, 29(12), págs.1735-1747.

Jones, N.W. et al., 2011. Evaluating the intra- and interobserver reliability of three-dimensional ultrasound and power Doppler angiography (3D-PDA) for assessment of placental volume and vascularity in the second trimester of pregnancy. Ultrasound in Medicine & Biology, 37(3), págs.376-385.

Kiserud, T., 2001. The ductus venosus. Seminars in Perinatology, 25(1), págs.11-20.

Kiserud, T. et al., 2006. Ductus venosus shunting in growth-restricted fetuses and the effect of umbilical circulatory compromise. Ultrasound in Obstetrics & Gynecology: The Official Journal of the International Society of Ultrasound in Obstetrics and Gynecology, 28(2), págs.143-149.

Kripfgans, O.D. et al., 2006. Measurement of volumetric flow. Journal of Ultrasound in Medicine: Official Journal of the American Institute of Ultrasound in Medicine, 25(10), págs.1305-1311.

Kupesic, S. & Kurjak, A., 2000. Contrast-enhanced, three-dimensional power Doppler sonography for differentiation of adnexal masses. Obstetrics and Gynecology, 96(3), págs.452-458.

Kurjak, A. et al., 1998. The assessment of ovarian tumor angiogenesis: what does three-dimensional power Doppler add? Ultrasound in Obstetrics & Gynecology: The Official Journal of the International Society of Ultrasound in Obstetrics and Gynecology, 12(2), págs.136-146.

Lai, P.K., Wang, Y.A. & Welsh, A.W., 2010. Reproducibility of regional placental vascularity/perfusion measurement using 3D power Doppler. Ultrasound in Obstetrics & Gynecology: The Official Journal of the International Society of Ultrasound in Obstetrics and Gynecology, 36(2), págs.202-209.

Li, X. et al., 2005. A novel method for the assessment of the accuracy of computing laminar flow stroke volumes using a real-time 3D ultrasound system: In vitro studies. European Journal of Echocardiography: The Journal of the Working Group on Echocardiography of the European Society of Cardiology, 6(6), págs.396-404.

Marín, R.C. et al., 2010. Use of 3-dimensional sonography for prenatal evaluation and follow-up of fetal goitrous hypothyroidism. Journal of Ultrasound in Medicine: Official Journal of the American Institute of Ultrasound in Medicine, 29(9), págs.1339-1343.

Martins, W.P. & Raine-Fenning, N J, 2010. Analysis and acquisition reproducibility of 3D power Doppler. Ultrasound in Obstetrics & Gynecology: The Official Journal of the International Society of Ultrasound in Obstetrics and Gynecology, 36(3), págs.392-393; author reply 393-394.

Morel, O. et al., 2010. Correlation between uteroplacental three-dimensional power Doppler indices and true uterine blood flow: evaluation in a pregnant sheep model. Ultrasound in Obstetrics & Gynecology: The Official Journal of the International Society of Ultrasound in Obstetrics and Gynecology, 36(5), págs.635-640.

Moskalik, A.P. et al., 2001. Analysis of three-dimensional Doppler ultrasonographic quantitative measures for the discrimination of prostate cancer. Journal of Ultrasound in Medicine: Official Journal of the American Institute of Ultrasound in Medicine, 20(7), págs.713-722.

Nardozza, L.M.M. et al., 2009. Evolution of 3-D power Doppler indices of fetal brain in normal pregnancy. Ultrasound in Medicine & Biology, 35(4), págs.545-549.

Negrini, R. et al., 2011. Assessment of placental blood flow between 22 and 34 weeks of gestation by 3D-sonography power Doppler vascular indices. Archives of Gynecology and Obstetrics, 284(1), págs.53-57.

Odeh, M. et al., 2011. Placental volume and three-dimensional power Doppler analysis in prediction of pre-eclampsia and small for gestational age between Week 11 and 13 weeks and 6 days of gestation. Prenatal Diagnosis, 31(4), págs.367-371.

Odibo, A.O. et al., 2011. Placental volume and vascular flow assessed by 3D power Doppler and adverse pregnancy outcomes. Placenta, 32(3), págs.230-234.

Pairleitner, H. et al., 1999. Three-dimensional power Doppler sonography: imaging and quantifying blood flow and vascularization. Ultrasound in Obstetrics & Gynecology: The Official Journal of the International Society of Ultrasound in Obstetrics and Gynecology, 14(2), págs.139-143.

Pemberton, J. et al., 2005. The use of live three-dimensional Doppler echocardiography in the measurement of cardiac output: an in vivo animal study. Journal of the American College of Cardiology, 45(3), págs.433-438.

Petersch, B. & Hönigmann, D., 2007. Blood flow in its context: combining 3D B-mode and color Doppler ultrasonic data. IEEE Transactions on Visualization and Computer Graphics, 13(4), págs.748-757.

Pomorski, M. et al., 2011. Comparative analysis of placental vasculature and placental volume in normal and IUGR pregnancies with the use of three-dimensional Power Doppler. Archives of Gynecology and Obstetrics. Available at: http://www.ncbi.nlm.nih.gov/pubmed/21744006 [Accedido Julio 17, 2011].

Raine-Fenning, N J, Nordin, N.M., Ramnarine, K.V., Campbell, B.K., Clewes, J.S., Perkins, A. & Johnson, I.R., 2008a. Determining the relationship between three-dimensional power Doppler data and true blood flow characteristics: an in-vitro flow phantom experiment. Ultrasound in Obstetrics & Gynecology: The Official Journal of the International Society of Ultrasound in Obstetrics and Gynecology, 32(4), págs.540-550.

Raine-Fenning, N J, Nordin, N.M., Ramnarine, K.V., Campbell, B.K., Clewes, J.S., Perkins, A. & Johnson, I.R., 2008b. Evaluation of the effect of machine settings on quantitative three-dimensional power Doppler angiography: an in-vitro flow phantom experiment. Ultrasound in Obstetrics & Gynecology: The Official Journal of the

International Society of Ultrasound in Obstetrics and Gynecology, 32(4), págs.551-559.

Richards, M.S. et al., 2009. Mean volume flow estimation in pulsatile flow conditions. Ultrasound in Medicine & Biology, 35(11), págs.1880-1891.

Rizzo, G. et al., 2009. First-trimester placental volume and vascularization measured by 3-dimensional power Doppler sonography in pregnancies with low serum pregnancy-associated plasma protein a levels. Journal of Ultrasound in Medicine: Official Journal of the American Institute of Ultrasound in Medicine, 28(12), págs.1615-1622.

Ruano, R. et al., 2006. Quantitative analysis of fetal pulmonary vasculature by 3-dimensional power Doppler ultrasonography in isolated congenital diaphragmatic hernia. American Journal of Obstetrics and Gynecology, 195(6), págs.1720-1728.

Rubin, J M, 1999. Flow quantification. European Radiology, 9 Suppl 3, págs.S368-371.

Rubin, J M et al., 1994. Power Doppler US: a potentially useful alternative to mean frequency-based color Doppler US. Radiology, 190(3), págs.853-856.

Rubin, J M et al., 1997. Normalizing fractional moving blood volume estimates with power Doppler US: defining a stable intravascular point with the cumulative power distribution function. Radiology, 205(3), págs.757-765.

Rubin, J M, Tuthill, T.A. & Fowlkes, J B, 2001. Volume flow measurement using Doppler and grey-scale decorrelation. Ultrasound in Medicine & Biology, 27(1), págs.101-109.

Sauders, J.B., Wright, N. & Lewis, K.O., 1980. Measurement of human fetal blood flow. British Medical Journal, 280(6210), págs.283-284.

Schulten-Wijman, M.J. et al., 2011. Re: Three-dimensional power Doppler: validity and reliability. Ultrasound in Obstetrics & Gynecology: The Official Journal of the International Society of Ultrasound in Obstetrics and Gynecology, 37(5), págs.620-621.

Sun, Y. et al., 1995. Estimation of volume flow rate by surface integration of velocity vectors from color Doppler images. Journal of the American Society of Echocardiography: Official Publication of the American Society of Echocardiography, 8(6), págs.904-914.

Tchirikov, M., Schröder, H.J. & Hecher, K., 2006. Ductus venosus shunting in the fetal venous circulation: regulatory mechanisms, diagnostic methods and medical importance. Ultrasound in Obstetrics & Gynecology: The Official Journal of the International Society of Ultrasound in Obstetrics and Gynecology, 27(4), págs.452-461.

Tuuli, M.G. et al., 2010. Validation of placental vascular sonobiopsy for obtaining representative placental vascular indices by three-dimensional power Doppler ultrasonography. Placenta, 31(3), págs.192-196.

Welsh, A., 2004. Quantification of power Doppler and the index «fractional moving blood volume» (FMBV). Ultrasound in Obstetrics & Gynecology: The Official Journal of the International Society of Ultrasound in Obstetrics and Gynecology, 23(4), págs.323-326.

Welsh, A.W. et al., 2005. Standardization of power Doppler quantification of blood flow in the human fetus using the aorta and inferior vena cava. Ultrasound in Obstetrics & Gynecology: The Official Journal of the International Society of Ultrasound in Obstetrics and Gynecology, 26(1), págs.33-43.

Yigiter, A.B. et al., 2011. Placental volume and vascularization flow indices by 3D power Doppler US using VOCAL technique and correlation with IGF-1, free beta-hCG, PAPP-A, and uterine artery Doppler at 11-14 weeks of pregnancy. Journal of Perinatal Medicine, 39(2), págs.137-141.

16

Thyroid Sonography in 3D with Emphasis on Perfusion

Roy Moncayo and Helga Moncayo
WOMED, Innsbruck, Austria

1. Introduction

Ultrasound examination of the thyroid gland is an essential diagnostic element in daily clinical practice. The aim of this chapter is to describe the advanced clinical value of conducting 3D ultrasound examinations putting emphasis on the quantitative evaluation of perfusion characteristics of the thyroid gland and to relate these results to therapeutic interventions aimed at diminishing inflammation.

2. Historical aspects of ultrasound

The term echo (Greek: Ηχώ, *Ēkhō*; "Sound") refers to the persistence of sound after its source has stopped. Greek mythology tells from an Oread (a mountain nymph) who pined away for love of Narcissus (in Ovid, Metamorphoses). The phenomenon of air being sent back by a wall was described by Aristotles (384-322 BCE). The Greek word echo came into German writings in the 16th century. Athanasius Kircher (1602 - 1680) used the principle of "Echometria" to determine the depth of a well. His book was entitled: "Neue Hall- und Thon-Kunst oder Mechanische Gehaim-Verbindung der Kunst und Natur durch Stimme und Hall" and appeared 1684. At this time he was able to measure the speed of sound propagation.

On May 25th, 1842 Christian Doppler (born in Salzburg, Austria) presented in Prague his talk on "Abhandlung Über das farbige Licht der Doppelsterne und einiger anderer Gestirne des Himmels" (Eng. *On the coloured light of the binary stars and some other stars of the heavens)* at the Prague Polytechnic [1]. The Doppler effect is a main stand of many examinations today.

In 1880 Pierre and Jacques Curie discovered the piezoelectric effect and postulated the generation of ultrasound waves [2]. They found that applying an electric current to a crystal would produce a vibration which could in turn produce sound waves. In turn, sound waves striking a crystal would produce an electric voltage. In 1917 Langevin constructed for the first time a piezoelectric ultrasound transducer based on quartz elements and which was called sandwich-style. This product was oriented towards military use in World War I, i.e. the detection of submarines. The Langevin-type transducers were utilized in depth sounding devices [3]. More details on the work of Langevin is found elsewhere [4]. In 1921 Behm in Vienna described the Echolot which was used to determine the water depth for ships [5].

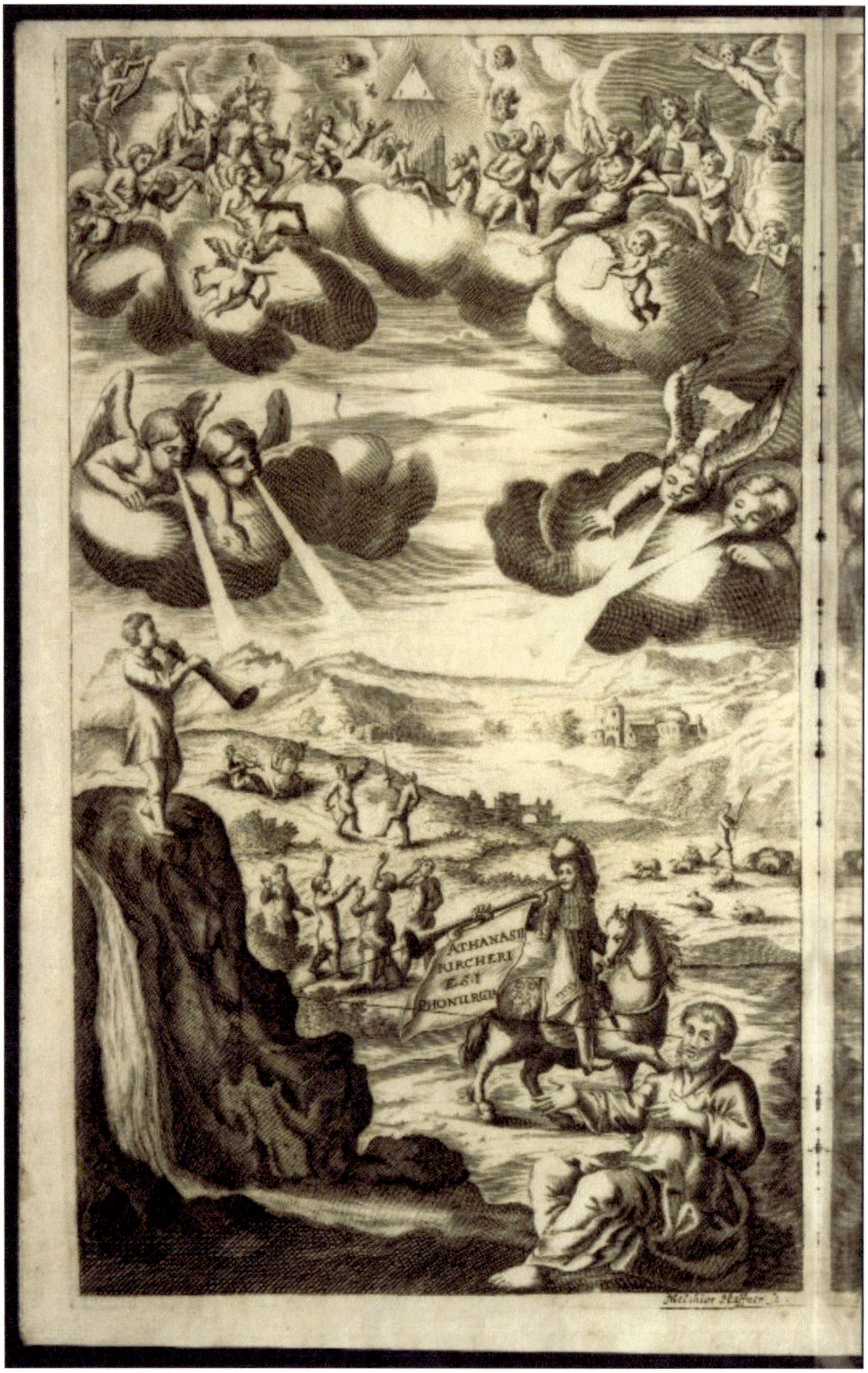

Source: http://echo.mpiwg-berlin.mpg.de/ECHOdocuView?url=/mpiwg/online/permanent/library/1EZGRF6Y/pageimg&viewMode=images&pn=6&mode=imagepath

Fig. 1. An image from Kircher's book depicting air reflection

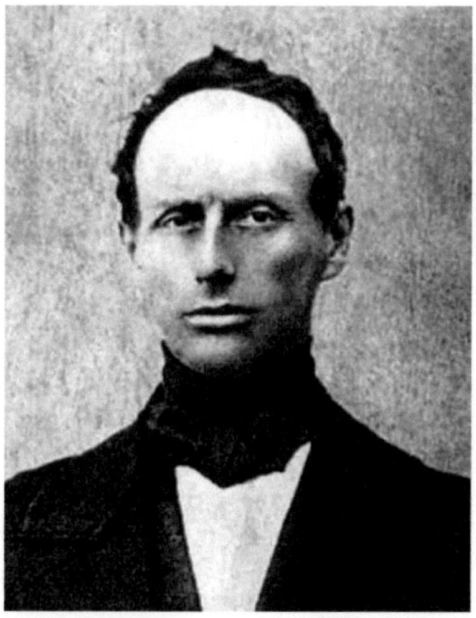

Source: http://en.wikipedia.org/wiki/File:Christian_Doppler.jpg

Fig. 2. C. Doppler, born november 29th, 1803 in Salzburg, public domain

Following these fundamental developments, clinical applications began to develop. The first clinical applications of ultrasound are credited to the Austrian neurologist Karl Theo Dussik [6]. In the introduction of his article he mentions that he was motivated to investigate the medical importance of ultrasound in 1937 after having read a review on use of underwater ultrasound techniques (Echolotung) as well as the use of ultrasound for the detection of material flaws in industrial settings by Sokolov [7]. He goes on to discuss the properties of auscultation, which in the end works because changes in tissue density, relative water content, and colloidal structure have occured. Further references on the basic physics of ultrasound can be found in the paper. The initial clinical indications according to Dussik were the ventricle system of the brain and the spinal bones in a procedure called hyperphonography. Further fields of application were liver, kidneys, testicles, and the extremities.

Some of the data mentioned above have been extracted from the publication by Frentzel-Beyme [8]. Additional information has been obtained via Wikipedia.

2.1 Modern history of ultrasound including thyroid examinations

General articles on the historical aspects and developments of ultrasound can be found in recent publications [8-10]. In addition to this some useful clinical publications on thyroid examinations are those of Ruchala and Szczepanek [11] and Sholosh and Borhani [12]. The physics of ultrasound have been presented by Kossoff [13].

In the 1950's Howry and Bliss presented their device which was used for the ultrasonic visualization of body soft tissue structures [14,15]. Some interesting images can be found in their publication [15]: Figure 3 shows the apparatus called "Somascope". Due to its use of a cattle drink tank it was also called the "cattle tank scanner". Figure 4 in shows the anatomical structures of the neck at the C5 level. Figure 5 depicts the findings of a case thyroid carcinoma where liver metastases were present.

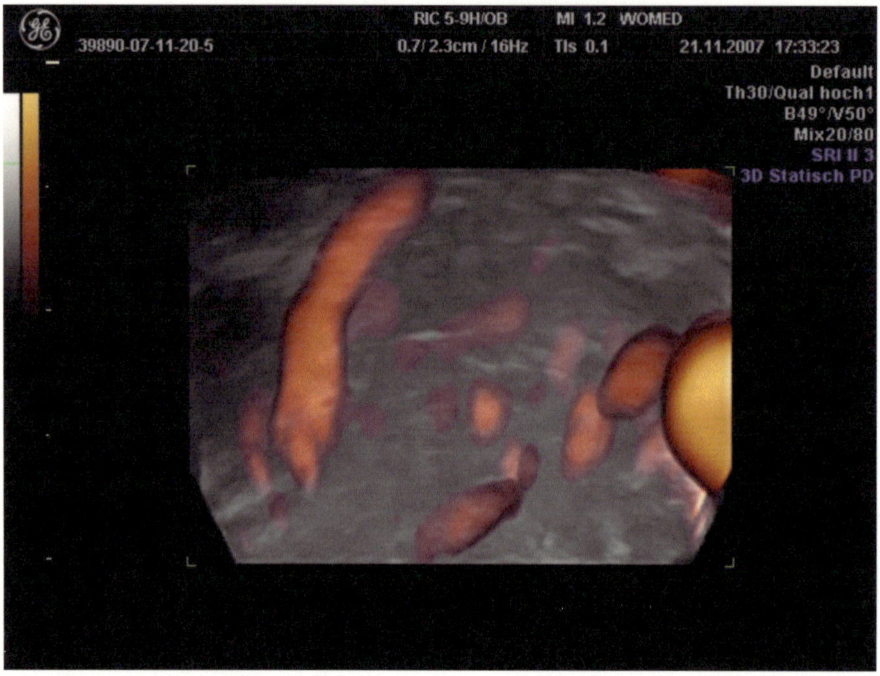

Fig. 3. Case 1. Normal thyroid seen in 3-D power Doppler modus using a vaginal transducer. The thick vessel corresponds to a laryngeal artery

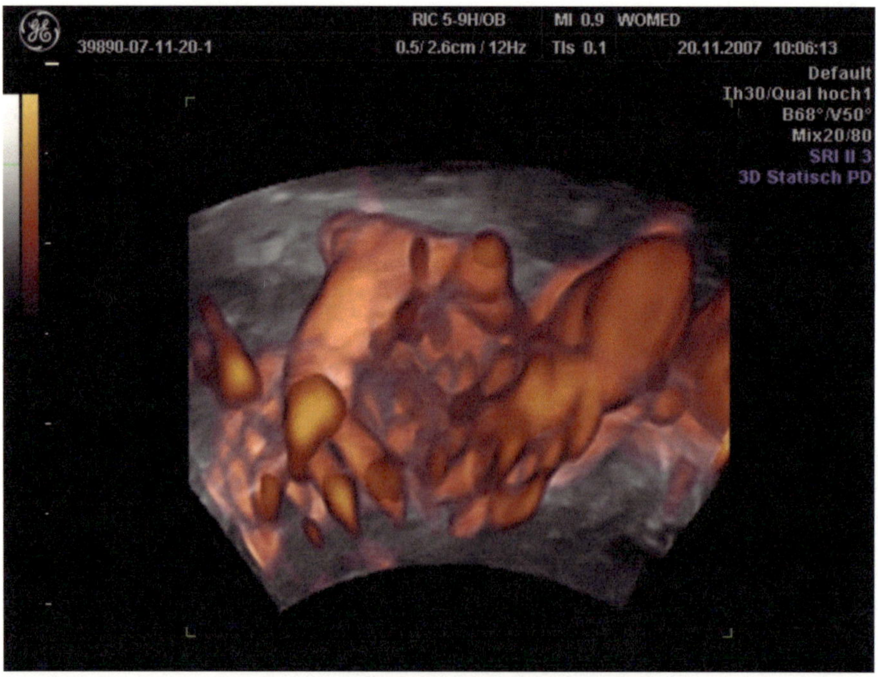

Fig. 4. Case 2. Chronic recurrent thyroiditis in 3-D power Doppler modus using a vaginal transducer. Note the increased vascularity as compared to Figure. 3

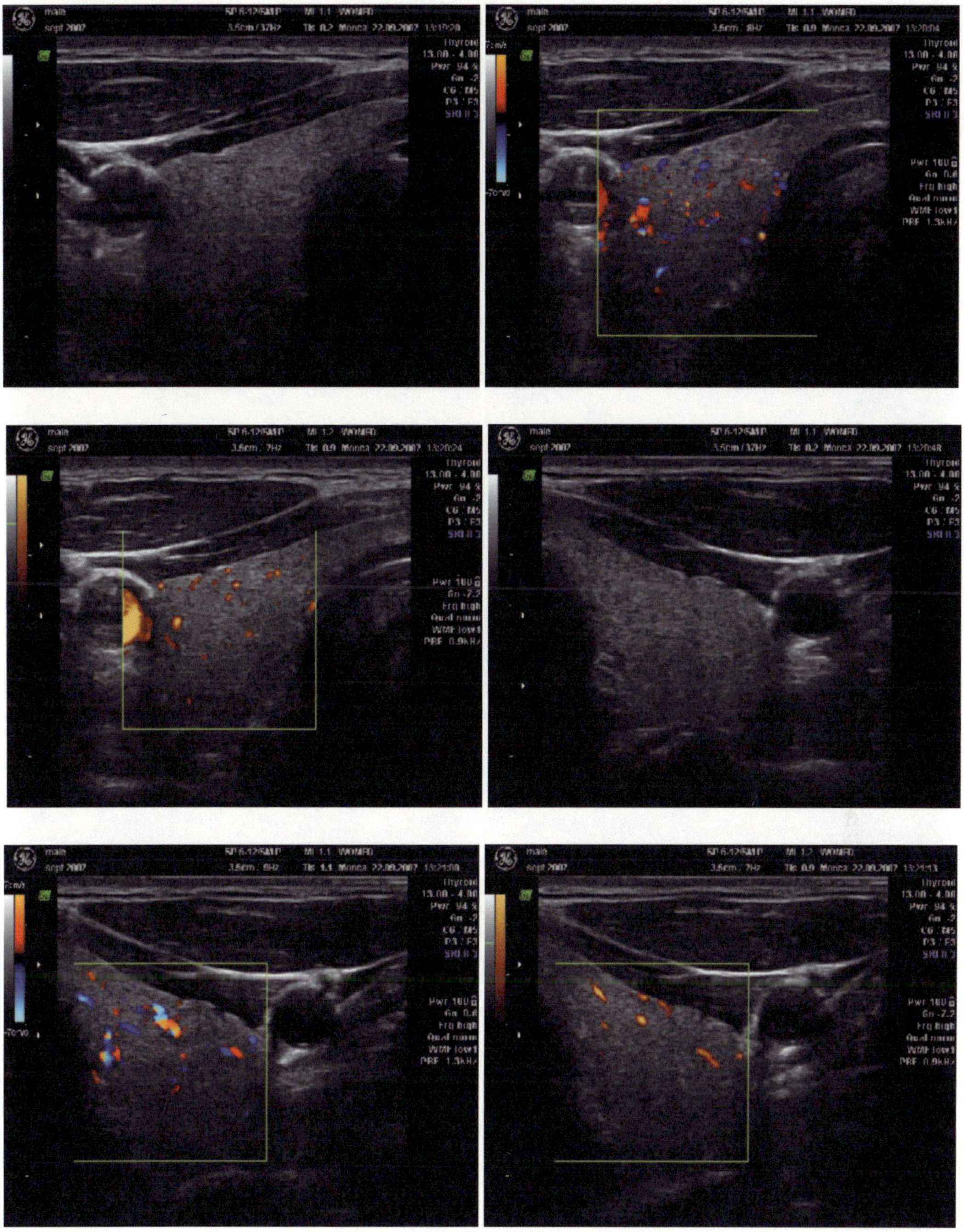

Fig. 5 (a-f). Case 3. Both lobes of a normal thyroid shown in gray, color, and power Doppler modus. The VFI value of 0.09 is reflected by the almost complete absence of perfusion signs. Such cases do not require quantitative evaluation of perfusion

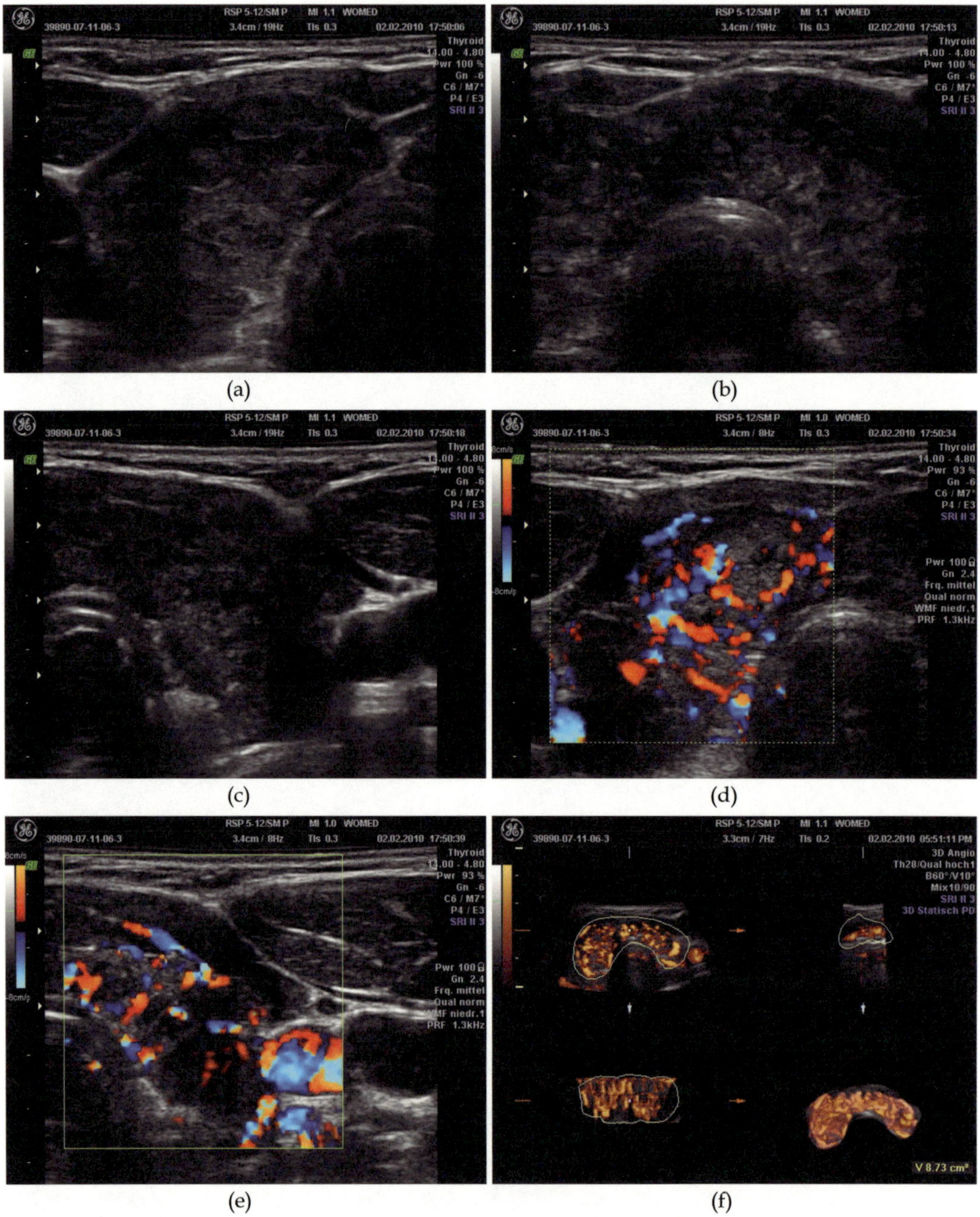

Fig. 6. (continues on next page) Case 4. The same patient shown in Figure. 4 examined with the RSP5-12 transducer. a-c: the hypoechogenic structure of the thyroid. d-e: single slice in color mode showing several vessels. f: the 3D image reconstruction using VOCAL. g: the final 3D image showing total thyroid vascularity. Note the almost total absence of underlying thyroid tissue. h-i: segmented imaging of the thyroid. This procedure is important in order to detect any nodular changes within the gland. j: The parameters obtained after the VOCAL analysis. The gray value is relatively low due to the increased vascular density

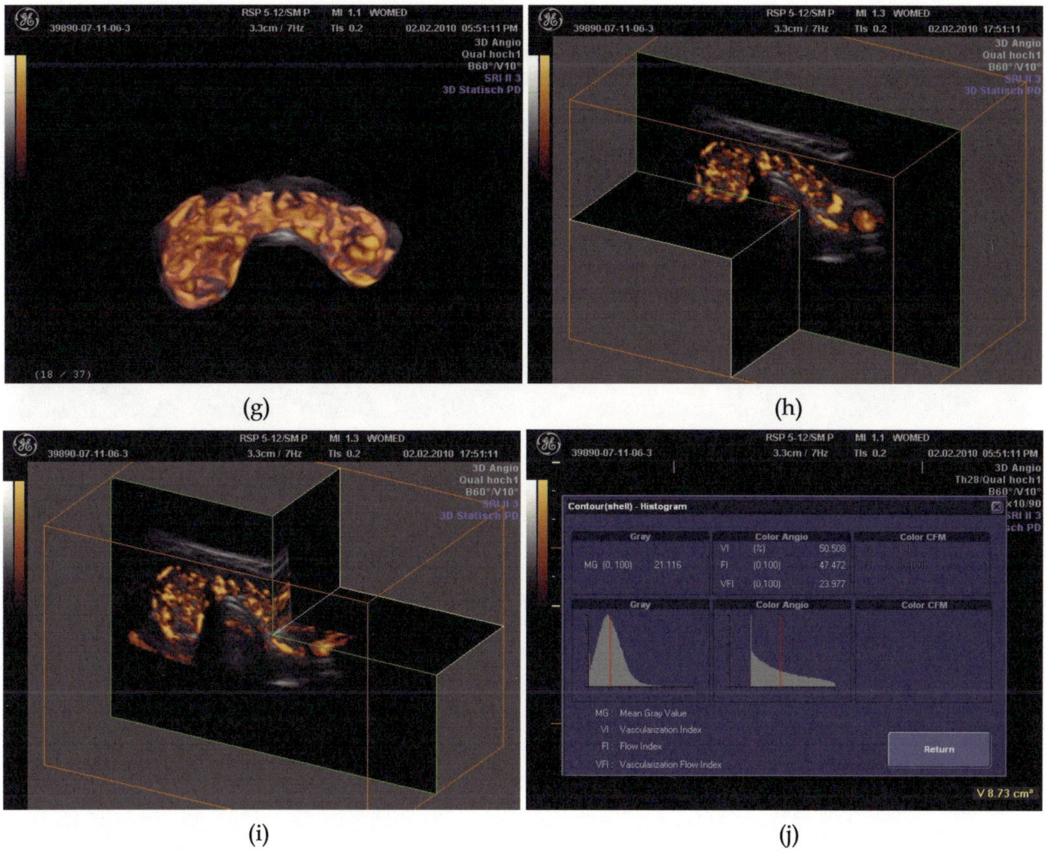

Fig. 6. (continued) Case 4. The same patient shown in Figure 4 examined with the RSP5-12 transducer. a-c: the hypoechogenic structure of the thyroid. d-e: single slice in color mode showing several vessels. f: the 3D image reconstruction using VOCAL. g: the final 3D image showing total thyroid vascularity. Note the almost total absence of underlying thyroid tissue. h-i: segmented imaging of the thyroid. This procedure is important in order to detect any nodular changes within the gland. j: The parameters obtained after the VOCAL analysis. The gray value is relatively low due to the increased vascular density

In 1967 Fujimoto et al. published their data on US examination of the thyroid [16]. The authors described 4 basic echo patterns: cystic, sparsely spotted, strong internal echoes, and the lack of internal echoes. In 1971 the first paper by Blum et al. documented the use of A-mode sonography [17]. In 1972 Blum [18] published an article entitled: "Clinical applications of thyroid echography" which described the data on 122 patients who had had thyroid surgery. Both A-mode and B-mode sonography was done with a 5 megahertz apparatus. In the one dimensional A-mode imaging a water-soluble gel was interposed between the transducer and the skin. For 2-dimensional B-mode imaging a mineral oil was used as coupling agent. During the examination the gain was changed in order to detect structures that had a maximal reflection while using low-sensitivity and finally high gain in order to detect lower amplitude echoes. Examples of these examinations can be seen in Figures 2-5 [18]. Acoustic dense structures were described in an adenoma (Fig. 6). Solid masses (benign or malignant) as well as thyroiditis appeared to be sonographically indistinguishable.

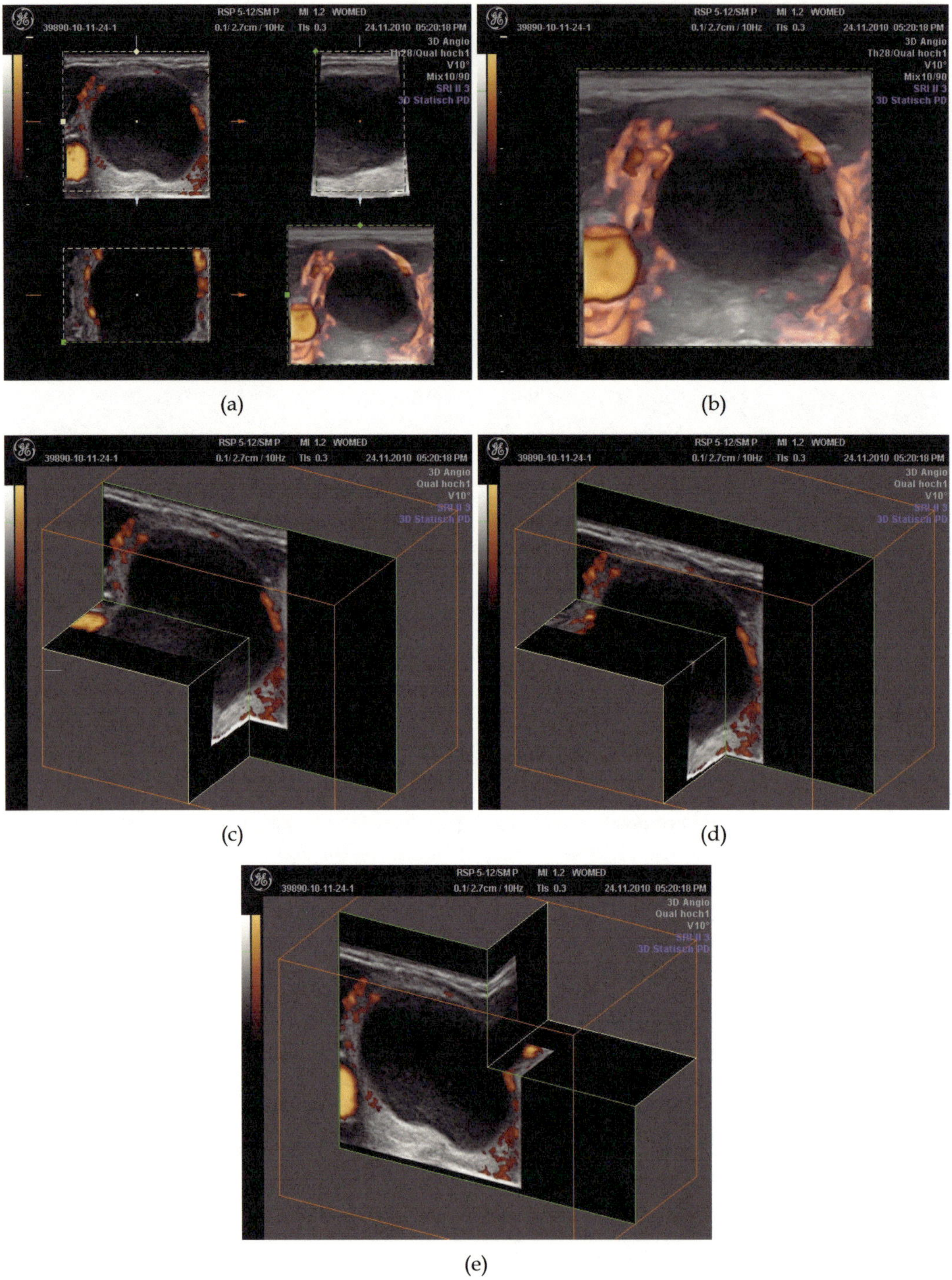

Fig. 7. Case 5. A female patient with a cystic nodule. The cyst has clear limits, no vessels penetrate the cavity. a: the 3D image set. b: enlarged view of the 3D reconstruction. c-e: segmentation of the cyst

In subacute thyroiditis and Graves' disease the authors found very uniform low-amplitude echoes which were only visible at high-gain setting in the A-mode. The image of B-mode was described as having a very fine stippling. According to Blum the basic purposes for conducting thyroid ultrasound examinations were: to determine whether a solitary cold nodule was cystic or solid, to document changes in size of solitary nodules even under suppressive therapy, to evaluate the depth dimension [18]. According to Australian specialists the development of ultrasound techniques for thyroid examinations is based on a breast ultrasound examination apparatus installed at the Royal North Shore Hospital in Sydney. The publication by Crocker and Jellins appeared in 1978 [19].

After the first definitions on the use of ultrasound for thyroid investigations, the notion of adding data on the depth of the nodule was presented by Thijs et al. [20]. The authors combined digital scintigraphy with ultrasound. The classification of nodules into hot, warm, cool, and cold was also advanced. The feature of sonolucent halo of adenomatous nodules was demonstrated by Scheible et al. in 1979 [21]. In 1988 Ralls et al. coined the term "thyroid inferno" to describe the characteristics of color-flow Doppler sonography in patients with Graves' disease [22]. Their study did not include patients with thyroiditis nor with latent hypothyroidism. In 1992 Miyakawa et al. described a pattern of decreased echogenicity in cases of silent thyroiditis. Such patients had a high T3 to T4 ratio [23].

In 1994-1995 Rubin reported the development of Power Doppler technology [24,25]. This development was considered an improvement of color Doppler which can detect fractional moving blood volume. A demonstration of the applicability of this technique for the detection of inflammatory changes in joints was already published 1994 [26]. The authors described increased blood flow as being suggestive of mild inflammation of the tendon examined, and marked hyperemia with vascular blush in severe changes (Fig. 2 in [26]).

The following general considerations on the characteristics of ultrasound investigations are taken from Rose and Nelson [27]. In brightness mode or gray scale US the velocity of US wave propagation in fluids and soft tissues is approximately 1540 meters per second. The time delay between the pulse sent and that of the returned wave is the basis for the determination of the reflector depth. The intensity of the reflected US wave is given as brightness of the image. Spatial resolution is dependent on the wavelength of the US wave. US attenuation increases with increased frequency. Deep structures require low frequencies in the range of 2.5-3.5 MHz, while superficial structures can be investigated within the range of 7-10 MHz. Signals are transmitted by the transducer and at the same time echo reflections are registered. According to the structure of the tissues, some portions of the sound is reflected back to the surface. Dense echoes are reflected from structures with different acoustic densities. Homogeneous liquids transmit sound without reflections. Air-filled structures do not transmit ultrasound. Attenuation of waves can be due to body fat and fascial structures [27]. In thyroid examinations such attenuation can occur due to the cervical fasciae.

2.2 Historical aspects of 3D ultrasound – The Kretz story

The beginnings of Kretz can be traced back to early 1947 when the company started the production of resistance-welded wired goods. The founder of the company was engineer Paul Kretz. Some of the products included glass balloon baskets, milk bottle carriers and potato baskets. The company started in the old rooms of the old brewery in Zipf, Austria. In 1952 the first own building was built.

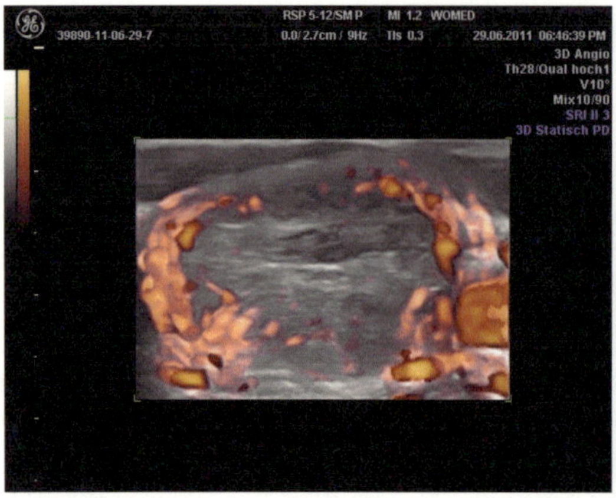

(a)

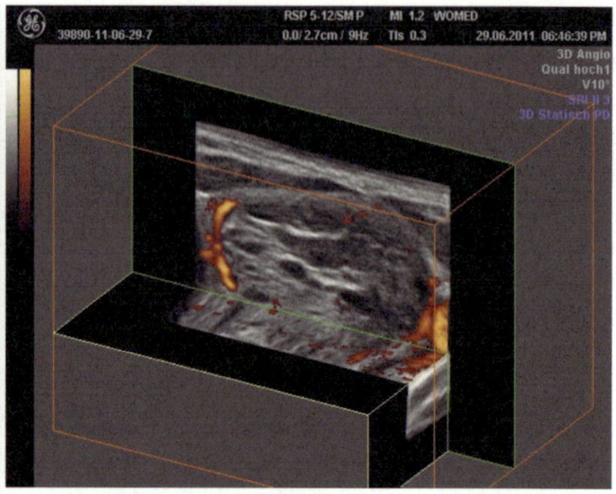

(b)

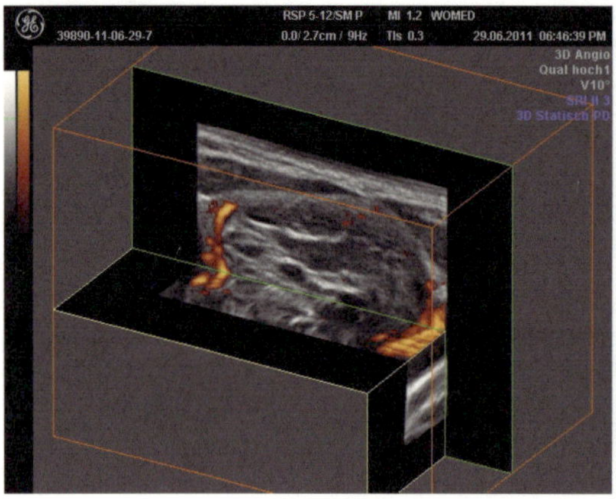

(c)

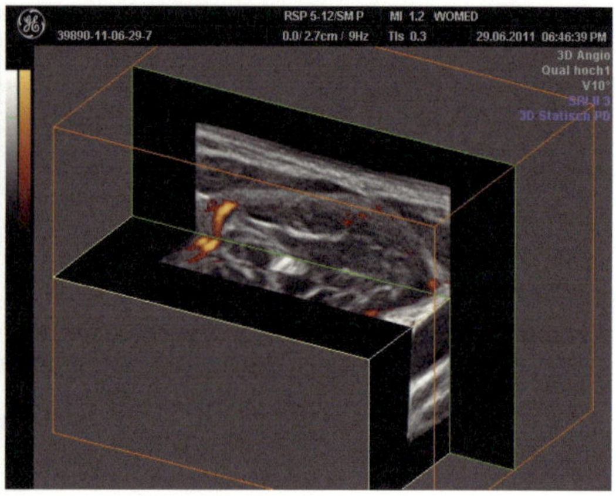

(d)

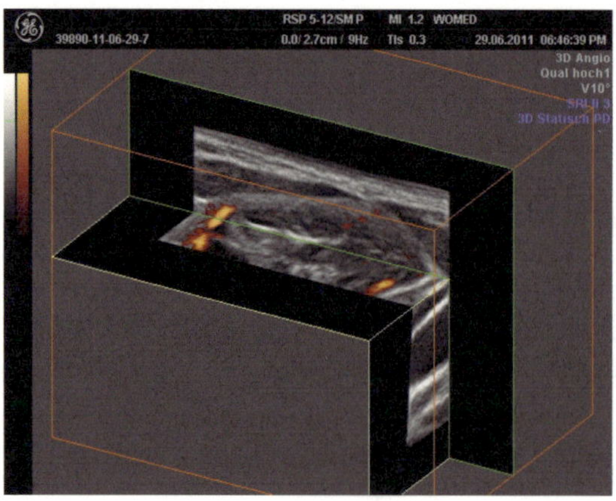

(e)

Fig. 8. Case 6. A female patient with a compensated autonomous adenoma. a: demonstration of the vessels surrounding the adenoma. In gray modus these vessels appear as a halo. b-e: segmentation of the nodule that shows lack of vascularity within the nodule

In 1950 the company started to develop Echolot (echo sounding) machines for the purpose of material testing. By 1957 the material testing machines became the main stand of the company.

In 1962 medical professionals start tests on the clinical use of the available material test apparatus. One of the first users was Prof. Kratochwil who used the technology for gynecological examinations, i.e. "ultrasonic placentography" (1962) [28]. In the time between 1967 and 1977 the ultrasound machines were used in gynecology, ophthalmology, neurology, and radiology based on A-mode, B-mode, time-motion and Doppler techniques. Some of the early models which were developed were: Combison 200 (1975-1978), and the improved Combison 202/R, the Minifason (1973-1977) - a hand-held Doppler for fetal heart investigations. The Combison 100 (1977) was the first real-time sector scanner of the world equipped with the first single element rotating transducer. The Combison 310 released in 1987 was a compact ultrasound machine. The following Combison 320 included computer technology.

In 1987 the first images of 3D scanning began. This technology was included in the first generation of 3D machines, having the Combison 330 in 1989. In 1992 the Combison 520 appeared. This was the 2nd generation of 3D machines to be produced in series. Between 1996 and 2001 Kretztechnik and Medison (Korea) fused and brought out the Voluson 530D in 1997. In 2001 Kretztechnik was taken over by G.E. The Austrian press reported: "Medical Systems, a subsidiary of US group General Electric (GE), acquired a 65.4% majority in Austrian Kretztechnik from Korean Medison. GE paid EUR 97.5mn, or EUR 12 per share, for Medison's stake. GE offers to buy widespread shares for EUR 17 per share in the coming two weeks. Zipf-based Kretztechnik is the world market leader for modern ultrasound systems, i.e. three-dimensional real-time imaging systems". The following models were those of the Voluson 730 series. In 2011 the Voluson S8 and S6 were released.

The accomplishments of Carl Kretz were honored in 1999 when he received the Ian Donald Gold Medal for Technical Development by the International Society of Ultrasound in Obstetrics and Gynecology [29]. The publication by Chiou et al. on 3D thyroid investigations provides some additional information as to the development of 3D imaging in general [30].

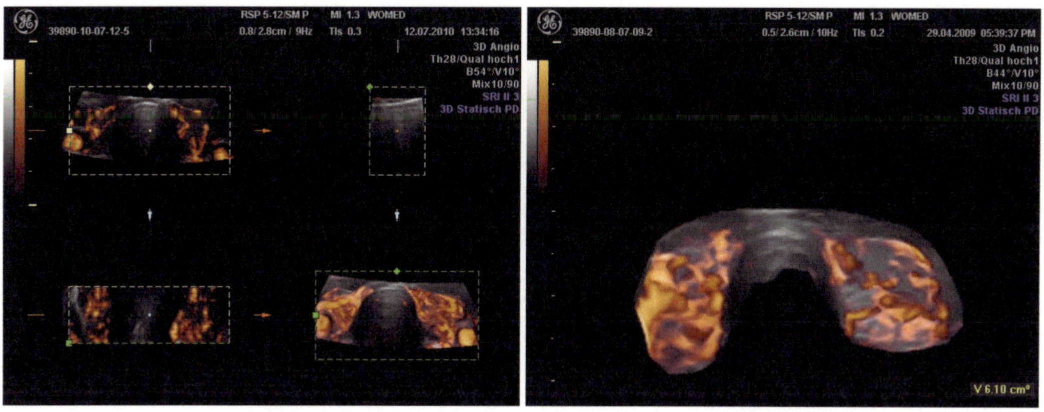

(a) (b)

Fig. 9. Case 7. A female patient with Graves' disease presenting bilateral thyroid associated ophthalmopathy. a: 3D reconstruction. b: detail of the 3D reconstruction. VFI 14.8

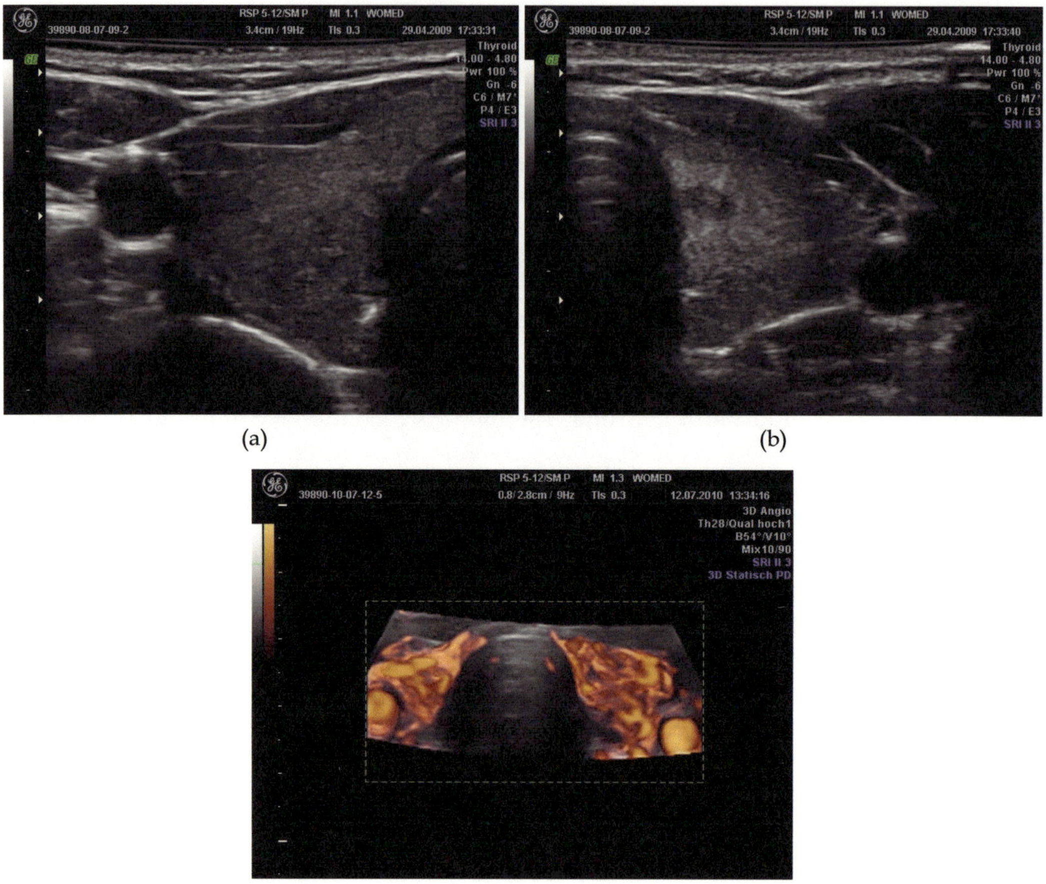

(a) (b)

(c)

Fig. 10. Case 8. A female patient with Graves' disease prior to treatment with selenomethionine and Mg. a-b: low echogenic signal of the thyroid. c: demonstration of increased total vascularity, VOCAL reconstruction, VFI 10.91

The paper describing the characteristics of quantified blood flow analysis using these machines was published by Pairleitner in 1999 [31]. The original definition of the indices states: "VI measures the number of color voxels in the cube, representing the vessels in the tissue (Figure 3). FI, a mean color value of all blood flow or induced flow intensities, represents the intensity of flow at the time of the three dimensional sweep. FI is not an indicator of perfusion, so it cannot give information on the volume of blood pumped through the vessels during a certain period of time. VFI is a combination of vascularization and flow information relating the weighted color values (weighted by their amplitudes) to the cube. Therefore, VFI represents both blood flow and vascularization". The automatic procedure for the quantification of vascularization indices was called VOCAL™. VOCAL stands for the 3D virtual organ computer-aided analysis program developed by Kretz. Data on the reliability of the VOCAL analysis as well as on the parametric setting for the examinations in gynecological applications have been presented by Bordes and Raine-Fenning [32,33].

3. 3D-Ultrasound thyroid examination

3D-Ultrasound examinations in this paper were done using a General Electrics Voluson 730 Pro ultrasound machine equipped with a RealTime 4D linear transducer (RSP5-12, GE Healthcare, Waukesha, WI 53188, USA). Data analysis was done using the VOCAL™ software (4DView Version 5.x, GE Medical Systems - Kretztechnik GmbH & Co OHG) installed on the ultrasound machine. Both the gray-scale values and the color values were normalized from 0 to 100, 100 being the highest intensity. The analysis of the 3D Doppler data sets provided the following indexes: VI, FI, and VFI [31]. The examination was done with the patients lying supine and with a light hyperextension of the neck. The transducer was placed on the midline of the neck having the whole gland inside the field of view. The mean time of data acquisition for the thyroid studies was approximately 20 seconds. The study had to be repeated only when movement artifacts arising from the patients (coughing or swallowing) had occurred. The drawing of the area of the thyroid gland was carried out using manual trace at 15° steps [34]. During drawing care was taken not to include laryngeal vessels which are typically seen on the medial border of the thyroid.

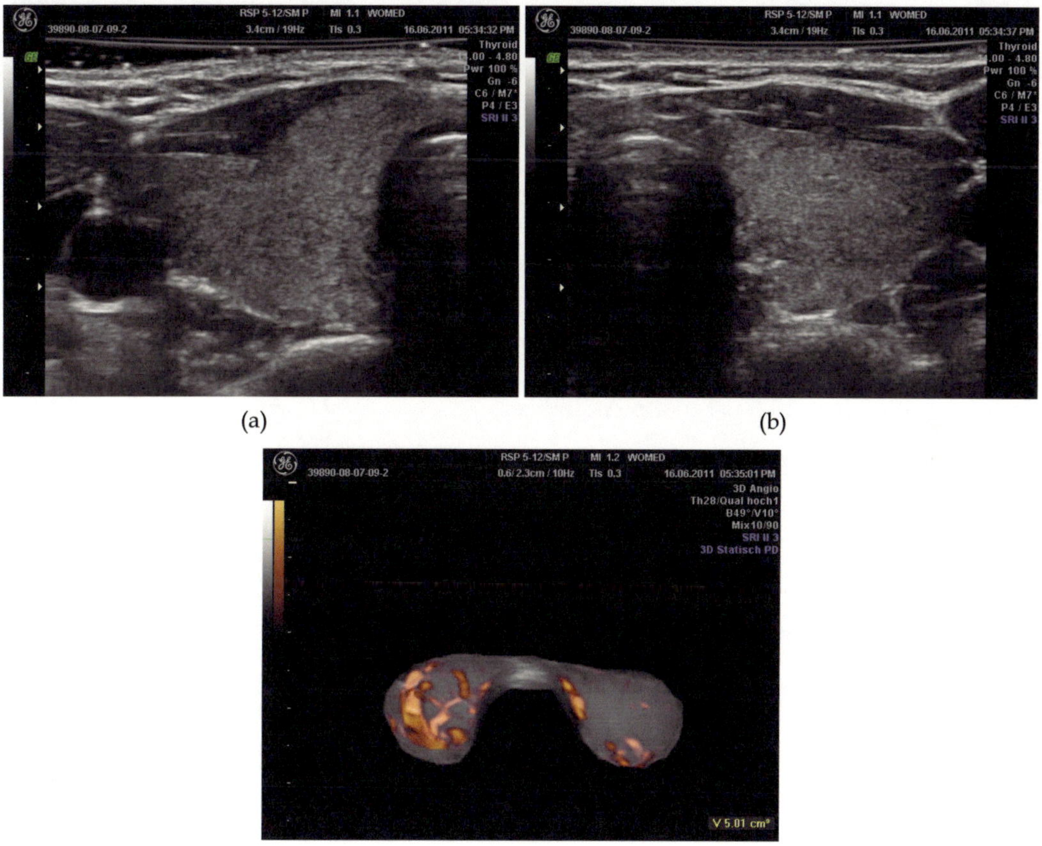

(a) (b)

(c)

Fig. 11. Case 8. A female patient with Graves' disease after treatment with selenomethionine and Mg. a-b: normal echogenic signal of the thyroid. c: demonstration of less total vascularity, VOCAL reconstruction, VFI 3.49

4. Clinical cases: Normal thyroid, nodular disease, cystic disease, latent hypothyroidism, hypothyroidism, hyperthyroidism

The ultrasound data presented here have been obtained during examinations carried out at our Institution WOMED in Innsbruck, Austria. A total of 140 examinations were carried out. The procedures were carried in accordance with the Declaration of Helsinki [35]. The list of representative demonstration cases presented in this chapter is shown in the Table. The initial ultrasound examinations (cases 1 and 2) were done by both authors based on the previous experience of HM in the field of reproductive medicine. These first 2 studies were carried out using a vaginal transducer. Two cases with nodular disease are presented in order to demonstrate the capability of 3-volume visualization of the thyroid. The most relevant perfusion parameter for hypo- and hyperthyroidism, i.e. VFI, is shown.

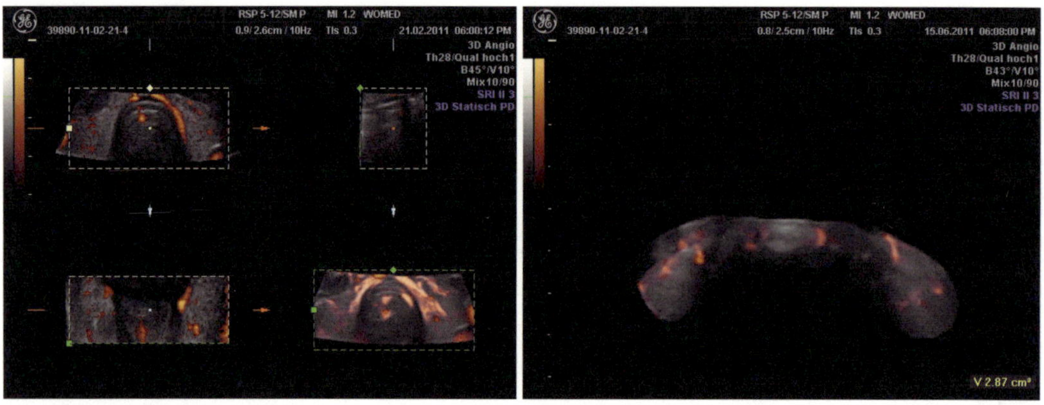

(a) (b)

Fig. 12. Case 9. A female patient with latent hypothyroidism prior to treatment with selenomethionine and Mg. a: 3D reconstruction. b: 3D VOCAL reconstruction, VFI 4.22. Compare with Figure 13 (post-treatment images)

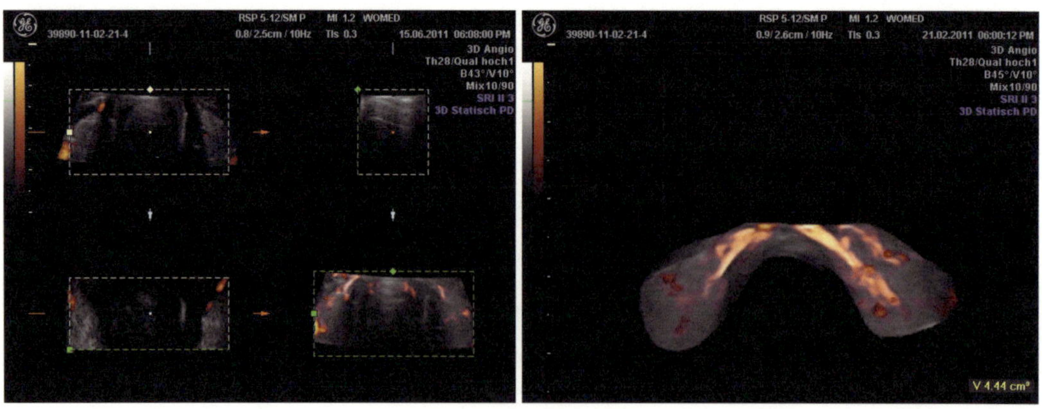

(a) (b)

Fig. 13. Case 9. A female patient with latent hypothyroidism after treatment with selenomethionine and Mg. a: 3D reconstruction. b: 3D VOCAL reconstruction, VFI 1.21. Compare with Figure 12 (pre-treatment images)

Case	Sex	Diagnosis	VFI
1	m	Normal thyroid – (study done with a vaginal transducer)	n.d.
2	f	Chronic recurrent thyroiditis – (study done with a vaginal transducer)	n.d.
3	m	Normal thyroid	0.09
4	f	Chronic recurring thyroiditis	23.97
5	f	Cystic adenoma	n.d.
6	f	Autonomous adenoma	n.d.
7	f	Graves' disease and thyroid associated orbitopathy	14.8
8	f	Graves' disease pre-treatment	10.91
9	f	Graves' disease after treatment	3.49
10	f	Latent hypothyroidism pre-treatment	4.22
11	f	Latent hypothyroidism post-treatment	1.21

Table 1.

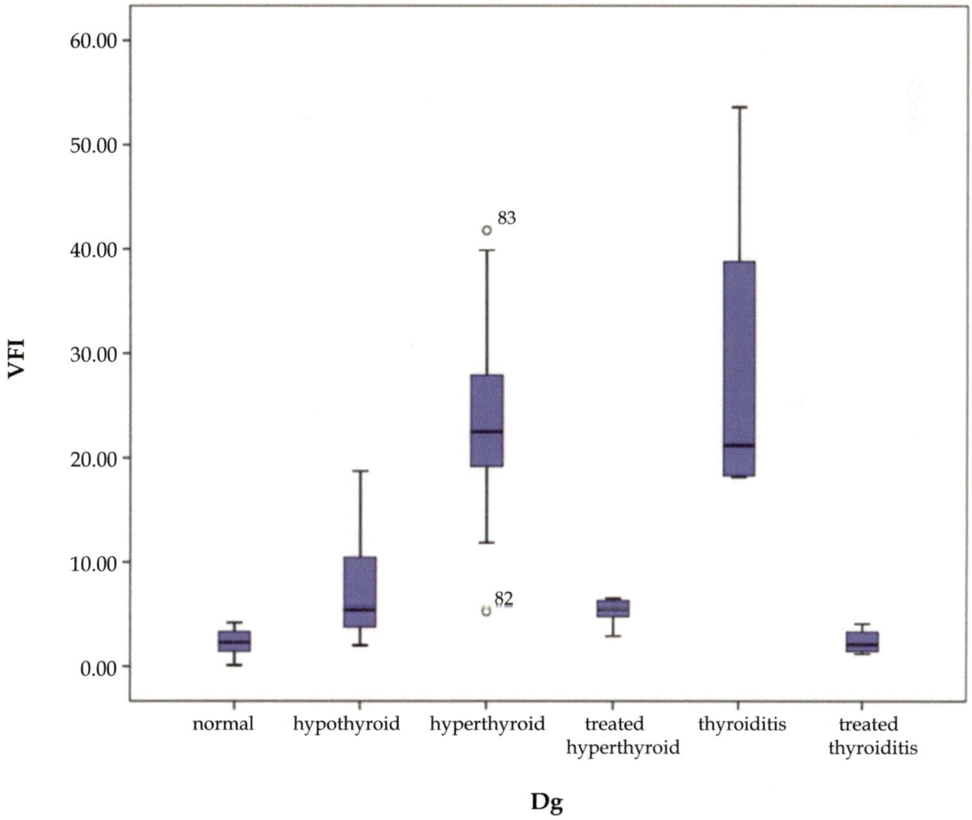

Fig. 14. The VFI value in different thyroid conditions. The first two bars correspond to single observations. The following groups of 2-bars each demonstrate the VFI changes following therapy with selenomethionine and Mg citrate ($p<0.01$)

Based on the results of previous investigations [36-40] supportive treatment included selenomethionine and Mg-citrate. Supplementation with selenomethionine (200 µg/d, Pure

Encapsulations ©, pro medico HandelsGmbH, Graz Austria) was prescribed if the serum levels were less than 80µg/l. Magnesium substitution was prescribed if the serum level was lower than 0.8 mmol/l (Magnesium Verla©, 60mg of Mg-citrate/Mg-L-glutamate, Kwizda Pharma GmbH, Vienna) at a dose of 360mg/day. This treatment was given over a period of 3 months in cases 8 and 10. The changes in thyroid morphology and VFI are given as cases 9 and 11. Statistical analysis of the 140 observations revealed that VFI was the most relevant parameter showing significant changes after our therapy approach (Figure 14).

5. Discussion

Studies with 3D technology concerning thyroid function are scarce. Only 2 publications have addressed this issue [30,41]. The paper by Chiou et al. is the first one in the literature to deal with the same technology as us [30]. This study included patients with Hashimoto's disease as well as Graves' disease. In Figure 1 the authors present the VFI value of a patient with Graves' disease (VFI = 30.7). This value is similar that the ones we have obtained. Unfortunately further individual data are not presented. The authors present exhaustive data on correlation analyses. The second publication on 3D ultrasound of the thyroid by Slapa et al. is centered on nodular thyroid disease [41]. This publication has no comparable data to our results. All together it can be said that 3D perfusion studies of the thyroid are rare.

3D perfusion studies, however, has found much wider application in the field of reproductive medicine since the original publication of the qualitative analysis method by Pairleitner et al. [31]. Data on the reliability of the VOCAL analysis as well as on the parametric setting for the examinations have been presented by Bordes and Raine-Fenning [32,33]. Concerns regarding power Doppler signal attenuation as discussed by Raine-Fenning [33] should not be relevant in thyroid examinations since the distance between the transducer and the organ is relatively constant (app. 1 to 1.5 cm).

Since more data is available from the gynecological field we will mention some data related to ovarian perfusion studies. Examination of the ovaries as reported by in Rainne-Fenning [33] revealed mean VFI values for the ovary of 2.076 and 2.074 (2 observers). Changes in ovarian vascularization during the menstrual cycle has been reported by Järvelä et al. [42]. In Table 2 of [42] a comparison of vascularization parameters between the right and left ovaries is shown. The mean values for VI, FI, VFI, and mean grayness were: 6.2/7.4, 43.4/46.5, 2.8/3.7, and 45.8/46.0, respectively. In 2002 Pan et al. compared the vascularization characteristics between patients with polycystic ovarian syndrome and controls [43]. The mean values for VI, FI, and VFI for normals and PCO patients were: 0.8/2.1, 44.44/50.26, and 1.44/3.99, respectively. In 2003 Pan et al. [44] described a stimulatory effect of HRT on the ovarian vascularization parameters in postmenopausal women (!). The mean values for VI, FI, and VFI before and after HRT were: 0.31/1.12, 30.47/38.41, and 0.13/0.59, respectively. This finding implies a stimulatory effect of conjugated equine estrogen on these parameters. The same group of investigators described increased vascularization parameters in women that showed a hyper-response to stimulation protocols for IVF [45]. Hyperresponders had higher levels of estradiol (>3000 pg/ml) or had more than 15 oocytes retrieved. The mean values for VI, FI, and VFI for patients with a "normal" and patients with an increased response to stimulation were: 1.25/2.27, 43.19/50.23, and 0.63/1.18, respectively.

Comparing the image material presented in the above mentioned citations with our images, it can be clearly recognized that the thyroid gland has a wider range of variation in the degree of vascularization. The VFI values seen in thyroiditis and Graves' disease are generally higher than in different conditions of ovarian function. These differences cannot be taken as absolute ones. Data variability between different publications has 2 main sources of error. The first one is the use of different Kretz machines (Combison, Voluson). The second one is the fact that each investigator or each machine has different examination settings for carrying out the studies. We recommend the continuous use of the same settings in order to produce comparable results. These facts have been mentioned by de Ziegler [46]. De Ziegler points out the weakness of early studies which were arbitrary and subjective in interpretation [46]. Some of the open expectations mentioned by de Ziegler included the "desire for an understanding of the mechanisms at play" as well as whether ovarian function had a relation to perfusion values. As we show in Figure 12, the relevant parameter VFI decreases significantly following the combined treatment with selenomethionine and magnesium. We postulate that the VFI represents an inflammatory process that is present in several thyroid entities. Initially we had described this as a "low grade connective tissue inflammation" in patients with thyroid associated ophthalmopathy [39]. In this publication we discussed amply the role of Se in inflammation. Data concerning Mg and inflammation can be found in the literature [47-60]. The initial invitation of the Editors of this book was indeed to elaborate on these pathophysiological connections.

6. Conclusions

Increased perfusion characteristics in 3D modus provide an exact picture of the underlying inflammatory changes in the thyroid. This description is better than that of indirect signs said to be associated with such changes (simple Doppler imaging, pulsed Doppler). This technical enhancement will allow the clinician to gain immediate access to the basic underlying processes of thyroid disease, i.e. inflammation. This process of inflammation is directly related to the available body resources of substances that regulate inflammatory processes. Effectiveness of treatment can be uniquely evaluated by the quantitative 3D power Doppler perfusion study of the thyroid.

7. Acknowledgements

Historical data on the development of GE Kretztechnik was kindly provided by GE Austria.

8. References

[1] Doppler C: Abhandlung Über das farbige Licht der Doppelsterne und einiger anderer Gestirne des Himmels. *Abh K Bohm Ges Wissen Prag* 1842, 465-482.

[2] Curie J, Curie P: Development par pression de l'electricite polaire dans les cristaus hemidres a faces inclinees. *C R Acad Sci Paris* 1880, 91: 294-295.

[3] Mason WP: Piezoelectricity, its history and applications. *J Acoust Soc Am* 1981, 70: 1561-1566.

[4] Paty P: Paul Langevin (1872-1946), la relativité et les quanta. *Bull Soc Fr Phys* 1999, 119: 15-20.

[5] Behm A: Das Behm-Echolot. *Ann Hydrogr* 1921, 49: 241-247.

[6] Dussik KT: Über die Möglichkeit, hochfrequente mechanische Schwingungen als diagnostisches Hilfsmittel zu verwerten. *Z Gesamte Neurol Psychatr* 1941, 174: 153-168.

[7] Sokolov SY: On the problem of the propagation of ultrasonic oscillations in various bodies. *Elek Nachr Tech* 1929, 6: 454-460.

[8] Frentzel-Beyme B: [From echo-sounding to color doppler sonography. The history of diagnostic ultrasonic diagnosis.]. *Radiologe* 2005, 45: 363-370.
[9] Jecker P, Frentzel-Beyme B: [The history of head and neck sonography]. *Laryngorhinootologie* 2002, 81: 900-905.
[10] Levine RA: Something old and something new: a brief history of thyroid ultrasound technology. *Endocr Pract* 2004, 10: 227-233.
[11] Ruchala M, Szczepanek E: Thyroid ultrasound - a piece of cake? *Endokrynol Pol* 2010, 61: 330-344.
[12] Sholosh B, Borhani AA: Thyroid ultrasound part 1: technique and diffuse disease. *Radiol Clin North Am* 2011, 49: 391-416.
[13] Kossoff G: Basic physics and imaging characteristics of ultrasound. *World J Surg* 2000, 24: 134-142.
[14] Howry DH, Bliss WR: Ultrasonic visualization of soft tissue structures of the body. *J Lab Clin Med* 1952, 40: 579-592.
[15] Holmes JH, Howry DH, Posakony GJ, Cushman CR: The ultrasonic visualization of soft tissue structures in the human body. *Trans Am Clin Climatol Assoc* 1954, 66: 208-225.
[16] Fujimoto Y, Oka A, Omoto R, Hirose M: Ultrasound scanning of the thyroid gland as a new diagnostic approach. *Ultrasonics* 1967, 5: 177-180.
[17] Blum M, Weiss B, Hernberg J: Evaluation of thyroid nodules by A-mode echography. *Radiology* 1971, 101: 651-656.
[18] Blum M, Goldman AB, Herskovic A, Hernberg J: Clinical applications of thyroid echography. *N Engl J Med* 1972, 287: 1164-1169.
[19] Crocker EF, Jellins J: Grey scale ultrasonic examination of the thyroid gland. *Med J Aust* 1978, 9: 244-248.
[20] Thijs LG, Roos P, Wiener JD: Use of ultrasound and digital scintiphoto analysis in the evaluation of solitary thyroid nodules. *J Nucl Med* 1972, 13: 504-509.
[21] Scheible W, Leopold GR, Woo VL, Gosink BB: High-resolution real-time ultrasonography of thyroid nodules. *Radiology* 1979, 133: 413-417.
[22] Ralls PW, Mayekawa DS, Lee KP, Colletti PM, Radin DR, Boswell WD *et al.*: Color-flow Doppler sonography in Graves disease: "thyroid inferno". *Am J Roentgenol* 1988, 150: 781-784.
[23] Miyakawa M, Tsushima T, Onoda N, Etoh M, Isozaki O, Arai M *et al.*: Thyroid ultrasonography related to clinical and laboratory findings in patients with silent thyroiditis. *J Endocrinol Invest* 1992, 15: 289-295.
[24] Rubin JM, Bude RO, Carson PL, Bree RL, Adler RS: Power Doppler US: a potentially useful alternative to mean frequency-based color Doppler US. *Radiology* 1994, 190: 853-856.
[25] Rubin JM, Adler RS, Fowlkes JB, Spratt S, Pallister JE, Chen JF *et al.*: Fractional moving blood volume: estimation with power Doppler US. *Radiology* 1995, 197: 183-190.
[26] Newman JS, Adler RS, Bude RO, Rubin JM: Detection of soft-tissue hyperemia: value of power Doppler sonography. *AJR Am J Roentgenol* 1994, 163: 385-389.
[27] Rose SC, Nelson TR: Ultrasonographic modalities to assess vascular anatomy and disease. *J Vasc Interv Radiol* 2004, 15: 25-38.
[28] Kratochwil A: [Possibilities of ultrasonic diagnosis in labor gynecology]. *Wien Klin Wochenschr* 1966, 78: 190-191.
[29] Kratochwil A: Presentation of the Ian Donald Gold Medal for Technical Development to Carl Kretz. *Ultrasound Obstet Gynecol* 2000, 16: 107-108.

[30] Chiou SC, Hsieh MH, Chen HY, Lin JD, Chen CC, Hsu WH *et al.*: The reproducibility of the virtual organ computer-aided analysis program for evaluating 3-dimensional power Doppler ultrasonography of diffuse thyroid disorders. *J Endocrinol Invest* 2009, 32: 139-146.

[31] Pairleitner H, Steiner H, Hasenoehrl G, Staudach A: Three-dimensional power Doppler sonography: imaging and quantifying blood flow and vascularization. *Ultrasound Obstet Gynecol* 1999, 14: 139-143.

[32] Bordes A, Bory AM, Benchaïb M, Rudigoz RC, Salle B: Reproducibility of transvaginal three-dimensional endometrial volume measurements with virtual organ computer-aided analysis (VOCAL) during ovarian stimulation. *Ultrasound Obstet Gynecol* 2002, 19: 76-80.

[33] Raine-Fenning NJ, Campbell BK, Clewes JS, Kendall NR, Johnson IR: The reliability of virtual organ computer-aided analysis (VOCAL) for the semiquantification of ovarian, endometrial and subendometrial perfusion. *Ultrasound Obstet Gynecol* 2003, 22: 633-639.

[34] Mercé LT, Gómez B, Engels V, Bau S, Bajo JM: Intraobserver and interobserver reproducibility of ovarian volume, antral follicle count, and vascularity indices obtained with transvaginal 3-dimensional ultrasonography, power Doppler angiography, and the virtual organ computer-aided analysis imaging program. *J Ultrasound Med* 2005, 24: 1279-1287.

[35] World Medical Association Declaration of Helsinki: ethical principles for medical research involving human subjects. *JAMA* 2000, 284: 3043-3045.

[36] Moncayo R, Moncayo H, Kapelari K: Nutritional treatment of incipient thyroid autoimmune disease. Influence of selenium supplementation on thyroid function and morphology in children and young adults. *Clin Nutr* 2005, 24: 530-531.

[37] Moncayo R, Rudisch A, Kremser C, Moncayo H: 3D-MRI rendering of the anatomical structures related to acupuncture points of the Dai mai, Yin qiao mai and Yang qiao mai meridians within the context of the WOMED concept of lateral tension: Implications for musculoskeletal disease. *BMC Musculoskelet Disord* 2007, 8: 33.

[38] Moncayo R, Rudisch A, Diemling M, Kremser C: In-vivo visualisation of the anatomical structures related to the acupuncture points Dai mai and Shen mai by MRI: A single-case pilot study. *BMC Med Imaging* 2007, 7: 4.

[39] Moncayo R, Moncayo H: A musculoskeletal model of low grade connective tissue inflammation in patients with thyroid associated ophthalmopathy (TAO): The WOMED concept of lateral tension and its general implications in disease. *BMC Musculoskelet Disord* 2007, 8: 17.

[40] Moncayo R, Kroiss A, Oberwinkler M, Karakolcu F, Starzinger M, Kapelari K *et al.*: The role of selenium, vitamin C, and zinc in benign thyroid diseases and of Se in malignant thyroid diseases: low selenium levels are found in subacute and silent thyroiditis and in papillary and follicular carcinoma. *BMC Endocrine Disorders* 2008, 8: 2.

[41] Slapa RZ, Jakubowski WS, Slowinska-Srzednicka J, Szopinski KT: Advantages and disadvantages of 3D ultrasound of thyroid nodules including thin slice volume rendering. *Thyroid Res* 2011, 4: 1.

[42] Järvelä IY, Sladkevicius P, Kelly S, Ojha K, Nargund G, Campbell S: Three-dimensional sonographic and power Doppler characterization of ovaries in late follicular phase. *Ultrasound Obstet Gynecol* 2002, 20: 281-285.

[43] Pan HA, Wu MH, Cheng YC, Li CH, Chang FM: Quantification of Doppler signal in polycystic ovary syndrome using three-dimensional power Doppler ultrasonography: a possible new marker for diagnosis. *Hum Reprod* 2002, 17: 201-206.
[44] Pan HA, Li CH, Cheng YC, Wu MH, Chang FM: Quantification of ovarian stromal Doppler signals in postmenopausal women receiving hormone replacement therapy. *Menopause* 2003, 10: 366-372.
[45] Pan HA, Wu MH, Cheng YC, Wu LH, Chang FM: Quantification of ovarian Doppler signal in hyperresponders during in vitro fertilization treatment using three-dimensional power Doppler ultrasonography. *Ultrasound Med Biol* 2003, 29: 921-927.
[46] de Ziegler D: Uterine Doppler studies: technology driven data, or answers to our pathophysiological queries? *Hum Reprod* 2004, 19: 2615-2618.
[47] Brautbar N, Carpenter C: Skeletal myopathy and magnesium depletion: cellular mechanisms. *Magnesium* 1984, 3: 57-62.
[48] Weglicki WB, Phillips TM: Pathobiology of magnesium deficiency: A cytokine/neurogenic inflammation hypothesis. *Am J Physiol* 1992, 263: R734-R737.
[49] Garcia LA, Dejong SC, Martin SM, Smith RS, Buettner GR, Kerber RE: Magnesium reduces free radicals in an in vivo coronary occlusion-reperfusion model. *J Am Coll Cardiol* 1998, 32: 536-539.
[50] Tejero-Taldo MI, Chmielinska JJ, Gonzalez G, Mak IT, Weglicki WB: N-methyl-D-aspartate receptor blockade inhibits cardiac inflammation in the Mg2+-deficient rat. *J Pharmacol Exp Ther* 2004, 311: 8-13.
[51] Bo S, Durazzo M, Guidi S, Carello M, Sacerdote C, Silli B *et al.*: Dietary magnesium and fiber intakes and inflammatory and metabolic indicators in middle-aged subjects from a population-based cohort. *Am J Clin Nutr* 2006, 84: 1062-1069.
[52] Guerrero-Romero F, Rodríguez-Morán M: Hypomagnesemia, oxidative stress, inflammation, and metabolic syndrome. *Diabetes Metab Res Rev* 2006, 22: 471-476.
[53] Almoznino-Sarafian D, Berman S, Mor A, Shteinshnaider M, Gorelik O, Tzur I *et al.*: Magnesium and C-reactive protein in heart failure: an anti-inflammatory effect of magnesium administration? *Eur J Nutr* 2007, 46: 230-237.
[54] Mazur A, Maier JA, Rock E, Gueux E, Nowacki W, Rayssiguier Y: Magnesium and the inflammatory response: potential physiopathological implications. *Arch Biochem Biophys* 2007, 458: 48-56.
[55] Evangelopoulos AA, Vallianou NG, Panagiotakos DB, Georgiou A, Zacharias GA, Alevra AN *et al.*: An inverse relationship between cumulating components of the metabolic syndrome and serum magnesium levels. *Nutr Res* 2008, 28: 659-663.
[56] Balage M, Averous J, Rémond D, Bos C, Pujos-Guillot E, Papet I *et al.*: Presence of low-grade inflammation impaired postprandial stimulation of muscle protein synthesis in old rats. *J Nutr Biochem* 2010, 21: 325-331.
[57] Nielsen FH: Magnesium, inflammation, and obesity in chronic disease. *Nutr Rev* 2010, 68: 333-340.
[58] Weglicki WB, Mak IT, Chmielinska JJ, Tejero-Taldo MI, Komarov AM, Kramer JH: The role of magnesium deficiency in cardiovascular and intestinal inflammation. *Magnes Res* 2010, 23: 199-206.
[59] Bo S, Milanesio N, Schiavone C, Villois P, Durazzo M, Gentile L *et al.*: Magnesium and trace element intake after a lifestyle intervention. *Nutrition* 2011, 27: 108-110.
[60] Nielsen FH, Johnson LK, Zeng H: Magnesium supplementation improves indicators of low magnesium status and inflammatory stress in adults older than 51 years with poor quality sleep *. *Magnes Res* 2011, 23: 158-168.

17

Dynamic Tissue Perfusion Measurement – Basics and Applications

Thomas Scholbach
Chemnitz Clinics, Chemnitz
Germany

1. Introduction

1.1 Rationale

Perfusion is a fundamental prerequisite for all living tissues to meet their needs in terms of supply of oxygen, nutrients, hormones, messenger substances and other necessary dilutes. Dynamic Tissue Perfusion Measurement (DTPM) was developed to quantify the perfusion of tissues and organs by means of colour Doppler sonography. Perfusion is perceived as a certain amount of blood passing through a defined region of interest (ROI) in a certain time.

Colour Doppler sonography is universally used to visualize blood flow inside tissues. The velocity of moving red blood cells is depicted as coloured pixels on the background of uncoloured, black and white pixels, which describe parts of tissues without detectable blood flow. The colouration differs according to the velocity and direction of flow. A colour scale within each image shows the spectrum of reddish and bluish colours used to differentiate the direction (reddish hues describe flow which is reversely directed to bluish flow, in most cases the machine is set to depict flow towards the transducer in red). In both directions, lighter shades describe higher velocities than darker shades. A wall filter is used to exclude extremely low velocity signals from imaging, which mostly emanate from vessel wall vibrations and do not add to real blood flow. The colour scale or colour bar thus gives a visual clue to assign velocity signals from zero to a maximum value to certain vessels inside a tissue. At both ends of the colour scale, the maximum flow velocities for red and blue colour are depicted. These values are determined by the actual pulse repetition frequency and the applied ultrasound frequency. They correspond to the outermost hue on each side of the colour bar whereas the minimum flow is determined by the hue next to the black line (indicating the wall filter) separating blue and red hues from each other.

To calculate perfusion in a certain ROI two parameters must be known:

1. The flow velocity in all vessels within the ROI
2. The area of all vessel transsections in this ROI

Both parameters change during the heart cycle. A third prerequisite is thus to take into account these rhythmic changes and to refer them to their basic rhythm which is a full heart cycle.

DTPM makes use of the data offered by any colour Doppler machine, namely the real time depiction of rhythmically changing coloured pixels and the colour scale to gauge them. To achieve this each hue at the scale is assigned a specific velocity value. This value is calculated by the DTPM-software (PixelFlux, Chameleon-Software, Germany [1]) from a linear correlation of all colours from zero (the lower end of the scale) to the actual maximum value (which is depicted numerically at the outer end of the scale and corresponds to the lightest reddish and bluish shades of the scale). The PixelFlux-software also calculates the area of all coloured pixels inside the ROI. Thus, each coloured pixel is evaluated by assigning a specific velocity and area to it. This is possible only after calibrating the image.

Distance calibration is also done automatically by use of the DICOM data, which are delivered along with the image by the ultrasound machine. A so-called DICOM- header file accompanying each image contains non-visible data such as the type of the ultrasound machine, the transducer, the preset information, the patient data and the distance calibration among many other data.

The mean flow intensity (Q) inside a ROI with the area (A_{ROI}) is then automatically calculated by assigning each colour pixel a velocity (v) and area (A) value according to the following equation:

$$Q\ [cm/s] = v\ [cm/s] * A\ [cm^2] / A_{ROI}\ [cm^2]$$

2. Standardized video acquisition

An indispensable precondition for reliable measurements is the use of comparable videos in terms of the imaging conditions applied to the investigated tissue. Only by keeping the fundamental circumstances of data acquisition constant, it is possible to compare the measurement results. Such parameters which need to be held constant are colour Doppler frequency and gain, type and software of the ultrasound machine, transducer type, persistence, wall filter, smoothing, type of the colour scale, preference for spatial versus time-resolution and others, depending on the actual configuration of the ultrasound machine. These parameters are summarized and stored as a certain preset of the machine and must be recalled at the beginning of an ultrasound investigation. This step is a widely used practice in order to maintain optimum imaging conditions also in examinations, where a measurement of image data is not a priori planned. The prepared preset is then re-instituted before recording videos for DTPM.

3. Setting the region of interest (ROI) and Doppler angle correction

The ROI is that area inside an ultrasound image, where tissue perfusion measurement is scheduled. The selection of the ROI depends on the type of tissue, structure of the organ and aim of the investigation. The following principles and physical restrictions should be kept in mind in defining the ROI.

In 2D-images, vessels are encoded in colour depending on the angle, which they have with the ultrasound wave. This propagation line of waves is oriented perpendicular to the transducer surface. The colouration represents the exact velocity value only in vessels running straight towards the transducer, i.e. parallel to the course of the sound wave propagation line. All other vessels are encoded with colour hues representing velocity values (v) which are a product of the cosine of the Doppler angle (α) and the true velocity (v_t), according to the Doppler principle:

$$fd = 2^* fo * v_t/c * \cos \alpha$$

with: fd: Doppler shift, fo: insonation frequency, c: sound velocity

This means that in many cases the tissue microvasculature colouration shows velocity values which are smaller than real. To overcome this, an angle correction for each vessel would be necessary. This cannot be done yet in two-dimensional images. With 3D imaging, such a correction is already feasible (see below in section "foetus"). In 2D images, thus an error occurs with DTPM, which must be kept constant to allow comparisons between investigations. This can be achieved under following circumstances:

1. A chaotic vessel architecture without predominant vessel diameters and Doppler angles (type tumour perfusion) (fig. 1)
2. A regular vessel architecture, which can be reliably retrieved (kidney type).

In the latter case, the orientation on anatomical landmarks offers a sufficient framework to find the vascular patterns, which are typical for a certain organ (fig. 2). An example how to choose relevant landmarks is given for the kidney below.

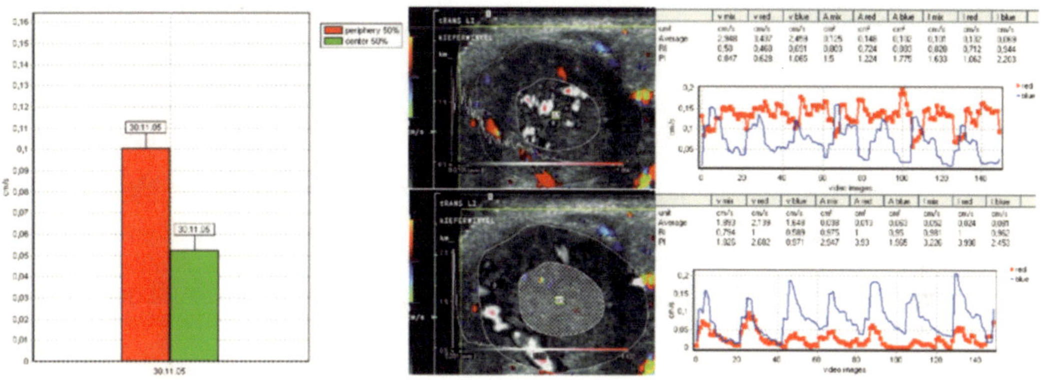

Fig. 1. Example of tumor perfusion measurement. Two concentric ROIs are separately investigated. The vessel architecture is irregular or chaotic (center). No specific prevailing vessel size or orientation can be stated. Left: comparisons of perfusion intensities in the periphery (red column) and the center (green column). Center: Display of the ROIs and false color maps with perfusion intensity curves. Right: time course of the relevant perfusion parameters (from [2])

In both cases, the inevitable error of impossible individual Doppler angle correction for each vessel is held constant. Comparisons of different examinations thus become possible.

For all these considerations, it is crucial to achieve comparable conditions for depicting the vessels in a certain ROI. In the kidney the ROI should be placed inside the outer cortex, in a layer stretching from the outer border of the medullary pyramids to the renal surface and laterally from the watershed of two neighbouring segments to the opposite watershed (see chapter: kidney). In the lymph node and thyroid lobes, a longitudinal section trough the centre of the ovoid shaped organ should be used as definite transsection plane. In the bowel wall, a longitudinal cut perpendicular to the proximal wall is the best. Tumours should be cut centrally in two perpendicular planes.

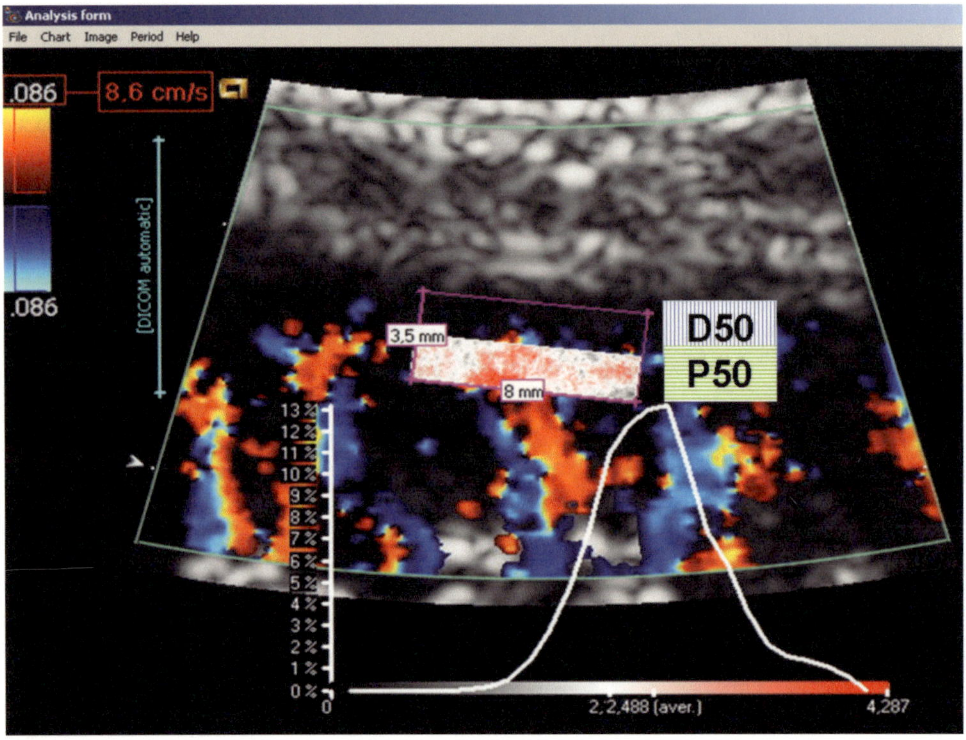

Fig. 2. Example for regular vessel architecture in a renal transplant - see also figure 3. The sub-ROIs are highlighted: P50 - proximal 50% of the outer cortex. D50- distal 50% of the outer cortex. False color map and distribution curve of perfusion intensities are displayed

4. Reading the results

Figure 3 gives an overview of the most important output features in a typical DTPM measurement. In DTPM all data are derived from the basic parameters mean flow velocity, mean perfused area and their change during the heart beat with reference to the entire ROI [2, 3]. In three-dimensional images, the spatial angle correction adds to the primary 2D measurement inside the horizontal plane.

In addition to mean perfusion intensity, calculation parameters are generated to describe the dynamics of perfusion. Examples are Tissue Resistance Index (TRI) and Tissue Pulsatility Index (TPI). TRI and TPI may refer to velocity, intensity and perfused area according to the following formulas:

TRI(velocity *or intensity or area*) = maximum mean velocity *or* intensity *or* area of the ROI during one heart cycle - minimum mean velocity *or intensity or area* of the ROI during one heart cycle divided by maximum mean velocity *or intensity or area* of the ROI during one heart cycle

TPI(velocity *or intensity or area*) = maximum mean velocity *or* intensity *or* area of the ROI during one heart cycle - minimum mean velocity *or intensity or area* of the ROI during one heart cycle divided by mean mean velocity *or intensity or area* of the ROI during one heart cycle

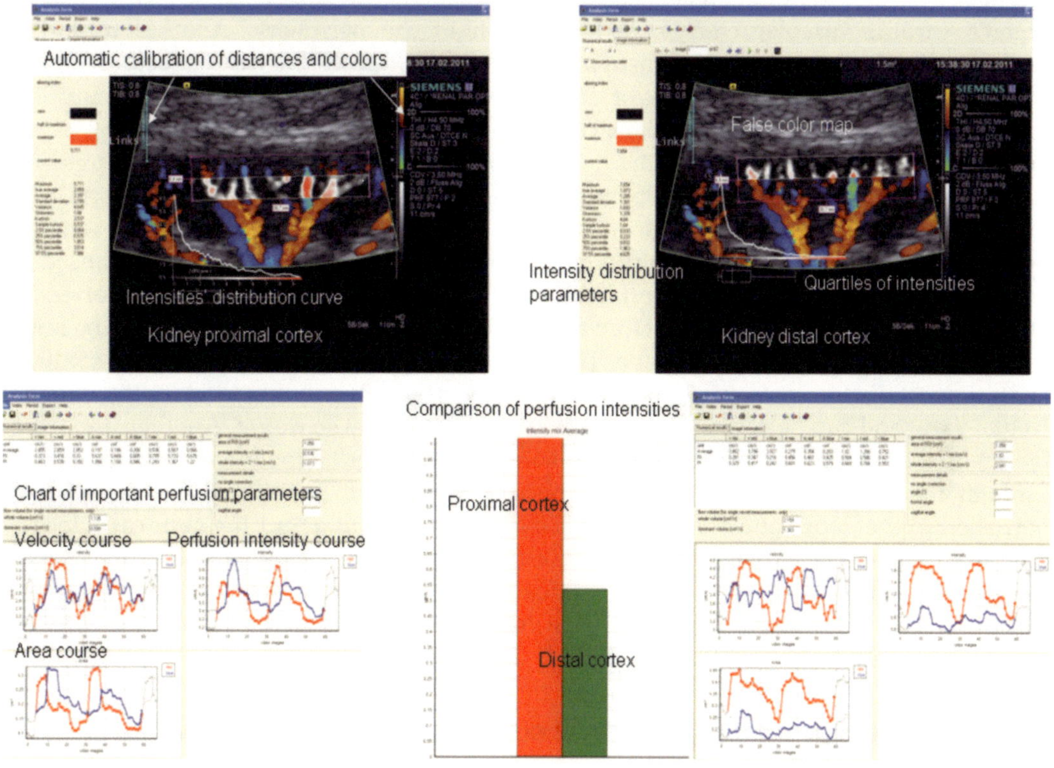

Fig. 3. Example of DTPM output. Overview of the most important output features of a DTPM measurement. Comparison of the proximal and distal cortical ROIs. False color maps (areas shaded in white, red and grey hues), perfusion intensities' distribution curves and additional parameters (upper line). Time curves of the basic perfusion parameters and perfusion intensities (below). Comparison of the overall perfusion intensities in both sub-ROIs (lower line center)

A dynamic perfusion map is generated to pinpoint the local perfusion in a sub-millimetre graded fashion numerically with false colours (fig. 2 and 13). Moreover, the distribution of perfusion intensities according to the whole spectrum of occurring intensities, which are assigned to one of 33 intensity classes, is calculated and diagrammatically displayed. Thus, tissues may be compared according to their content of stronger or weaker perfused areas and vessels (fig. 2, fig. 11). This allows insights into the microarchitecture of a tissue's vascular tree and its changes over time, which is helpful in chronic diseases and tumours. These intensity distribution curves are further described mathematically with the parameters kurtosis and skewness according to their bulging and asymmetry.

Altogether more than 50 parameters are calculated to describe the tissue perfusion numerically. The most important is perfusion intensity to give a general measure of tissue perfusion. Very instructive too is the distribution curve, outlined below the false colour map (fig. 11). Here shifts within the microvessel population can be reviewed at a glance. This is further underlined with the distribution parameters skewness and kurtosis, which describe the shape of this curve numerically. Statistical comparison of microvessel arrangement thus becomes feasible, permitting the follow up of slight changes of an organ's chronic vascular changes, which begin in the periphery. Another important feature is the false colour map. This map stains the ROI according to the local perfusion intensities over the entire length of the colour Doppler sonographic video clip. The information added to the anatomical structures displayed by the ultrasound image can be helpful in differentiating parts of the tissue with respect to their vascular structures. The flow of the hepatic artery can be separated from the same coloured flow of the portal vein in this way, which might be welcome in the follow up of liver transplants. Another possible application might be the differentiation of local tissue disturbances, as caused by tumour infiltration or scarring or inflammation. To perform an automatic angle correction of all vessels 3D images are used. Here the spatial angel is calculated from both the angle in the frontal and in the sagittal plane. This angle then is applied to calculate true spatially angle corrected flow velocities and vessel diameters. Both are distorted in the original frontal view and can be corrected for 3D flow calculations in so doing. Another important feature is the use of predefined relational sub-ROIs to describe the blood flow on its way through the tissue. Gradients of perfusion can be used to quantify the dampening of perfusion in the depth of a vascular tree. This can be used to detect the very early loss of the tiniest vessels in a tissue, which are often the first to be damaged due to their small lumen. So a chronic pathological process can be discovered in the very beginning and treatment can be started preventing further damage in stages, where the organ's compensatory capacity is still strong enough to recover.

5. Differences to existing methods of sonographic perfusion evaluation

Today RI and PI calculations are the most widely used techniques to quantify flow velocity changes [4-10]. They do not allow conclusions as for the perfusion intensity or volume since the perfused area of the vessel under investigation is not included in the calculation. Even the exact velocities of flow do not need to be measured since the formula refers to two (RI) or three (PI) velocities only which are related to each other to define the velocity change throughout the heart cycle instead of exact velocities. RI = peak systolic velocity - end diastolic velocity / peak systolic velocity and PI = peak systolic velocity - end diastolic velocity / mean velocity of the entire heart cycle.

Contrast enhanced ultrasound (CEUS) can describe the perfusion of larger regions inside organs and thus deliver precise images of typical perfusion patterns of e.g. liver tumours or renal transplant cortical perfusion [11-13]. External influences are relevant concerning the reproducible influx of the contrast enhancer from the injection site to the ROI [14, 15]. The perfusion in CEUS is calculated as the velocity of contrast saturation. The pulsatility of perfusion is not depicted. CEUS thus delivers two parameters to measure: level of saturation and the velocity to reach this level.

The advantages of dynamic tissue perfusion measurement over conventional resistance index measurements and contrast-enhanced sonography (CEUS) are summarized below:

Dynamic tissue perfusion measurement	RI measurement	Contrast enhanced sonography
Measurement of perfusion intensity in all vessels of a larger ROI	Single point measurement in colored vessels	Measurement of contrast enhancement in a larger ROI
Measurement of flow velocities of all pixels in all vessels' transsection	Measurement of flow velocities only in some pixels of a vessel (sample volume)	No flow velocity measurement
Appreciation of heart beat specific flow dynamics	Appreciation of heart beat specific flow dynamics	Loss of heart beat dynamics - saturation curves are calculated
All relevant raw data (i.e. velocities and areas of perfusion) are measured directly during complete heart cycles	Only systolic and enddiastolic velocities are measured	Perfusion intensity is evaluated indirectly from contrast enhancer influx curves (steepness of influx and level of saturation)
Use of unmodified flow data	Use of unmodified flow data	Contrast enhancer as additional source of error
Non-invasive	Non-invasive	Injection necessary
No side effects	No side effects	Rarely side effects
No running costs	No running costs	Additional costs for contrast enhancer (about 92 € per vial)
No age limitation	No age limitation	Not universally licensed for paediatric use

6. Comparison to RI measurements

Resistance index (RI) measurements are widely used to extract a handy quantitative measure from PW (pulsed wave) - Doppler investigations by using to velocity measurements, peak systolic (vs) and enddiastolic velocity (vd) from a single site inside a vessel according to the equation: RI = vs-vd/vs. Despite its broad use the theoretical basis for perfusion quantification remains weak and not surprisingly leads to misleading conclusions. A high RI is commonly linked to a high downstream resistance against flow - often raising the suspicion of a suppressed perfusion while normal RI measurements are referred to as a sign of normal perfusion. Figure 4 clearly demonstrates that this fundamental theoretical misconception also might have obvious practical implications. In the upper line spectral analysis of three peripheral arterial branches of a renal transplant with a stark reduction of peripheral cortical microvessels are shown - averaging to a RI of 0.66. The same value is calculated in the lower line, which stems from another transplant with much better function (serum creatinine 70 vs. 231 µmol/l in the upper line) and abundant vascular signals in the outer cortical periphery. A decision based on RI would attest both transplants a normal "perfusion". DTPM brings out the difference clearly (fig. 5): Perfusion intensity is eight times higher in the proximal cortex in the transplant with a normal function. The insufficient transplant has no peripheral perfusion at all.

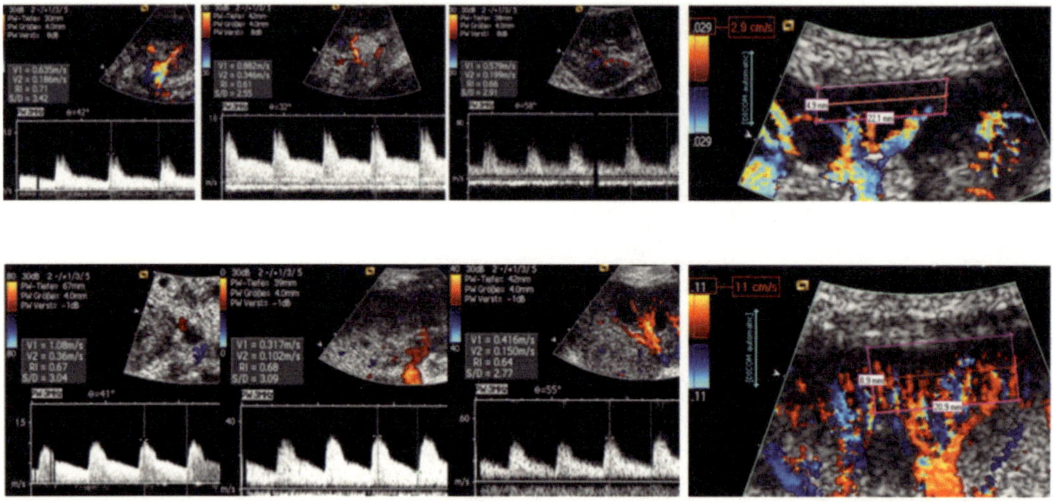

Fig. 4. Two renal transplants compared: upper line insufficient kidney with serum creatinine of 231 µmol/l and normal kidney with a serum creatinine of 70 µmol/l in the lower line. Left: RI measurement in three cortical arteries. Right: Color Doppler sonograms. Insufficient kidney displays a pronounced loss of peripheral perfusion despite more sensible color Doppler setting compared to the kidney below. RI mean values are 0,66 for both transplants

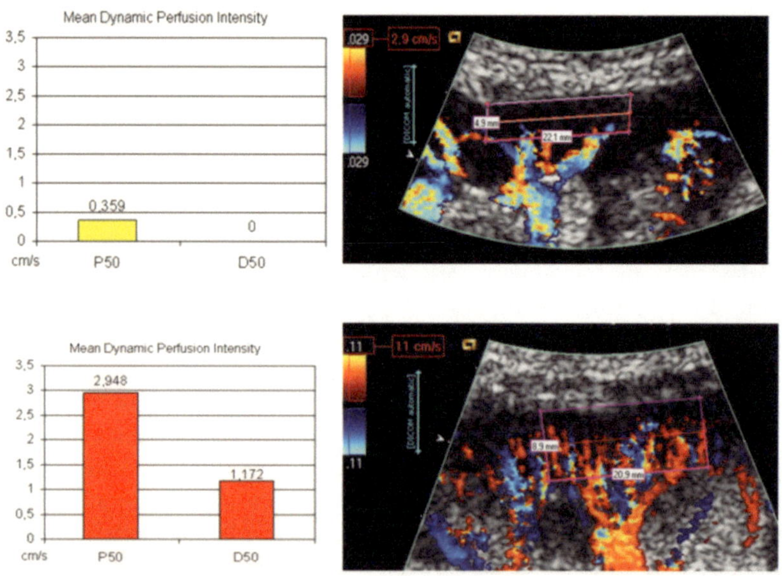

Fig. 5. Same transplants as in fig. 3. DTPM is able to demonstrate a massive difference of tissue perfusion in contrary to RI measurements

Another example for the low power of RI evaluations is figure 6. In a child with acute renal insufficiency due to a hemolytic-uraemic syndrome (HUS), two neighbouring cortical arteries demonstrate vastly different RIs. Depending on which arteries the investigator selects, contradictory conclusions must be drawn from such evaluations. Another seldom-considered drawback of RI measurements inside tissues is that thin arteries can only be located to interrogate the flow as long as the vessel is still coloured. If perfusion drops significantly, colour signals become weak and disappear at all. These vessels, the most affected, are excluded from evaluation by RI altogether. This must distort the overall evaluation of tissue perfusion if RI measurements are its basis.

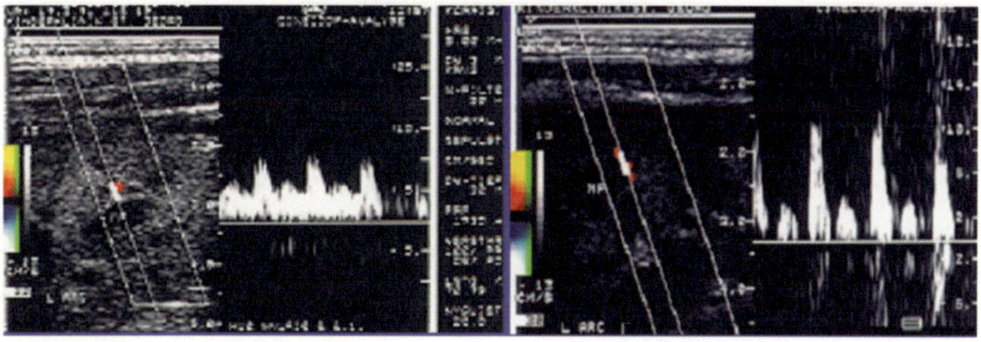

Fig. 6. Misleading RI measurements in a kidney af a child affected by haemolytic-ureamic syndrome. During the same investigation strikingly different RIs are found in intimate neighborhood

The only way out of this dilemma is a method that takes into account simultaneously all flow signals in all vessels inside a larger ROI instead of single vessels, which also takes into account non-perfused areas. These are the fundamentals of DTPM, referring all flow signals inside an entire ROI thus reflecting properly vessel and flow intensity loss in chronic disease. It is just in chronic disease where remaining vessels amidst fibrosed tissue try to compensate the loss of neighbouring vessels by dilatation to feed the "thirsting" periphery and thus exhibit a lower RI than under normal conditions (fig. 5).

7. Phantom flow measurements

A phantom was built to measure the volume flow under externally controlled conditions consisting of a Teflon tube with an internal diameter of 2.0 mm that was placed into a water basin and fixed in a way that the tube was running straight in a steep angle towards the ultrasound transducer that was fixed to a tripod. The tube was perfused with a watery homogeneous rice starch solution.

Colour Doppler videos were recorded under standardized imaging conditions (ultrasound device: S2000, Siemens, Germany, linear transducer, colour Doppler frequency 4 MHz, the angle of the tube towards the ultrasound propagation line was 36°). The pump rate was changed; repeated colour Doppler recordings were made and measured by DTPM.

Two separate investigators independently performed these PixelFlux-measurements from 87 datasets (mean values based on altogether 191 recordings) at 22 different pump rates.

Phantom flow measurements showed an excellent correlation to pump rates (fig. 7) with a Pearson correlation coefficient of pump rate and investigator 1 of 0,987 and 0,991 for investigator 2. Both investigators measurements correlated with 0,997.

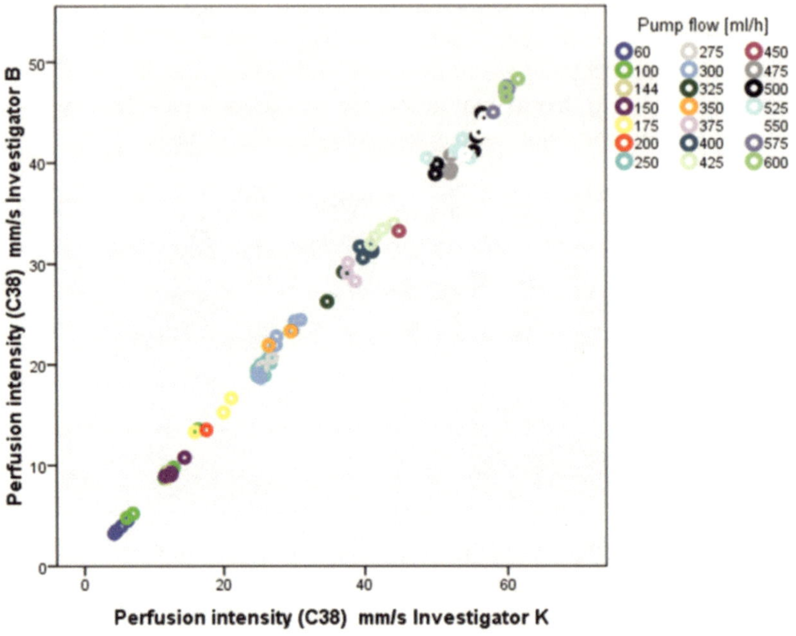

Fig. 7. In a perfusion phantom* DTPM measurements of two investigators were compared. An excellent correlation in-between both investigators and of both investigators to the externally measured flow rate was found. * Homogenized rice starch solution pumped by a precision laboratory pump, Flow volumes measured constantly by a laboratory balance

8. Dynamic tissue perfusion measurement – Applications

8.1 Kidneys

Kidneys are abundantly perfused and are second only to the brain with respect to their blood supply in the systemic circulation [16, 17]. Perfusion measurement is important to detect changes, which precede function loss - the so-called creatinine blind stage of renal insufficiency [18]. For reliable kidney perfusion measurements, it is necessary to adjust the ROI to the typical anatomical pattern of the renal microvessel architecture. The kidney consists of segments, each with an individual blood supply via an interlobar artery. This vessel is crossing the inner parenchyma in-between two neighbouring medullary pyramids to branch off symmetrically into arcuate arteries from which in a brush-like manner interlobular arteries emanate. Such a segment is chosen as the ROI in a way that the feeding interlobar artery runs straight towards the transducer.

The ROI itself is a parallelogram adjusted to the individual kidney's anatomical landmarks, which are as follows: the left upper corner of the parallelogram lies at the renal surface on the watershed line between two segments (i.e. where the interlobular arteries from two neighbouring segments seem to touch each other). The right upper corner then is fixed at the right border of the segment under investigation with the same premises as the first corner. The right lower corner then lies on the right watershed line, which is extended to the surface of the medullary pyramid and ends at the centre of the outer edge of the pyramid. From there the lower border of the ROI extends to the left pyramid to reach its centre point on its outer border. This is the left lower corner of the parallelogram. This way a symmetric distribution pattern of all branches of this vascular segment is achieved [19]. This parallelogram is divided into horizontal layers (e.g. p50 and d50) encompassing the proximal 50% (p50) or distal 50% (d50) of the ROI's height. Any other layer thickness can be chosen to meet the needs of the investigation (for instance 10 layers with the thickness of 1/10 of the ROI (fig. 13)). These layers thus have a thickness that refers to the overall dimensions of the ROI and are therefore relational layers. In thicker cortices, the layers are thicker than in thinner cortices. Nevertheless, the layers of different kidneys are comparable to each other since they comprise the comparable level of the cortical vascular tree (fig. 8).

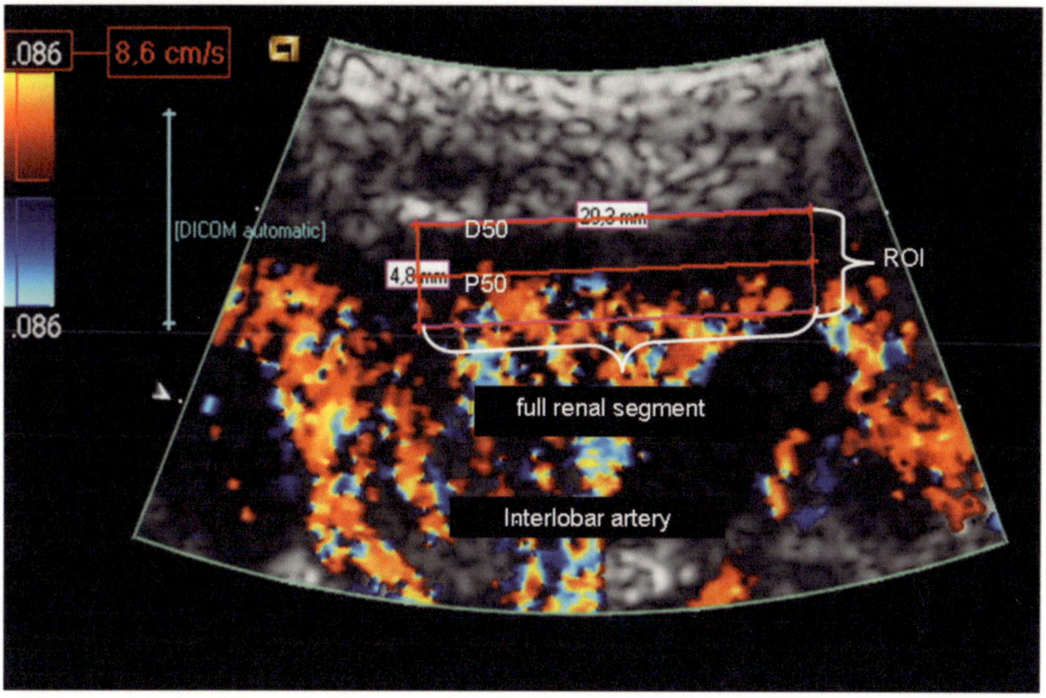

Fig. 8. Example of placing of a ROI in a kidney with indication of the anatomical landmarks to guide the setting

Own investigations yielded a decline of renal cortical perfusion with compromised creatinine clearance (fig. 9). Normal kidneys display a decline of cortical perfusion intensity from central to peripheral cortex (fig. 10) [19]. Inflammation causes a strong hyperperfusion (fig. 11). DTPM can help to differentiate the affection of either right or left kidney - helpful in children and non-communicating patients. Moreover, the different effects of hydronephrotic perfusion loss even in a state of general hyperperfusion due to inflammation can be demonstrated (fig. 11). In kidneys with vesico-ureteral reflux, we found a decline of perfusion inside the peripheral cortical layers, which corresponded to the reflux degree (low grade vs. high-grade reflux) (fig. 12).

In nutcracker phenomenon, a frequent anatomical variant of the course of the left renal vein with sharp narrowing of the vessel between the superior mesenteric artery and the

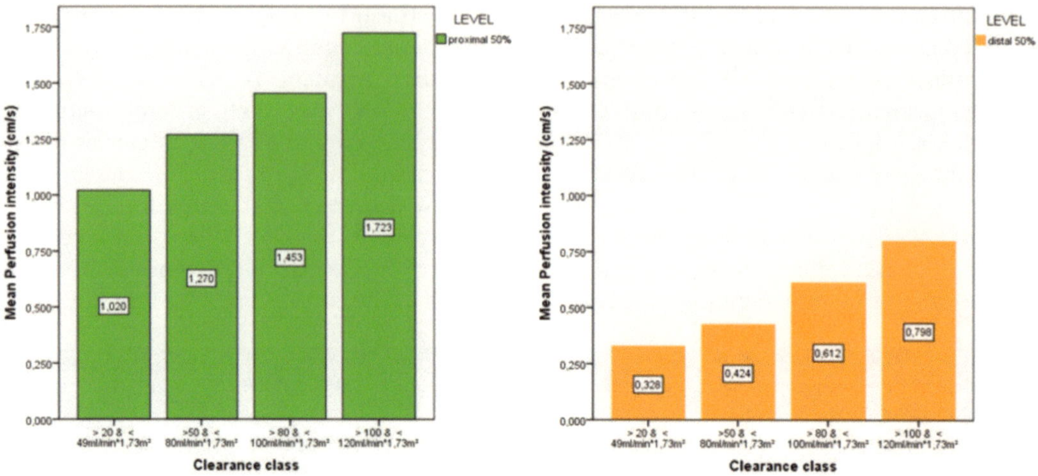

Fig. 9. Constant decline of cortical perfusion with progression of renal insufficiency. Left: proximal cortex. Right: distal cortex

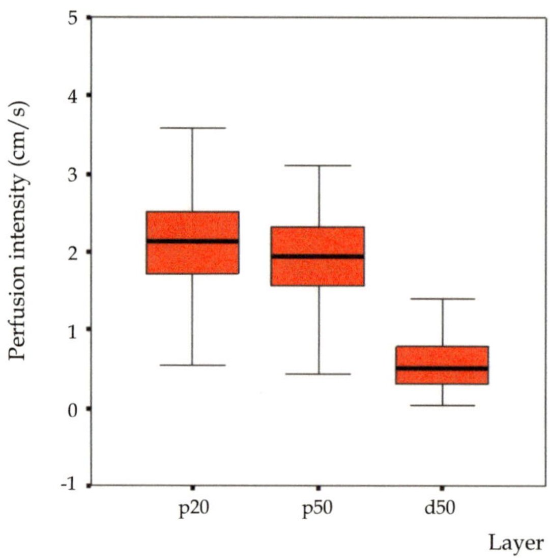

Fig. 10. Decline of renal cortical perfusion from the inner to the outer cortex

abdominal aorta, a venous congestion of the left kidney ensues. Its consequences are often misinterpreted from conventional imaging alone but are nonetheless often disabling for the affected ones. Many patients suffer from chronic and exacerbating abdominal fits of cramping pain. The congested kidney is often swollen and less perfused than the right one. This can be easily demonstrated by DTPM (fig. 13). Perfusion diminution is a signal of insufficient collateral pathways to drain the renal blood from the left side. A treatment with aspirin can either alleviate or often abolish pain and functional disturbances of the congested organs, which have to deal with the massive venous overflow from the left renal vein. Simultaneously with the clinical improvement, a significant increase of left kidney's perfusion can also be measures by DTPM (fig. 14) [20].

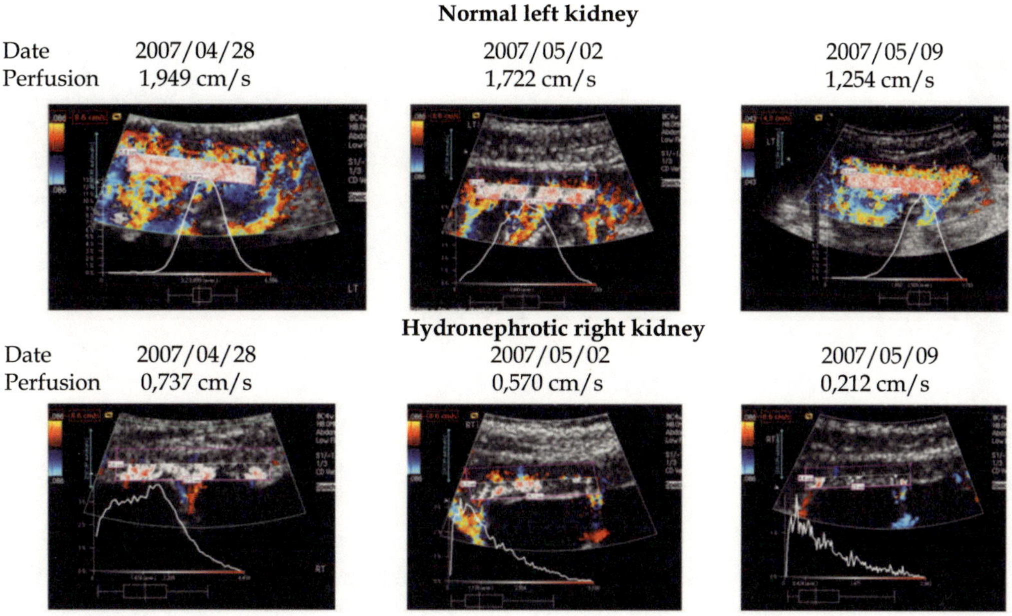

Fig. 11. Differing response of both kidneys towards an bacterial infection in a patient with a right sided hydronephrosis Perfusion intensity in the proximal cortex. MAG3 scintigraphy right kidney: 30% of both kidneys' function. Renal perfusion in a child with a normal kidney on the left and a hydronephritc kidney on the other side. Inflammation due to bacterial infection causes an initial perfusion increase (2007/04/28). With recovery perfusion drops in both kidneys (from 2007/05/02 to 2007/05/09). The decline is more pronounced in the hydronephrotic kidney. Perfusion intensity distribution curves differ markedly between both kidneys pointing to the damage of the microvasculature in the hydronephrotic kidney and a compensatory hyperperfusion trough dilated microvasculature on the left side

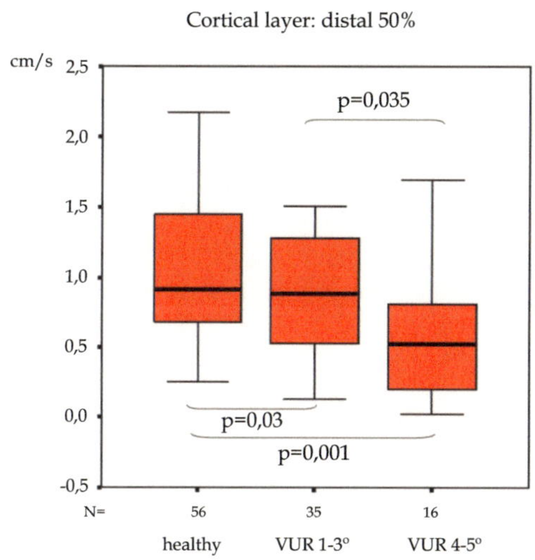

Fig. 12. Diminished perfusion of kidney in vesico-ureteral reflux compared to healthy ones. Compromise of perfusion dependent on degree of reflux

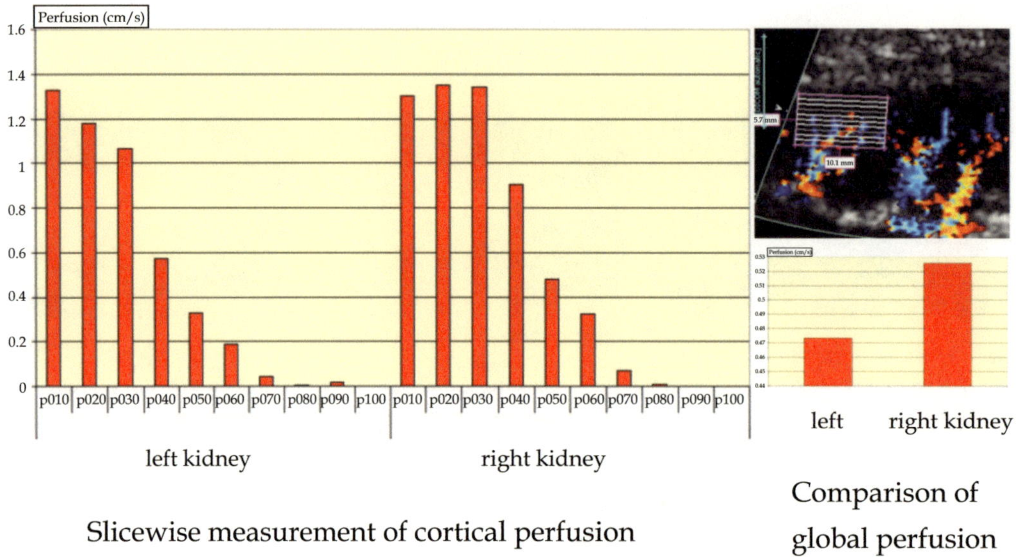

Fig. 13. The nutcracker phenomenon of the left kidney often causes depression of left renal perfusion. Left: Sub-millimeter layers show very precisely the potential of DTPM to describe microvascular perfusion in an unprecedented subtlety. Right: Heavily depressed perfusion of the left kidney in nutcracker phenomenon

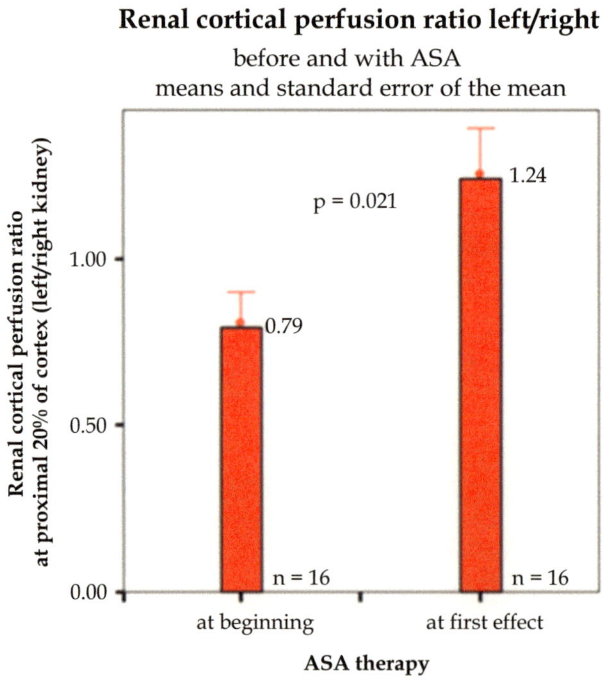

Fig. 14. Effect of aspirin (acetylsalicylic acid: ASA) onto the perfusion of the left kidney. The ratio of left to right kidney perfusion is displayed. After aspirin treatment a significant increase of this ratio can be stated. From [21]

In a preliminary study, we compared kidneys from children with juvenile diabetes of varying duration of disease to kidneys from healthy children with respect to the perfusion drop from central to peripheral cortical layers. Even in an early stage of disease, (no child had microalbuminuria) a highly significant peripheral perfusion loss could be demonstrated in diabetic kidneys (fig. 15).

Report

Data origin		Perfusion gradient from proximal 50 % to distal 50%	Perfusion gradient from proximal 20 % to distal 50%
healthy	Median	3,1813	3,5306
	Std Deviation	1,91990	2,31465
	N	110	110
diabetic	Median	5,5230	6,9531
	Std Deviation	16,10524	28,99295
	N	57	57

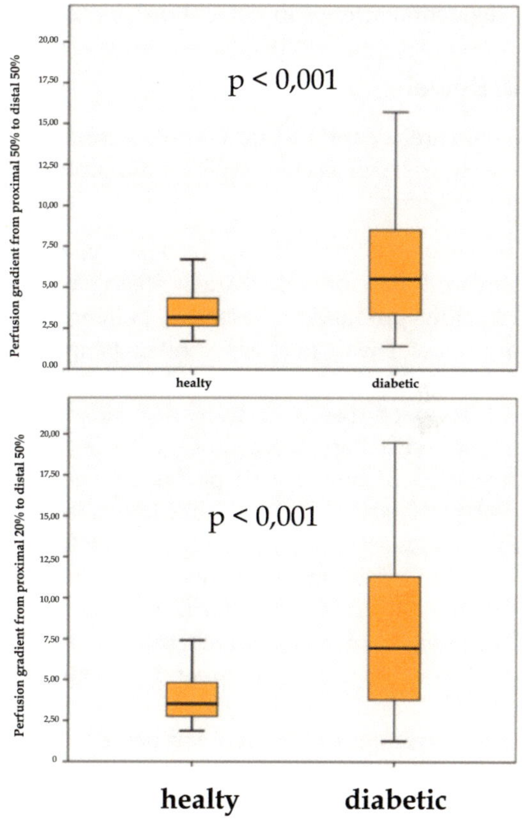

Fig. 15. DTPM discloses a significant reduction of peripheral to central cortical perfusion in diabetic children compared to healthy ones. The effect is more pronounced when comparing the proximal 20%/distal 50%-ratio (lower diagram) then in proximal 50%/distal 50%-ratio (upper diagram)

9. Renal transplants

Renal transplants are subject to chronic immunological attacks as well as toxic effects of immunosuppressive treatment. Repeated biopsies are today the only way to clarify the creeping changes within the renal parenchyma. We conducted a study on 75 renal transplant recipients, which had a DTPM immediately before their biopsy. Banff criteria were correlated to DTPM results. Some of the very important histological features correlated significantly with perfusion changes [21], pointing to the potential of DTPM for renal transplant long term follow up. RI values were much less instructive (insignificant differences) than DTPM measurements (significant differences) to discriminate varying stages of peritubular inflammation. Varying grades of transplant Polyomavirus infection were marked with significant increases of cortical tissue perfusion [21]. In another study, we found in children a marked decline of cortical perfusion in allograft cortices beginning already one year after transplantation [22] while the pulsatility of cortical perfusion rose significantly [23]. Recently, it was shown, that intrinsic donor-derived factors are associated with GFR and cortical parenchymal perfusion intensity, measured by DTPM, but not the RI of segmental arteries in renal allografts [24].

10. Bowel

A main area of interest for DTPM is chronic inflammatory bowel diseases. In Crohn disease as well as in ulcerative colitis inflammatory hyperperfusion of the bowel wall could be demonstrated.

Patients with Crohn disease irrespective of disease activity had higher blood flow intensity compared to healthy probands. Mean small bowel wall perfusion intensity was 0.025 cm/s in healthy probands whereas in patients with Crohn disease 0.095 cm/s was found [25]. Large bowel wall perfusion intensity in healthy probands was distinctively less than in patients with Crohn disease (0.012 cm/s vs. 0.082 cm/s, $p < 0.001$) [25]. Conventional evaluation of disease activity by means of activity indices did not clearly distinguish patients with high from those with less pronounced inflammatory hyperperfusion. The correlation of bowel wall perfusion and PCDAI-values was weak albeit significant ($r = 0.349$, $p = 0.001$) [25]. The individual effect of TNF alpha antibody treatment can be closely followed and treatment regimes can be tailored according to DTPM. Inflammatory activity in fistulas can be measured even after closure of the cutaneous orifice. DTPM can also be used to locate the focus of an abdominal inflammatory process by comparing the perfusion of different structures, which may be involved, but in different extent and activity. So lymph nodes, vermiform appendix, cecum and terminal ileum can be evaluated separately and clear decisions on the main source of complaints can be made. Unnecessary appendectomies can be avoided based on an imaging and perfusion measurements guided approach.

In ulcerative colitis, 14 histological criteria (changes of crypt architecture, depletion of goblet cells, Paneth cells distal of the left colon flexure, lymphocyte infiltration, plasma cells, eosinophils, unspecific inflammatory infiltrates, granulocytes in the lamina propria and lamina epithelialis, crypt abscesses, oedema, erosions or ulcerations, regenerative epithelium , fibrosis, increased cryptal distance to muscularis mucosae) of disease activity were compared to the local perfusion state of the bowel wall. Scores of neutrophil as well as lymphocytic invasion of the wall, crypt abscesses and wall oedema were significantly correlated (in oedema inversely) to the local wall perfusion (fig. 16) [26]. DTPM can add more differentiated and important numerical data, which make imaging data comparable and thus a tool for decision making in a clinical setting. Figure 17 compares histological images, colonoscopic photographs, colour Doppler sonographic images and the results of DTPM at the site where the images stem from. A convincing differentiation of these three bowel segments can be demonstrated by the different perfusion intensities.

Faingold et al. found a trend to decreased intestinal wall perfusion (0.040 ± 0.015 cm/s vs. 0.052 ± 0.029 cm/s) in neonates that died due to hypoxic ischemic injury [27].

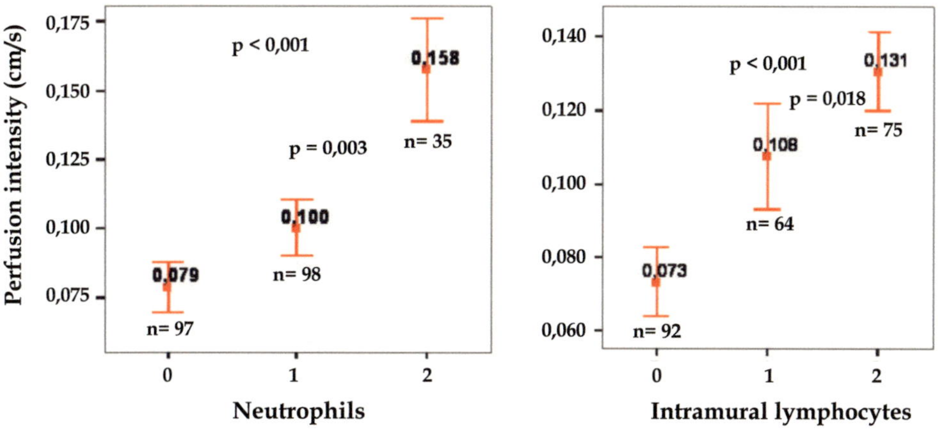

Fig. 16. Large bowel wall perfusion in ulcerative colitis. In ulcerative colitis an increasing score of granulocytic (left) and lymphocytic (right) wall infiltration is reflected by significant increase in wall perfusion

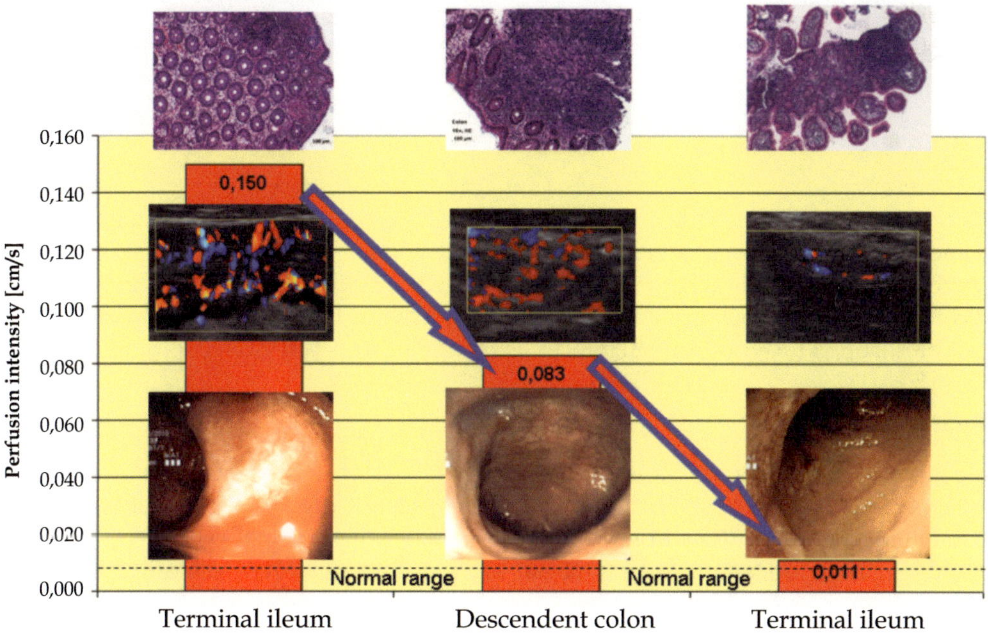

Fig. 17. Synopsis of DTPM measurements (red columns) histological images, color Doppler sonograms and colonoscopic images from three IBD patients and different sites. DTPM differentiates better than all other methods between acutely inflamed and resting bowel segments in IBD patients

11. Lymph nodes

Lymph node perfusion measurement helps to tell inflammatory changes and can provide insight into the dynamics of progression or retreat of the underlying process. Normal lymph nodes in the neck have a minute but always detectable perfusion, which can be measured accurately. In upper airway infections, lymph nodes do not react with a hyperperfusion whereas lymphotropic EBV infection resulted in a marked increase of perfusion (fig. 18) [28].

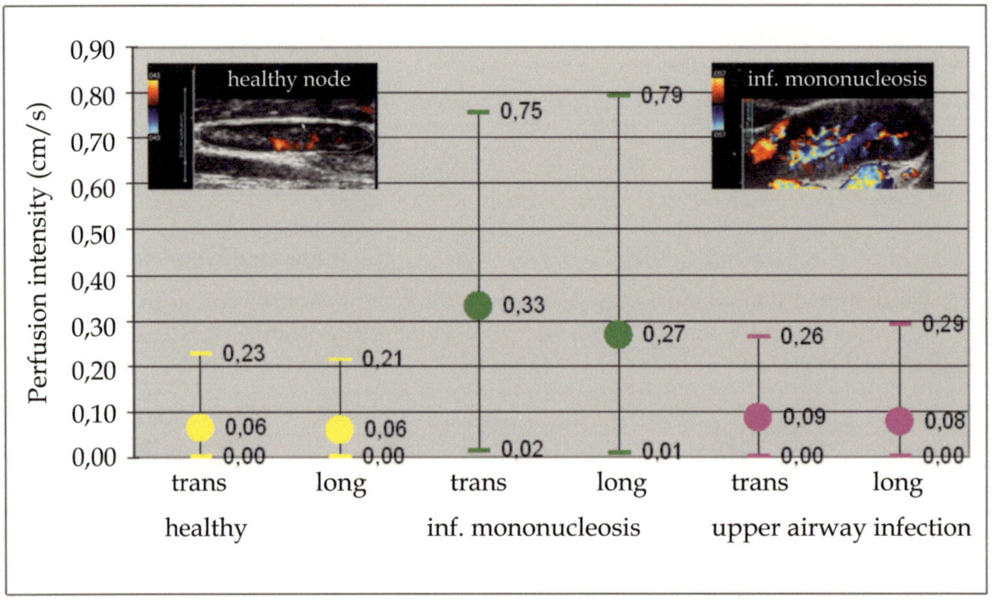

Fig. 18. Lymph node perfusion as seen in DTPM: no differences exist between longitudinal (long) and transverse (trans) sections of the nodes. Infectious mononucleosis raises cervical node perfusion significantly (green symbols) compared to nodes from healthy probands (yellow) in contrast to nodes in acute upper airway infections (pink). Insets: left: normal node in color Doppler Right: Node in infectious mononucleosis (EBV-infection)

12. Muscle

A muscle perfusion measurement is feasible with the demonstration of a marked increase during exercise and steep decline afterwards in athletes (fig. 19). The perfusion was measured in the M. rectus femoris in a horizontal section before during and after exercise along with the measurement of serum lactate and a self-estimation of subjective workload (fig. 20).

In aged patients, an increase of muscle perfusion of the M. biceps brachii was demonstrated during an exercise program to foster rehabilitation.

13. Thyroid

Reproducibility of thyroid DTPM between two investigators is significant (fig. 21).

Thyroid perfusion is strongly increased in thyreoiditis (fig. 22). It is not yet clear however, if the amount of perfusion is paralleled by conventional laboratory parameters or clinical symptoms.

Thyroid nodules differed with respect to their distribution of perfusion according to their biological behaviour. Comparison of perfusion intensities obtained from peripheral and central parts of the nodules revealed that, in non-neoplastic nodules the peripheral flow was more intense than the central flow and, on the contrary central flow was more prominent than the peripheral flow in neoplastic nodules (p<0.005) [29].

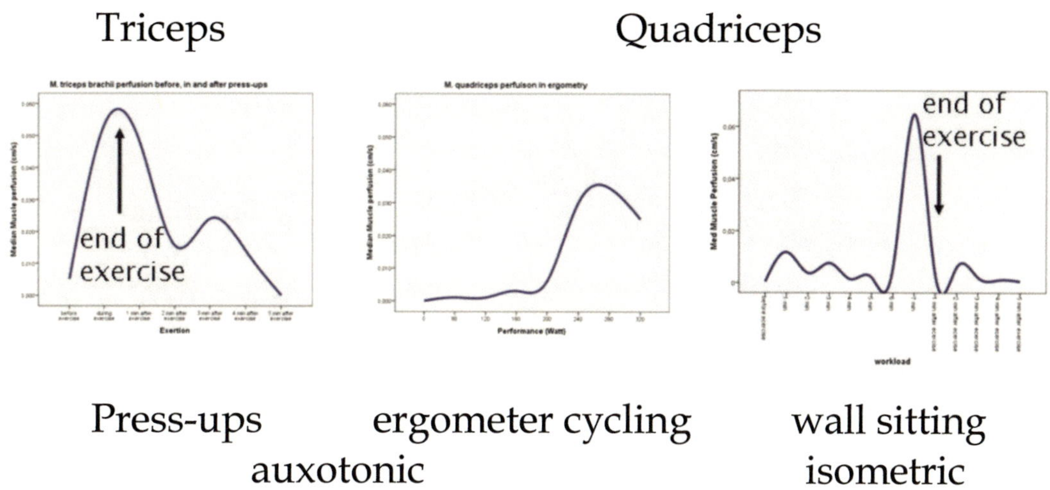

Fig. 19. Significant muscle perfusion increase in 13 athletes - maximal exercise. DTPM reflects the perfusion in muscles before, during and after physical exercise in various settings. Auxotonic as well as isometric exercises cause a strong perfusion increase. After exercise perfusion drops sharply

		Duration of exercise	Heart rate
Muscle Perfusion	Spearman corr. Coeff.	**,535**	**,469**
	Sig. (2-tailed)	**,000**	**,000**
	N	61	61

Fig. 20. Correlation of quadriceps perfusion during ergometer cycling. Exercise induced muscle perfusion correlates significantly to duration of exercise and heart rate

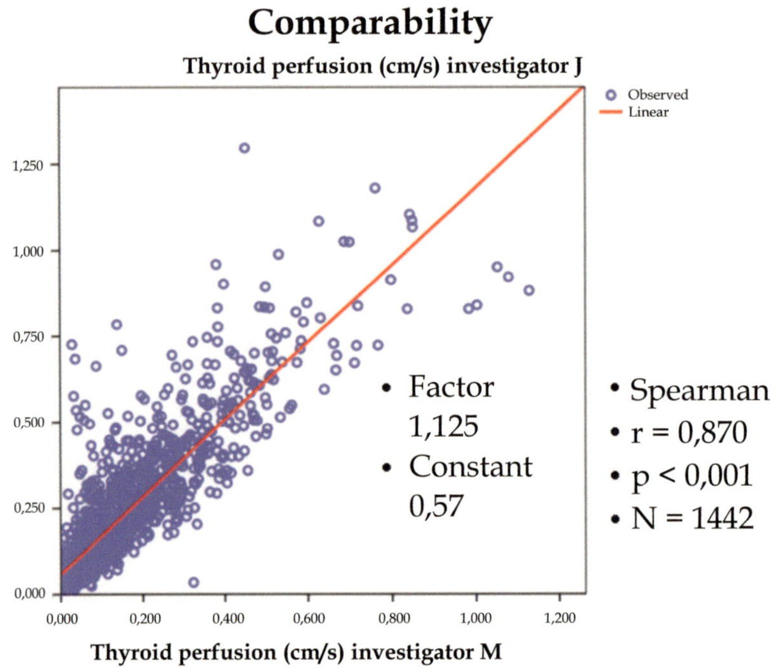

Fig. 21. Thyroid perfusion in 1142 measurements – low interobserver variation and highly significant correlation between both investigators

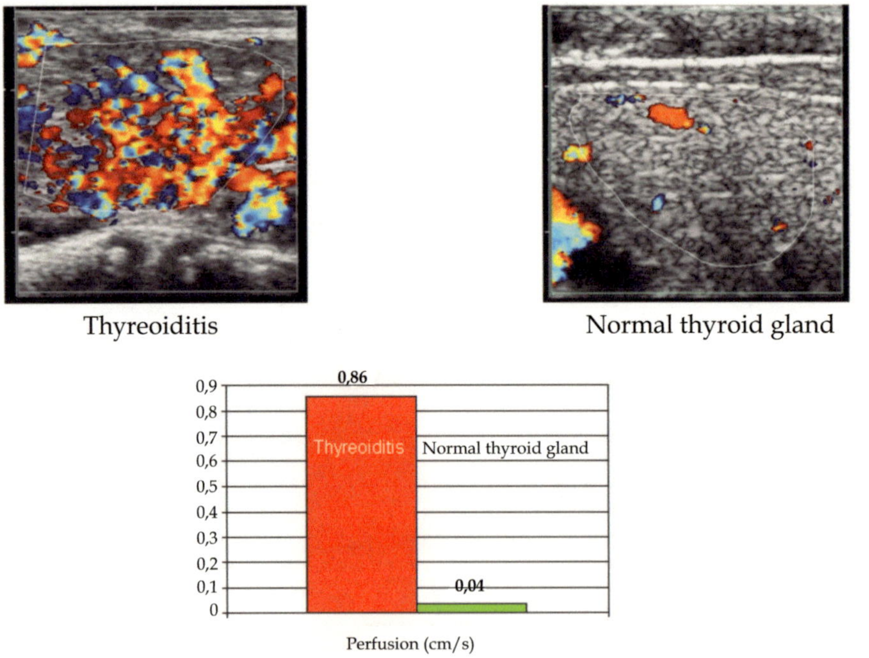

Fig. 22. Example of ample perfusion increase in thyroiditis – color Doppler sonograms and corresponding DTPM values are displayed

14. Tumours

Tumour perfusion evaluation by DTPM is also feasible and defined regions such as tumour core and periphery, whose size can be predefined, e.g. as concentric regions. This can uncover central tumour necrosis or ischemia, which might be relevant for treatment decisions. Hypoxia due to ischemia is a factor of chemo- and radioresistance of tumours [30-32]. Therefore, it might be useful to monitor tumour perfusion in separated shells.

In a series of metastatic tumours of the neck, a direct correlation of tumour perfusion measured by means of DTPM and directly measured tumour oxygenation could be demonstrated (fig. 23) [33]. In hypoxic tumours perfusion was significantly lower compared to normally oxygenated ones (fig. 24). Moreover, the pulsatility of tumour perfusion differed significantly between groups with different stages of metastasis (fig. 25) [33]. These results may be interpreted as a change of tumour stroma. The more densely packed the stroma is the higher the pulsatility is, since the distension of small vessels is influenced by the pressure change during a heart cycle on the one hand but on the other hand by the resistance against the widening of a vessel by the surrounding structures and their stiffness.

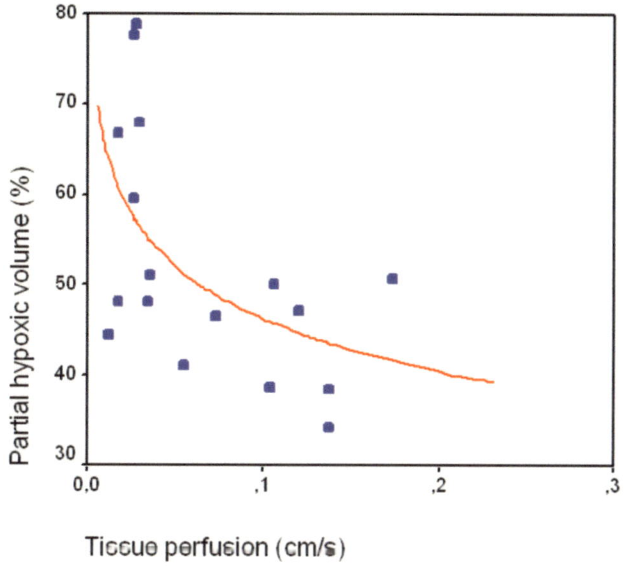

Fig. 23. Significant correlation between directly measured hypoxic volumes in metastatic lymph node tumors of the neck (Eppendorf histiograph) and DTPM (from [2])

15. Foetus

The foetal perfusion has to meet the needs of the rapidly growing organism, to deliver oxygen and nutrients in order to permit a normal intrauterine growth. Among other causes placental insufficiency is an important reason for disturbed intrauterine growth, resulting in intrauterine growth retardation (IUGR) and postnatal complications. The evaluation of foetal perfusion today is based in daily practice on the calculation of RI and PI in large arteries, mainly the umbilical, the cerebral arteries and the aorta, sometimes supplemented by flow pattern evaluations in the venous duct [34, 35]. In the eighties of the last century, first

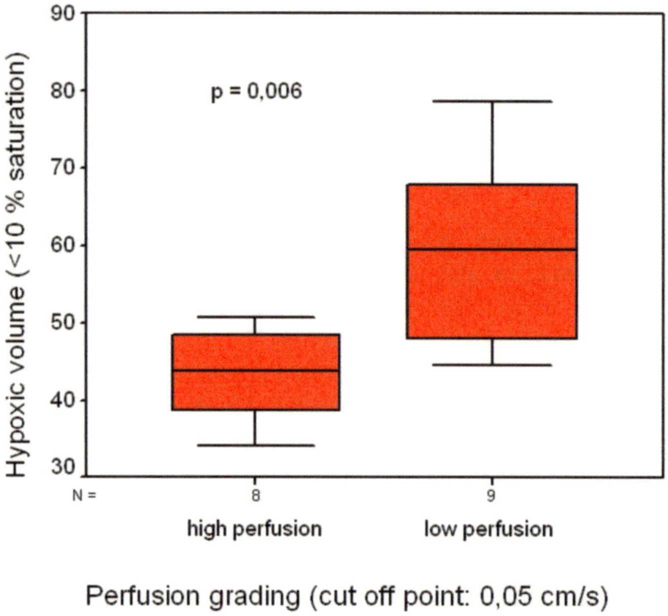

Fig. 24. Oxygenation differences in relation to tumor perfusion. Less perfused metastatic lymph nodes in the neck (cut off in DTPM: 0,05 cm/s) have a significantly higher hypoxic volume than well perfused nodes (from [2])

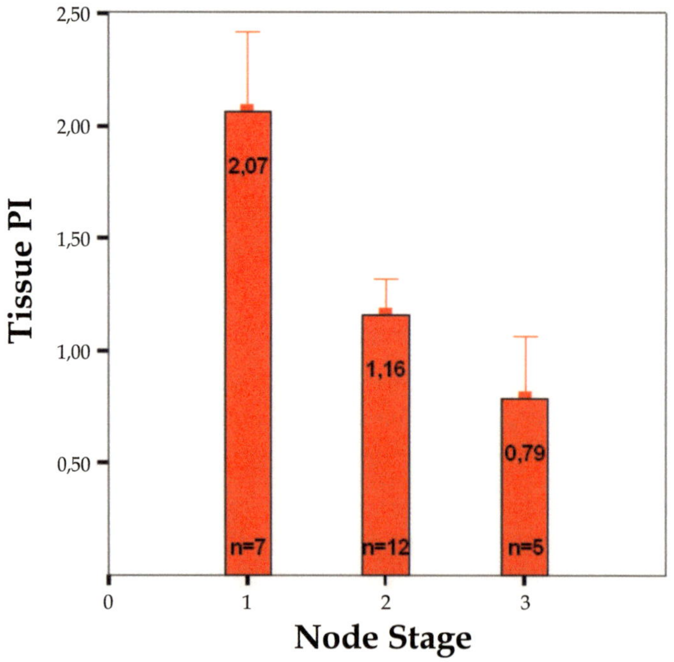

Fig. 25. The Tissue Perfusion Pulsatility Index (TPI) falls significantly with increasing N-stages of the nodes (from [2])

attempts tried to quantify the umbilical venous flow volume with the aim to evaluate the foetal perfusion in quantitative terms [36, 37]. These studies were not continued because of limited reproducibility [38]. Nevertheless, these studies targeted at a parameter - volume flow -, which has a much better rationale than the popular and easy to measure RI and PI. The early studies were flawed mainly by two limitations, which could not be overcome with two-dimensional sonographic techniques. First the angle correction of flow velocity in space and second the non-circular shape of the transsection of the umbilical vein (UV).

Spatial angle correction is but pivotal in this setting, because the UV is continuously winding around the umbilical arteries and the whole cord is irregularly bent within the amniotic cavity. Two-dimensional images thus may allow an angle correction within the frontal plane but this can be vastly misleading. Depending on the sagittal angle the true and only relevant spatial angle can differ substantially thus leading to unpredictable errors of the volume flow calculation, when unknown. The second source of error was the universal assumption, that the UV is a round tube. The investigators tried to depict a straight running venous segment with parallel borders to apply the formula for circular area calculation in order to multiply this area with the mean flow velocity which was traced with a pulsed-wave- Doppler instrument in the centre of the vein.

These sources of error combined in an unpredictable manner and caused the refusal of this approach.

The technique of DTPM combined with the modern three-dimensional imaging techniques can resolve all of these imponderabilities. We developed the three-dimensional, spatial angle corrected umbilical vein flow volume measurement, which is outlined below.

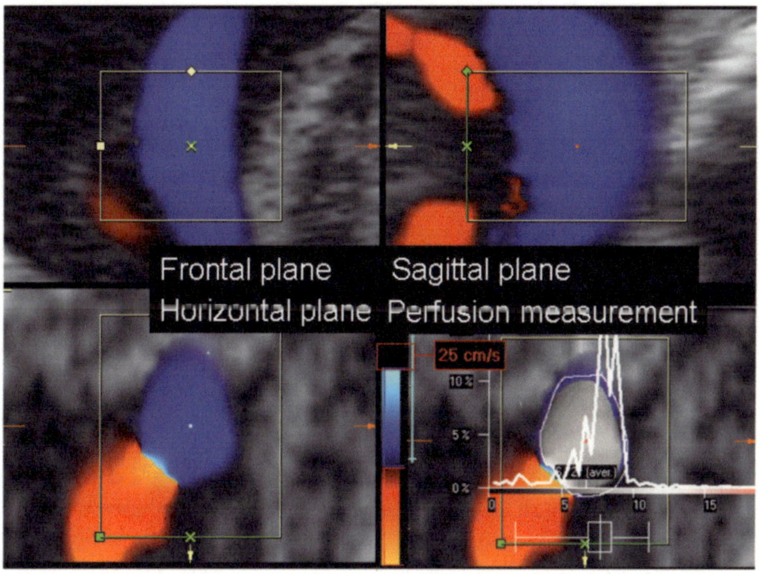

Fig. 26. Example of a spatially angle corrected fetal volume flow measurement in the umbilical vein. A 3D-dataset is shown displaying three perpendicular imaging planes. The horizontal plane is used for DTPM (right lower quarter): False color map of the venous flow. From these data the flow volume is directly calculated by the PixelFlux-software

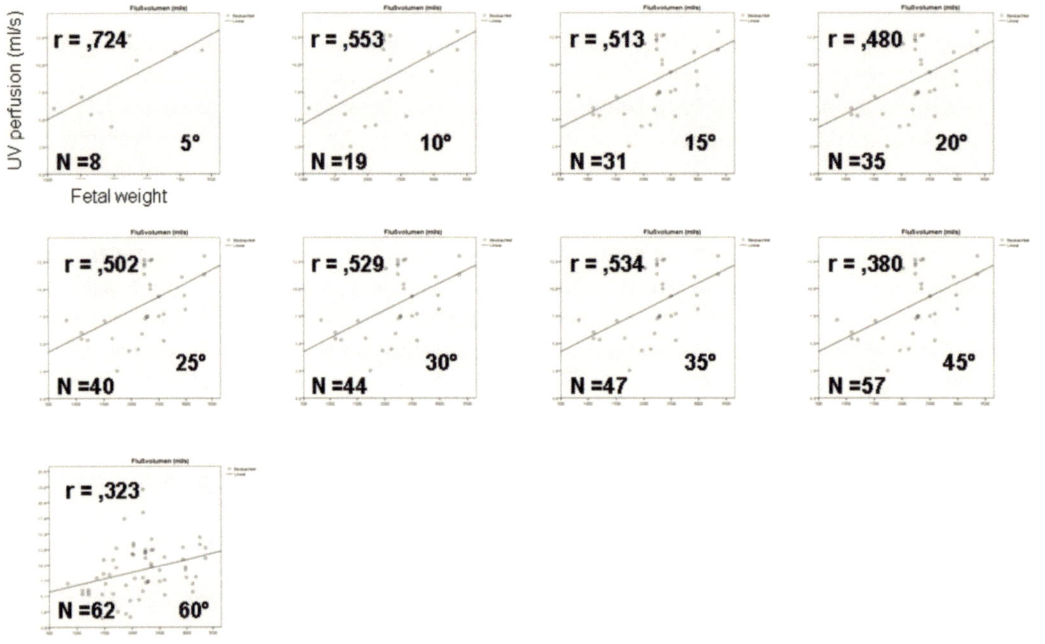

Fig. 27. DTPM reveals a significant correlation of fetal volume flow and fetal weight. This correlation improves significantly with reduction of the spatial angle (specified within each diagram)

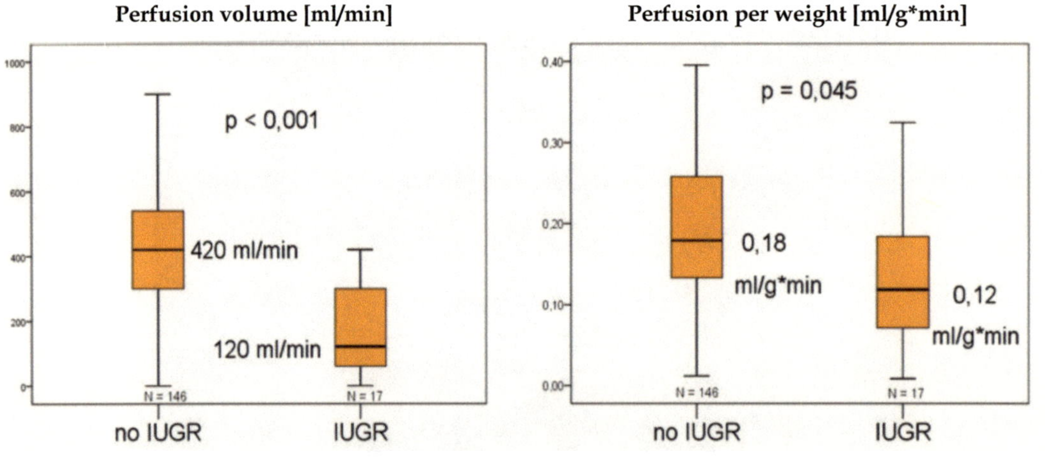

Fig. 28. A significant reduction of fetal perfusion per gram fetal weight could be demonstrated by DTPM in fetuses with intrauterine growth retardation (IUGR) compared to normal children

To achieve best results the umbilical cord should be recorded in a 3D-colour Doppler sweep so that the vein is running in a steep angle towards the transducer. The data block is then scanned with a 3D-manipulation software (4Dview, GE) by parallel shifts of the frontal and sagittal images to search for a transsection of the UV in the horizontal plane, which is clearly cut, has distinct borders and is not taken from a segment of the vein with strong bending (fig.

26). In this plane both velocity as displayed by a certain colour hue and shape of the vessel's cross section are distorted by a stretching factor which is equal to the cosine of the spatial angle between vessel's course and the ultrasound waves' propagation line - the so called Doppler angle α. While the area is stretched by the reciprocal of cos α the velocity is virtually reduced by the by multiplication with cos α (proof see chapter 18. Addendum on page 27). Therefore, direct calculation of true flow volumes directly from measurements within the horizontal plane is possible. This is accomplished by the DTPM software PixelFlux. The reproducibility of these measurements in a clinical situation lies in the range of around 6 % and less, if exclusively data with steep spatial Doppler angles are allowed (own unpublished data).

A significant correlation of such volume flow measurements with fetal weight could be demonstrated (fig. 27) [41] that was the better the steeper the spatial angle could be arranged. Moreover, in a preliminary study a significantly diminished flow volume per gram fetal weight could be shown (fig. 28).

16. Miscellaneous

In animal models, numerous reports underscore the interest in DTPM, especially in the field of theriogenology. The functional status of the bovine ovary (evaluated by the plasma progesterone concentration during the oestrous cycle) could be better correlated to luteal blood flow than to luteal size ([39]. The course of luteal perfusion mirrored progesterone levels much more readily than the sheer size of the corpus luteum. The perfusion measurement of the ovary in cows could differentiate between varying courses of progesterone plasma levels [41]. Perfusion measurements of the follicle, the corpus luteum and the uterus yielded differing responses in cows undergoing synchronization of ovulation [42]. They helped to explain the effect of human chorionic gonadotropin onto the progesterone synthesis and luteal blood flow [43], were useful in monitoring luteal perfusion during pregnancy and after embryonic loss [44] and could be used to tackle a variety of interactions between hormone production, luteal blood flow and gene expressions in luteal tissue [45].

In another study on the regulation of follicular development in cows DTPM demonstrated significant correlation with the follicular NO concentration and Estradiol (E2)/Progesterone (P4) ratio in those follicles, which developed to the dominant follicle in the ovary [46].

In milking of cows, a significant increase of utter perfusion was measured after 15 - 30 min to settle down after 45 min to the basic, pre-milking values. These basic values but differed considerably among the animals [47].

DTPM helped to describe the periurethral vascularity in women [3], was used to estimate the effect of periprostatic vascularity on the effect of HIFU in prostate cancer [48], proved to be more sensitive than computer assisted B-mode image analysis in testicular torsion and showed clearly a perfusion decline within two hours after torsion [49].

Perfusion measurements of the basal ganglia using DTPM in neonates with hypoxic ischemic encephalopathy (HIE) treated with therapeutic hypothermia demonstrated significantly higher perfusion values in neonates that died compared to the survivors (0.226± 0.221 cm/s vs. 0.111±0.082 cm/sec; p=0.02) (fig. 29). DTPM values also were higher in nine neonates with MRI showing moderate to severe injury (0.142±0.070 cm/s vs. 0.072±0.080 cm/s; p=0.04). DTPM opens a window to better understand reperfusion injury in HIE [49].

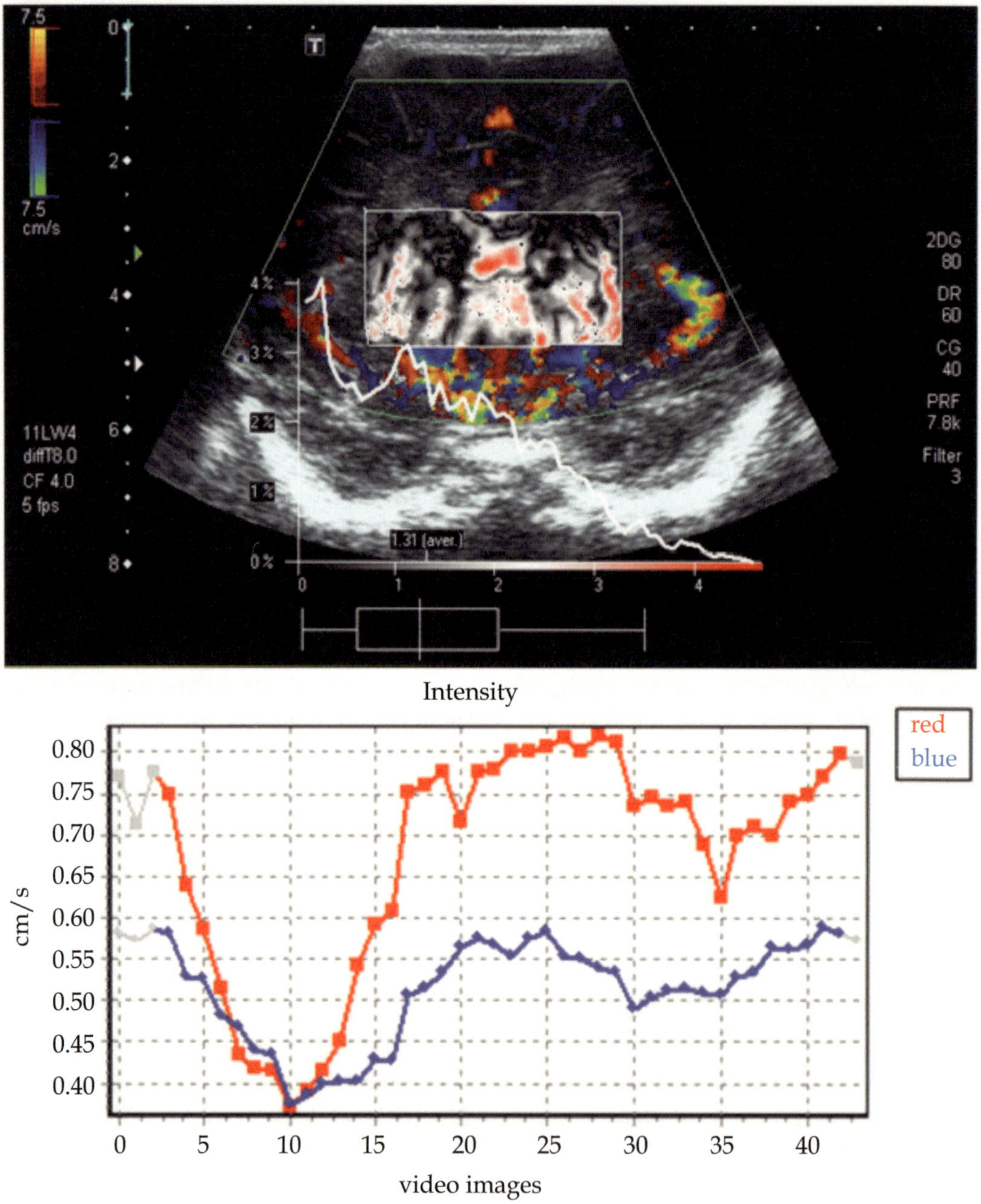

Fig. 29. Example of a DTPM of basal ganglia in a newborn. Upper part: false color map of the basal ganglia and distribution curve. Lower part: Perfusion intensity course during one examination. (Image and measurement courtesy of Dr. Ricardo Faingold, Montreal)

17. Summary

DTPM offers a universally applicable approach to tissue perfusion measurement as far as sonographic depiction of tissues is possible. So far, inaccessible details of perfusion intensity, perfusion distribution, perfusion gradients within a certain vasculature open a widow to an individualized evaluation of the specific pathophysiological situation. Treatment efforts can be evaluated according to their effect on perfusion. Besides these intrinsic advantages, the technique requires no additional hardware, is non-invasive, needs no specific preparation of the patient and thus can be recommended for a broad array of clinical applications.

18. Addendum: Proof of the congruence of the true flow volume and the flow volume calculated from the horizontally projected velocity and area of any vessel

True volume flow calculation becomes feasible with three-dimensional colour Doppler data.

True volume flow calculation means the exact calculation of the blood flow volume running through any vessel which is cut perpendicularly.

Our method of true volume perfusion measurement in vessels cut by the horizontal plane in any spatial angle is described and proven below.

The spatial angle, which is the angle between the vessel and the ultrasound propagation line, influences simultaneously the stretching of the shape of the vessels' cross-sectional area as well as the change of the recorded flow velocity. Figure 30 displays the respective situation schematically. The blood vessel (yellow rectangle) runs with the Doppler angle α towards the ultrasound propagation line (blue line). The horizontal imaging plane, which is calculated during the three-dimensional ultrasound imaging, cuts the vessel. Line a' is the stretched vessel's diameter as it can be seen in the horizontal plane. Vector b is the original flow velocity within the vessel. Due to the Doppler angle α the recorded velocity is displayed with the value for vector b'. This means, the color hue of b' is darker, representing a lower velocity as if vector b would be displayed in its appropriate color. This is the well known Doppler effect $\left(fd = 2 * fo * v_t / c * \cos\alpha\right)$, which reduces the recorded velocity according to the cosine of α.

The real flow volume per time (V) of a circular vessel is calculated as

$$V/t = \pi/4 * a * a * \vec{b} \tag{1}$$

// $\pi/4 * a * a$ calculates the circular area of the perpendicularly cut vessel

The oblique transsection of a round vessel, a vessel running not perpendicularly towards the horizontal plane, results in stretching of the circular vessel's round cross-sectional area in the direction of the projection vector of the spatial angle of this vessel with the horizontal plane. This results in an ellipse which longer axis is represented by a', the stretched projection of a onto the horizontal plane (Fig. 30). The shorter axis is equal to the original diameter of the vessel. It remains unstretched since no angulation occurs.

It is therefore possible to consider the change of diameter a towards a', the long axis of the ellipse in order to describe the change of the horizontally projected cross-sectional area of the vessel. The change of the circular area towards the elliptical area is thus equal to the stretching factor a'/a .

The other relevant change is the reduction of the displayed flow velocity compared to the original velocity b, the reduction factor is b'/b .

It is now claimed, that the flow volume V′ per time, which is passing through the horizontal plane in direction of the vessel, calculated by multiplying the elliptical area $(A = \pi/4 * a * a')$ with the flow velocity b′ of the vessel in the horizontal plane is equal to V per time, the flow volume passing through the perpendicularly cut vessel in the same time.

Claim:

$$V' = V \tag{2}$$

Proof:

$$V'/t = \pi/4 * a * a' * \vec{b'} \tag{3}$$

// $\pi/4 * a * a'$ calculates the elliptic area of the horizontally cut vessel
a : short axis of the ellipse
a' : long axis of the ellipse

The depiction of the horizontally cut vessel shows the velocity $\vec{b'}$ and a stretched vessel diameter a' .

The triangle ABC is rectangular, since the blood vessel is a rectangle, a perpendicularly cut circular straight vessel. Doppler angle α is complemented to 90° by the angles DAB and FAC since the ultrasound propagation line (blue line running through F) runs perpendicular to the transducer's surface and thus the horizontal imaging plane. Both angles are thus equal and named β. Angles FAC and CAB add to 90° since again the ultrasound propagation line runs perpendicular to the horizontal imaging plane. Thus angle CAB is α again, the Doppler angle.

$$a' = a / \cos\alpha \tag{4}$$

$$\vec{b'} = \vec{b} * \cos\alpha \tag{5}$$

by inserting (3) and (4) into (2) results (5)

$$V' = \pi/4 * a * a/\cos\alpha * \vec{b} * \cos\alpha \tag{6}$$

which is (6) after cancelling cos α

$$V' = \pi/4 * a * a * \vec{b} = V \text{ see (1)} \tag{7}$$

thus

$$V' = V \tag{8}$$

q.e.d.

This means, that it is possible to calculate the true flow volume of all vessels cut horizontally from the depicted flow velocities[1] and the pixelwise calculated cross-sectional areas[2] directly, thus compensating any spatial angle. Both measurements ([1] and [2]), are carried out automatically by the PixelFlux-software, which delivers thus true flow volumes of all vessels in any tissue section cut horizontally in three-dimensional color Doppler ultrasound data.

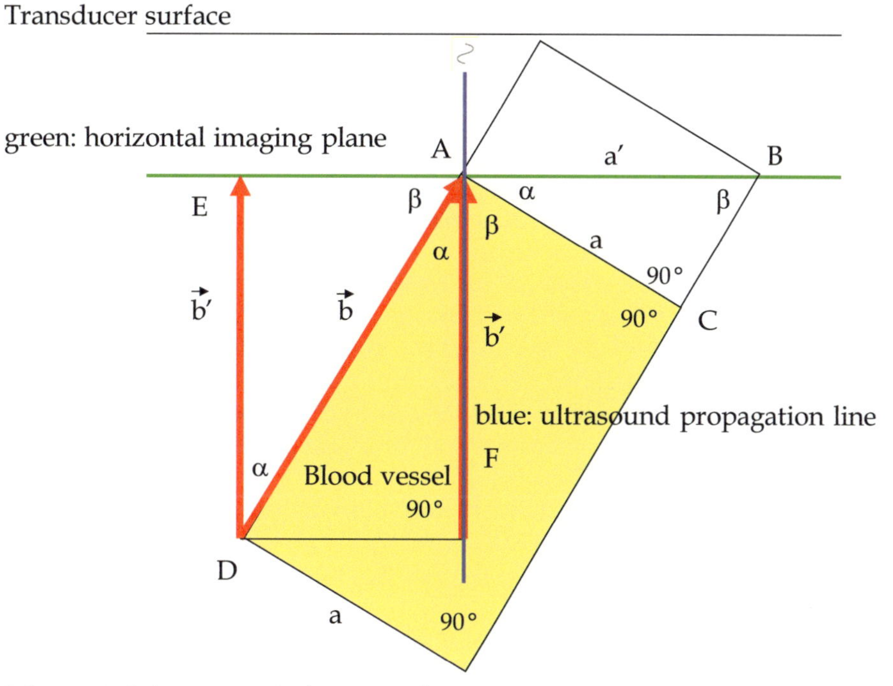

Fig. 30. Schematical depiction of a horizontally cut vessel in a 3D-color Doppler sonographic dataset

19. References

[1] Chameleon-Software, *PixelFlux*. 2011. http://www.chameleon-software.de/index-de.html.

[2] Scholbach T., DiMartino E., Scholbach J. "Dynamic color Doppler sonographic tissue perfusion measurement in tumors" in Cancer imaging (2 volumes) (Elsevier/ Academic Press, 2008) ed by M.A. Hayat

[3] Scholbach, T. and J. Scholbach, Can We Measure Renal Tissue Perfusion by Ultrasound? *Journal of Medical Ultrasound*, 2009. 17(1): p. 9-16.

[4] Wieczorek, A., et al., The assessment of normal female urethral vascularity with Color Doppler endovaginal ultrasonography: preliminary report. *Pelviperineology* 2009. 28: p. 59-61.

[5] Masulli, M., et al., Measurement of the intrarenal arterial resistance index for the identification and prediction of diabetic nephropathy. *Nutr Metab Cardiovasc Dis*, 2009. 19(5): p. 358-64.

[6] Radermacher, J., et al., The renal arterial resistance index and renal allograft survival. *N Engl J Med*, 2003. 349(2): p. 115-24.

[7] Ozelsancak, R., et al., Relationship between renal resistive index and inflammation in untreated hypertensive patients. *Int Heart J*, 2009. 50(6): p. 753-61.

[8] Crutchley, T.A., et al., Clinical utility of the resistive index in atherosclerotic renovascular disease. *J Vasc Surg*, 2009. 49(1): p. 148-55, 155 e1-3; discussion 155.

[9] Soria Galvez, F., et al., [Usefulness of renal resistive index in the diagnosis and evolution of the obstructive uropathy. Experimental study]. *Actas Urol Esp*, 2007. 31(1): p. 38-42.

[10] Onur, M.R., et al., Role of resistive index in renal colic. *Urol Res*, 2007. 35(6): p. 307-12.

[11] Krumme, B. and M. Hollenbeck, Doppler sonography in renal artery stenosis--does the Resistive Index predict the success of intervention? *Nephrol Dial Transplant*, 2007. 22(3): p. 692-6.

[12] Braun, B., Focal liver processes: "better is the enemy of good": CEUS in the fast lane. *Ultraschall Med*, 2009. 30(4): p. 329-32.

[13] D'Onofrio, M., et al., Focal liver lesions: sinusoidal phase of CEUS. *Abdom Imaging*, 2006. 31(5): p. 529-36.

[14] Trojan, J., et al., Contrast-enhanced ultrasound in the diagnosis of malignant mesenchymal liver tumors. *J Clin Ultrasound*. 38(5): p. 227-31.

[15] Dietrich, C.F., et al., Pitfalls and artefacts using contrast enhanced ultrasound. *Z Gastroenterol*. 49(3): p. 350-6.

[16] Hocke, M., et al., Contrast-enhanced endoscopic ultrasound in discrimination between benign and malignant mediastinal and abdominal lymph nodes. *J Cancer Res Clin* Oncol, 2008. 134(4): p. 473-80.

[17] O'Connor, P.M., Renal oxygen delivery: matching delivery to metabolic demand. *Clin Exp Pharmacol Physiol*, 2006. 33(10): p. 961-7.

[18] Wolff, C.B., Normal cardiac output, oxygen delivery and oxygen extraction. *Adv Exp Med Biol*, 2007. 599: p. 169 - 82.

[19] Ikee, R., et al., Correlation between the resistive index by Doppler ultrasound and kidney function and histology. *Am J Kidney Dis*, 2005. 46(4): p. 603-9.

[20] Scholbach, T., I. Dimos, and J. Scholbach, A new method of color Doppler perfusion measurement via dynamic sonographic signal quantification in renal parenchyma. *Nephron Physiol*, 2004. 96(4): p. p99-104.

[21] Scholbach, T., From the nutcracker-phenomenon of the left renal vein to the midline congestion syndrome as a cause of migraine, headache, back and abdominal pain and functional disorders of pelvic organs. *Med Hypotheses*, 2007. 68(6): p. 1318-27.

[22] Scholbach, T., et al., Correlation of histopathology and dynamic tissue perfusion measurement (DTPM) in renal transplants. http://www.postersessiononline.com/173580348_eu/congresos/48era/aula/poster_43104.pdf, 2011(ERA-EDTA Congress 2011).

[23] Scholbach, T., E. Girelli, and J. Scholbach, Dynamic tissue perfusion measurement: a novel tool in follow-up of renal transplants. *Transplantation*, 2005. 79(12): p. 1711-6.

[24] Scholbach, T., E. Girelli, and J. Scholbach, Tissue pulsatility index: a new parameter to evaluate renal transplant perfusion. *Transplantatio*n, 2006. 81(5): p. 751-5.

[25] Marti, E., et al., Donor effect on cortical perfusion intensity in renal allograft recipients: a paired kidney analysis. *Am J Nephrol*. 33(6): p. 530-6.

[26] Scholbach, T., I. Herrero, and J. Scholbach, Dynamic color Doppler sonography of intestinal wall in patients with Crohn disease compared with healthy subjects. *J Pediatr Gastroenterol Nutr*, 2004. 39(5): p. 524-8.

[27] Scholbach, T., J. Hormann, and J. Scholbach, Dynamic tissue perfusion measurement of the intestinal wall - correlation to histology in ulcerative colitis. *Journal of Medical Ultrasound* 2010. 18(2): p. 62-70.

[28] Cassia, G., et al., Hypoxic ischemic injury: intestinal appearances and perfusion measurements using ultrasound and dynamic color Doppler sonography in neonates submitted to therapeutic hypothermia. *Pediatr Radiol*, 2011. 41(Suppl 1): p. S250-S310 FN-9.

[29] Schäfer, M., Dynamische farbduplexsonografische Gewebeperfusionsmessung an cervicalen Lymphknoten (Dissertationsschrift). Katalog der Deutschen Nationalbibliothek, 2009: p. http://d-nb.info/1002591465

[30] Oktar, S., et al., Quantitative Color Doppler Evaluation of Perfusion in the Differential Diagnosis of Benign and Malignant Thyroid Nodules Using a Dedicated Software Program. http://rsna2007.rsna.org/rsna2007/v2007/conference/event_display.cfm?am_id=3&em_id=5008569, 2007.

[31] Vaupel, P., et al., Hypoxia in breast cancer: role of blood flow, oxygen diffusion distances, and anemia in the development of oxygen depletion. *Adv Exp Med Biol*, 2005. 566: p. 333-42.

[32] Vaupel, P. and A. Mayer, Hypoxia and anemia: effects on tumor biology and treatment resistance. *Transfus Clin Biol*, 2005. 12(1): p. 5-10.

[33] Vaupel, P., Prognostic potential of the pre-therapeutic tumor oxygenation status. *Adv Exp Med Biol*, 2009. 645: p. 241-6.

[34] Scholbach, T., et al., New method of dynamic color doppler signal quantification in metastatic lymph nodes compared to direct polarographic measurements of tissue oxygenation. *Int J Cancer*, 2005. 114(6): p. 957-62.

[35] Ebrashy, A., et al., Middle cerebral/umbilical artery resistance index ratio as sensitive parameter for fetal well-being and neonatal outcome in patients with preeclampsia: case-control study. *Croat Med J*, 2005. 46(5): p. 821-5.

[36] Figueras, F., et al., Umbilical artery pulsatility index: reliability at different sampling sites. *J Perinat Med*, 2006. 34(5): p. 409-13.

[37] Eik-Nes, S.H., K. Marsal, and K. Kristoffersen, Methodology and basic problems related to blood flow studies in the human fetus. *Ultrasound Med Biol*, 1984. 10(3): p. 329-37.

[38] Gill, R.W., et al., Umbilical venous flow in normal and complicated pregnancy. *Ultrasound Med Biol*, 1984. 10(3): p. 349-63.

[39] Erskine, R.L. and J.W. Ritchie, Quantitative measurement of fetal blood flow using Doppler ultrasound. *Br J Obstet Gynaecol*, 1985. 92(6): p. 600-4.

[40] Scholbach T., Stolle J., Scholbach J. Three dimensional volumetric spatially angle corrected pixelwise fetal flow volume measurement. *Eur J Ultrasound* (2011 accepted for publication)

[41] Herzog, K., et al., Luteal blood flow is a more appropriate indicator for luteal function during the bovine estrous cycle than luteal size. *Theriogenology*. 73(5): p. 691-7.

[42] Luttgenau, J., et al., Low plasma progesterone concentrations are accompanied by reduced luteal blood flow and increased size of the dominant follicle in dairy cows. *Theriogenology*. 76(1): p. 12-22.

[43] Bollwein, H., et al., Effects of a shortened preovulatory follicular phase on genital blood flow and endometrial hormone receptor concentrations in Holstein-Friesian cows. *Theriogenology*. 73(2): p. 242-9.
[44] Beindorff, N., et al., Effects of human chorionic gonadotropin on luteal blood flow and progesterone secretion in cows and in vitro-microdialyzed corpora lutea. *Theriogenology*, 2009. 72(4): p. 528-34.
[45] Herzog, K., et al., Luteal blood flow increases during the first three weeks of pregnancy in lactating dairy cows. *Theriogenology*. 75(3): p. 549-54.
[46] Luttgenau, J., et al., Plasma progesterone concentrations in the mid-luteal phase are dependent on luteal size, but independent of luteal blood flow and gene expression in lactating dairy cows. *Anim Reprod Sci*. 125(1-4): p. 20-9.
[47] Pancarcı, Ş.M., et al., Changes in follicular blood flow and nitric oxide levels in follicular fluid during follicular deviation in cows. *Animal Reproduction Science*, 2011. 123 (3-4): p. 149-156.
[48] Kuchler, K., et al., Measuring the blood flow of teats of dairy cows by using Color-Angiography. *Reproduction in Domestic Animals*, 2011. 46(S1): p. 25 http://onlinelibrary.wiley.com/doi/10.1111/j.1439-0531.2011.01755.x/pdf.
[49] Rouviere, O., et al., Can color doppler predict the uniformity of HIFU-induced prostate tissue destruction? *Prostate*. 2004 60(4): p. 289-97.
[50] Aslan, M., et al., Quantitative Analysis of Ultrasonographic Textures with Software in Experimental Testicular Torsion. *Turkish Association of Pediatric Surgeons*, 2011. http://www.tccd.org.tr/abstract/yayinlanan_bildiri.php?bid=77.
[51] Faingold, R., et al., Cerebral perfusion measurements using dynamic color Doppler sonography in neonates with hypoxic ischemic encephalopathy (HIE) treated with therapeutic hypothermia. *Pediatr Radiol* 2011. 41(Suppl 1): p. S250-S310 NE2-3.

18

Fetal Yawning

Olivier Walusinski
Family Physician. Private Practice
France

1. Introduction

The introduction of ultrasound exploration during pregnancy has led to very important conclusions concerning fetal behavioural milestones. For example, the development of oral sensorimotor functions such as swallowing (essential for survival) can be assessed from normal or abnormal neurobehavioral development during the fetal period. While the assessment of these functions takes a long time, another daily behaviour can be detected during an ultrasound examination: yawning. Before the development of real-time imaging techniques, it was impossible to assess facial movements, swallowing and thus yawning. Only the overall movements of the trunk and limbs could be perceived by the mother or by someone touching her belly with their hand. In this chapter, we will show the usefulness of ultrasound in exploring facial mobility, particularly yawning, and in drawing conclusions on harmonious fetal cerebral development.

The phenomenon of yawning is just as intriguing and fascinating as sleep, yet understanding of its causes and consequences has defied the human mind for centuries. Phylogenetically and ontogenetically primitive, this motor behaviour has been remarkably well preserved during evolution and is nearly universal in vertebrates. It appears closer to an emotional stereotypy than to a reflex. Yawning is a stereotyped and often repetitive motor act characterized by gaping of the mouth accompanied by a long inspiration of air or fluid, followed by a brief acme and a short expiration. It is not merely a simple opening of the mouth, but a complex coordinated movement bringing together a flexion followed by an extension of the neck, a wide dilatation of the laryngopharynx with strong stretching of the diaphragm and anti-gravity muscles. Highly stereotypical because no environmental input changes the sequence of movements, it is observed in cold-blooded and warm-blooded vertebrates, from reptiles with rudimentary 'archaic' brains to human primates, in water, air and land environments. The ethology, neurophysiology and neuropsychology literature describes yawning as a transitional behaviour associated with wake/sleep rhythms and hunger/satiety fluctuations, where it externalizes a group of possible vigilance-stimulating mechanisms and attests to the central role of the diencephalon and notably the hypothalamus in homeostasis (Walusinski, 2004; Guggisberg, 2010).

All the movements that a newborn is able to produce originate during the fetal phase and are performed throughout the life span. The fetus exhibits a wide range of behaviours starting with slow flexion and extension of the spine and limbs at around 7 weeks gestation. The variety of movements increases rapidly over the next three to four weeks and many different movement patterns have been described, including breathing, truncal rotation, limb flexion/extension, sucking and yawning (de Vries, 1982).

2. How to recognize a fetal yawn during ultrasound examination

During ultrasound facial examination, yawning can be seen accidentally. Yawning consists of a slow opening of the mouth with simultaneous downward movements of the tongue and is usually combined with retroflexion of the head. This phase occupies 50 to 75% of the

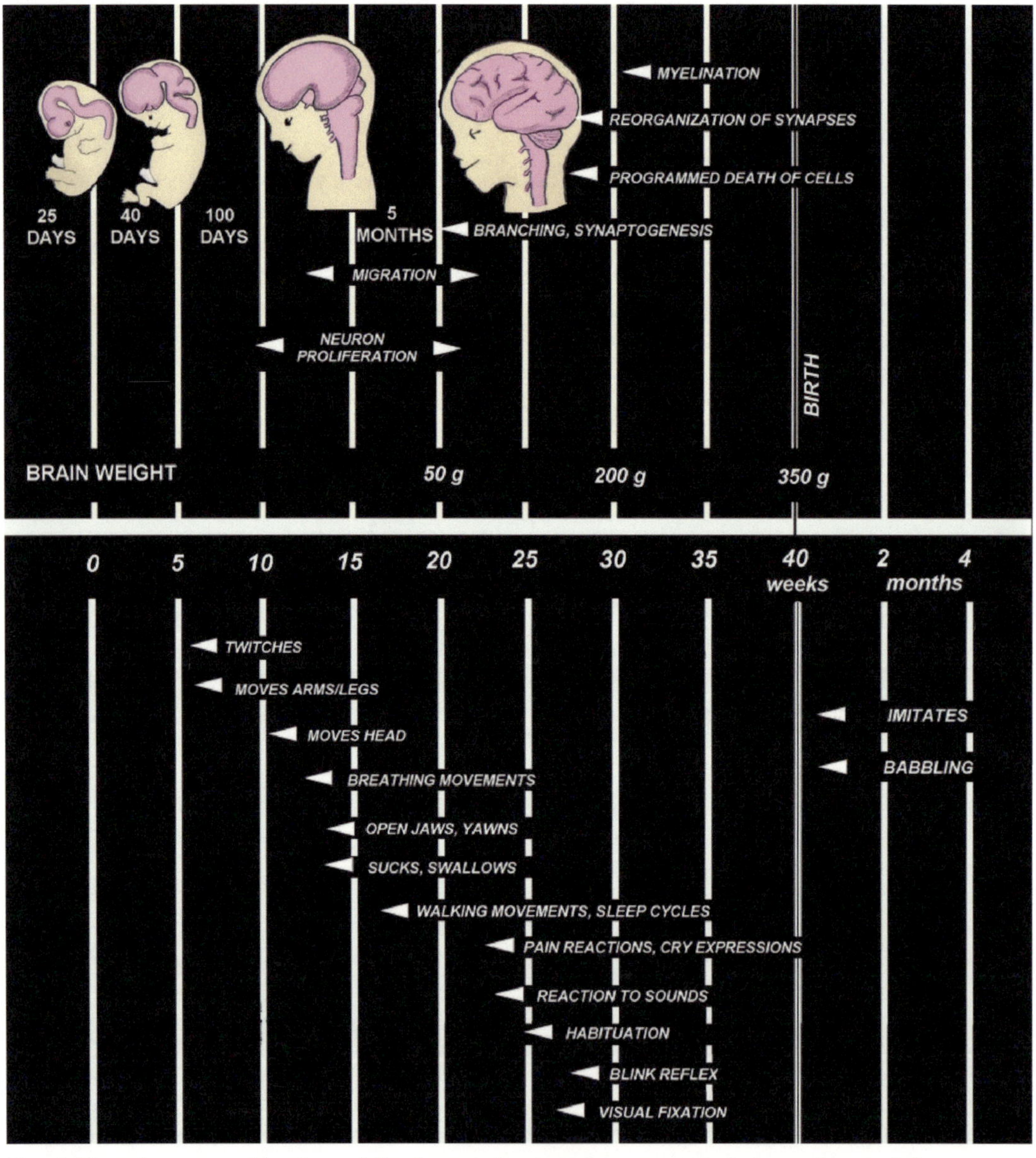

Fig. 1. Development of brain and fetal central nervous system and chronology of the functional development of fetal movements

yawning cycle. After reaching its maximum opening, the mouth remains wide open for 5 to 15 s and returns to its resting closed position within seconds. This harmonious sequence is markedly different from a brief swallowing episode. Using a colour Doppler technique, it is possible to observe the flow of amniotic fluid through the fetal mouth, oropharynx and trachea to the lungs. Contrary to adults, yawning is non-repetitive in the fetus. It is part of a generalized stretch, not just a matter of opening one's mouth. It especially involves the muscles of the respiratory tract (diaphragm, intercostals), face and neck. Fetal yawning can be recognized as one of the movement patterns consistently present starting at around 11-12 weeks of pregnancy (fig. 2). The frequency of yawning gradually increases between 12 and 24 weeks (fig. 3 and 4). During this time, it is possible to observe 40 to 60 yawns per day, and it is the best time to assess yawning with ultrasound examination. A plateau is reached, after which the number of yawns decreases slightly until term. Thus, yawning occurs regularly at a rate of about 1 to 3 yawns per hour. It is obviously by chance or after a long investigation that a yawn can be observed. Furthermore, occiput anterior fetal position unfortunately impedes adequate observation of yawning (Sepulveda, 1995; Masuzaki, 1996).

3. Yawning and neurodevelopmental assessments

Yawning is a phylogenetically old, stereotyped phenomenon. Its survival without evolutionary variations suggests a particular importance as far as development. The strong muscular contraction during yawning has a metabolically high cost. If we agree with Darwin's evolutionary propositions, the costs of brain activity must be outweighed by the developmental advantages. Thus, one structural hypothesis is activation of neurotrophins, which leads to a cascade of new synapse formation or recruitment as well as activation through the diencephalon, brainstem and spinal cord. Activity-dependent development has been clearly shown to be one mechanism by which early sensory or motor experience can affect the course of neural development. This mechanism may be a ubiquitous process in brain maturation, by which activity in one brain region can influence development of other regions. Fetal yawning can be seen as a mechanism that influences functional determination of the moving parts of the musculoskeletal system and contributes to joint development and maintenance.

Fetal movements become more regular and coordinated as a result of increased maturation of the nervous system. At the beginning of the third month, the embryo becomes a fetus with the occurrence of the first oral and pharyngeal motor sequences, controlled by neurological brainstem development and the development of the suction-swallowing activity and yawning. Indeed, suction and yawning have the same embryological origin, which shows the importance of the brainstem in the neurophysiological development of oropharyngeal activity coordinated by respiratory, cardiac and digestive regulations, which have the same neuroanatomical location. The cephalic pole comprises an original embryological encephalo-facial and encephalo-cervical segmentation with a strict topographical correspondence: the naso-frontal and premaxillary structures are connected to the forebrain; the maxillo-mandibular and anterior cervical structures are connected to the 41 brainstem and its nerves. The major structures of the brainstem are formed by the 7-8th postconceptional week, although brainstem maturation continues until the 8th postconceptional month. In addition to its many subnuclei, the brainstem gives rise to a variety of descending spinal motor tracts and hosts the nuclei of five cranial nerves (VIII-XII). Formation of the pons begins almost simultaneously, but its maturation is more prolonged. The structures of the pons include cranial nerves V-VIII and the medial

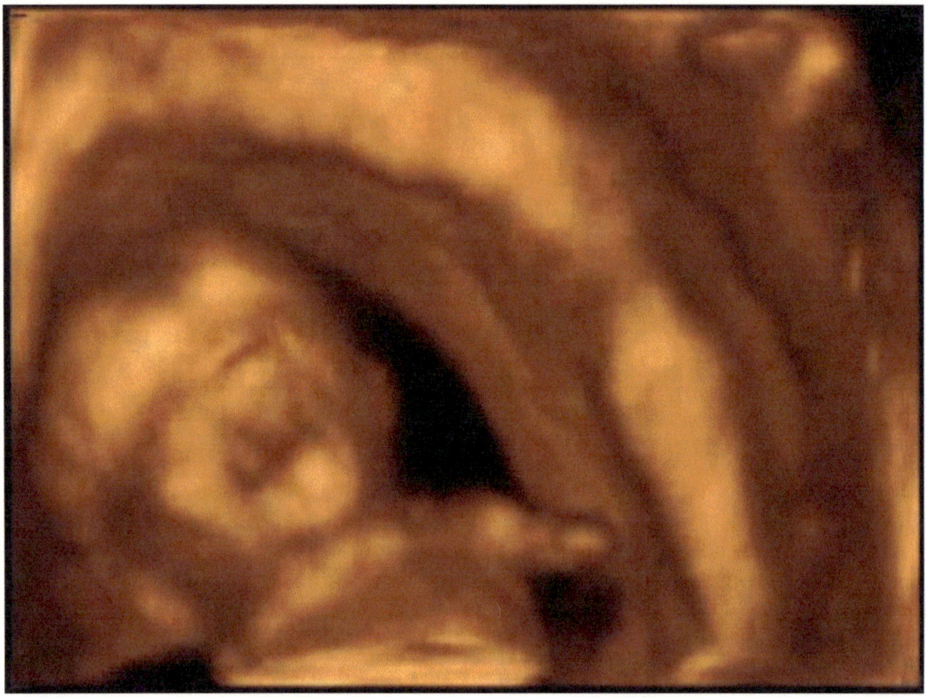

Fig. 2. Fetal yawn at 12 weeks of pregnancy (3D). Fetus weighing 80g

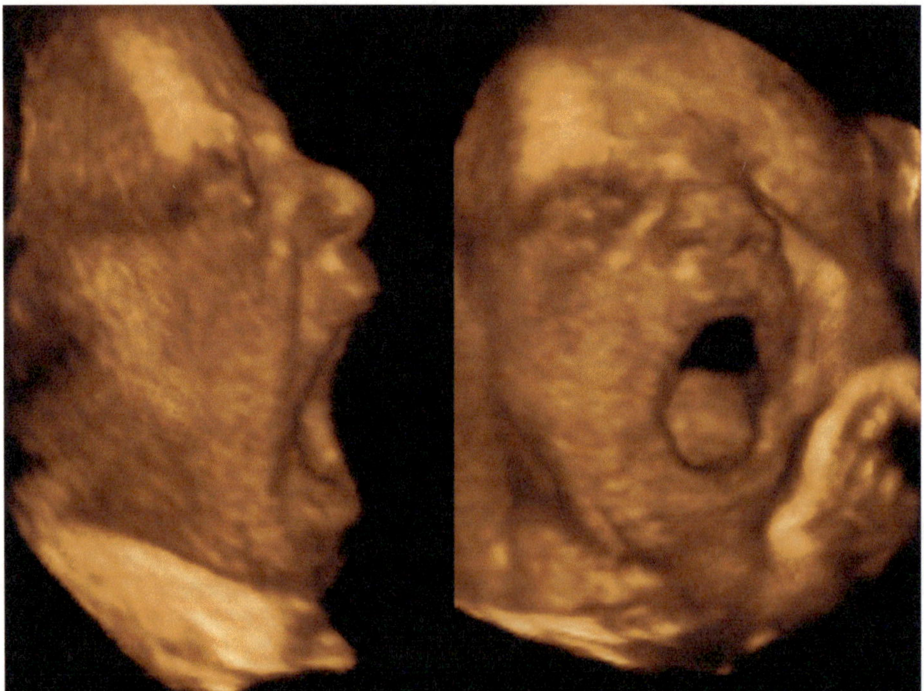

Fig. 3. Fetal yawn at 23 weeks of pregnancy (3D). Fetus weighing 200g

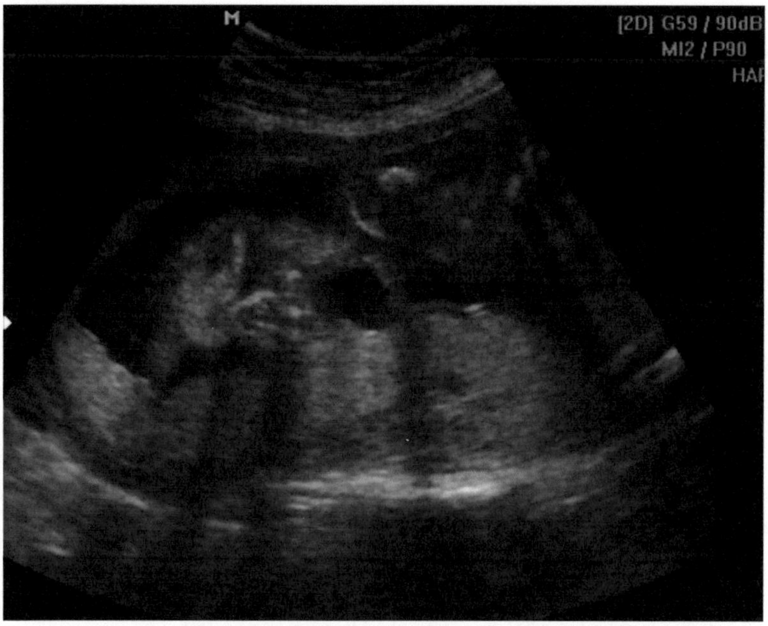

Fig. 4. Fetal yawn at 23 weeks of pregnancy (2D). Fetus weighing 200g

longitudinal fasciculus (MLF), pontine tegmentum, raphe nucleus and locus coeruleus, which exert widespread influence on arousal, including the sleep-wake cycle. Therefore, these structures exert tremendous influence on gross body movements, head turning, heart rate, and respiratory movements, as well as swallowing, yawning, suckling, hiccups, and 7 facial grimacing movements (Santagati, 2003; Kontges, 1996; Jacob, 2000; Sadler, 2009) (Fig. 1).

The emergence of different behavioural states is one of the most significant aspects of early brain maturation in the fetus. In early intra-uterine life, a diffuse collection of phasic and cyclic motor events occur that gradually coalesce. For the fetus, wakefulness and sleep are reliably characterized, respectively, by periods of myoclonic twitching and movements of the limbs against a background of muscle atonia. Periods of twitching are almost always followed by the abrupt onset of high-amplitude, wakeful behaviours. The emergence of distinct states is followed by dramatic changes in the level, duration and cyclicity. An ultradian rhythm may be observed: during a 60 to 90 minute period, there is an alternation of movement characterized by motor activity and movement characterized by rest, as in newborns. The switchover from periods of rest to periods of activity is accompanied by a yawn. Thus, a periodicity of one or two yawns per hour can be seen. Repetitive motions gradually determine the shape and composition of moving structures, as well as their associated neural control pathways. The precociousness and stability of yawning suggest that these characteristics contribute to such development. Furthermore, since a forced inspiration is a critical component of yawning, a potential role for expanding fetal terminal alveoli by the inspired fluid is possible (Marder, 2005).

4. Yawning as a testimony to safe neurological development

In pregnant women, the methods of assessing fetal wellbeing include the biophysical profile; however, this method is limited. Thus, infants must develop safe and effective respiration and oral feeding skills after birth if they are to survive. For this to occur, infants must have the necessary anatomical structures and adequate central control to coordinate swallowing, ventilation, sleep and arousal. Yawning is associated with all of these behaviours and thus is useful to observe. Fetal facial expressions and movements are known to be an indirect expression of cerebral functional maturity during the fetal period. Facial expressions during this period correspond to facial expression during the neonatal period. Ultrasound has become essential for assessing neurophysiological development as well as detecting anatomical pathology. 4D ultrasound makes it straightforward to comprehend morphological dynamics such as yawning or sucking. As we have seen, yawning can provide information about neurodevelopment and the development of behavioural rhythms (alternation between motor activity, rest and sleep). When fetal activity appears abnormal, nervous system development may be disturbed. Yawning indicates harmonious development of both the brainstem and the peripheral neuromuscular function, testifying to the induction of an ultradian rhythm of vigilance (Rogers, 2005; Einspieler, 2005; Kurjak, 2008). (Ultradian rhythms are recurrent periods or cycles repeated throughout a 24-hour circadian day. In contrast, infradian rhythms, such as the human menstrual cycle, have periods longer than a day. The descriptive term ultradian is used in sleep research in reference to the 90–120 minute cycling of the sleep stages during human sleep).

5. Fetal pathologies assessed by yawning exploration

Yawns recur regularly, about one or two per hour. When a yawn is observed during a 4D US examination, it is obviously by chance or after very long investigation. Yawning appears preferentially after a period of rest, and indicates waking. If normal swallowing is seen (much more frequent), yawning seems of no additional interest with regard to harmonious brainstem maturation. Inversely, the lack or dysfunction of swallowing requires taking the time to understand the set of phasic and cyclic motor events characterizing the ultradian fetal rhythm, thereby increasing the opportunity to observe a yawn. If the ultrasound examination suggests the absence of yawning and swallowing, it is imperative to search for developmental and anatomical abnormalities (van Woerden, 1988).

The lack of fetal yawning, frequently simultaneous to the lack of associated swallowing may be a key to predicting brainstem dysfunction after birth. It is thus imperative to search for mandibular hypoplasia and glossoptosis, often associated with cleft palate (Luedders, 2011; Palit, 2008). For example, Pierre Robin sequence is characterized by a posterior U-shaped cleft palate, retrognatia and glossoptosis. Several arguments favour an embryonic origin consisting of an anomaly in caudal hind brain development. Feeding disorders are the most important functional symptom. Mother testimonies are consistent with the lack of yawning at birth and its progressive appearance during the first year of life, simultaneous to the acquisition of the swallowing reflex necessary for feeding. Pierre Robin syndrome can be seen as the prenatal brainstem dysfunction responsible for orofacial maldevelopment, which can be diagnosed at 23 weeks gestation during a 4D ultrasound examination (Bromley, 1994; Rotten, 2001).

Petrikovsky et al. (1999) report that clusters of yawns were observed in a series of anaemic fetuses and suggest that yawning repetitiveness helps to track fetal anaemia, although fetal yawning has no effect on O2 pressure. Yawning can be seen as the exteriorization of a homeostatic process, the balance between adrenergic and cholinergic stimulation of the autonomic nervous system. We believe this function is already active in the fetus.

Although no data has actually been collected, we have made a non-exhaustive inventory of congenital pathologies in which yawning research is relevant:

- Mandibular hypoplasia is a frequently encountered craniofacial difference and can be classified into congenital and developmental types:
    - Mandibulofacial dysostosis with a variety of limb abnormalities
- Any syndrome (primary bilateral or unilateral growth anomalies), associated or not with temporo / mandibular joint ankylosis, aglossia / microglossia: Francheschetti syndrome, Goldenhar syndrome, Richner-Hanhart syndrome.
- Moebius syndrome comprises a congenital facial diplegia and bilateral abducens nerve palsies by degenerative and involved nuclei of the VI, VII, and XII nerves. Simultaneous occurrence of limb malformations with cranial nerve dysfunction suggests a disruption of normal morphogenesis during a critical period in embryonic brainstem development, most likely starting at 4 to 7 weeks of gestation. Instances of bilateral paresis of the soft palate and scattered instances of dysphagia (some of which resolve in infancy) have been reported. In this type of functional problem, the inability to close the mouth is constant.
- Watershed infarcts in the fetal and neonatal brainstem are clinically expressed as multiple cranial neuropathies, failure of central respiratory drive and dysphagia.
- Goldenhar Syndrome includes malformations primarily involving the jaw, mouth and ears and, in most cases, affects one side of the body. It represents defects in the embryonic first and second brachial arches, the first pharyngeal pouch and brachial cleft, and the primordia of the temporal bone.
- Joubert syndrome is a rare, genetic disorder characterized by absence or underdevelopment of the cerebellar vermis and a malformed brainstem. The most common features include ataxia, an abnormal breathing pattern, sleep apnea, abnormal eye and tongue movements, and hypotonia.
- It is possible to complete this catalogue by referring to Congenital trismus, Crisponi syndrome, Stüve-Wiedemann syndrome, etc.

6. Conclusion

An entirely new paradigm has emerged in fetal medicine, given that the advances in prenatal imaging allow one to see and diagnose disease not previously detected. Clinicians can better plan for the delivery of the neonate, with identified anomalies being optimally managed and the impact on the neonate's health minimized. There exists a sound rationale for including systematic observations of spontaneous motor activity in the neurological assessment of fetuses. Yawning, as spontaneous motility linked to brainstem activities, appears to be a good parameter for indicating such wellbeing and harmonious development. Thus, brainstem maturation could be associated with changes in the yawning pattern. A difficult task is qualitative evaluation of general and partial movements in order to distinguish normal from abnormal performance. Yawning is a basic behaviour that is easy to recognize and highly valuable in assessing brainstem activity. It is advisable to include the fetal yawning examination in the systematic week 23 ultrasound scan. Future studies will improve its diagnostic value in detecting neuromuscular developmental abnormalities as well as fetal behavioural abnormalities.

A complete review on yawning can be founded in the book: "The Mystery of Yawning in Physiology and Disease". Walusinski O. ed. Basel. Karger. 2010. 160p.

7. References

Bromley B, Benacerraf BR. Fetal Micrognathia: Associated Anomonalies and Outcome. *J Ultrasound Med.* 1994;13:529-533.

de Vries JI, Visser GH, Prechtl FM. The emergence of fetal behaviour. *Early Hum Dey* 1982;7:301-322.

Einspieler C, Prechtl HF. Prechtl's assessment of general movements: a diagnostic tool for the functional assessment of the young nervous system. *Ment Retard Dev Disabil Res Rev.* 2005;11:61-67.

Guggisberg AG, Mathis J, Schnider A, Hess CW. Why do we yawn? *Neurosci Biobehav Rev.* 2010;34:1267-1276

Jacob J, Gutrhie S. Facial visceromotor neurons display specific rhombomere origin and axon pathfinding behavior. *J Neuosci* 2000;20:7664-7671.

Kontges G, Lumsden A. Rhombencephalic neural crest segmentation is preserved throughout craniofacial ontogeny. *Development* 1996,122:3229-3242.

Kurjak A, Tikvica A, Stanojevic M, Miskovic B, Ahmed B, Azumendi G, Di Renzo GC. The assessment of fetal neurobehavior by three-dimensional and four-dimensional ultrasound. *J Matern Fetal Neonatal Med.* 2008;21:675-684.

Luedders DW, Bohlmann MK, Germer U, Axt-Fliedner R, Gembruch U, Weichert J. Fetal micrognathia: objective assessment and associated anomalies on prenatal sonogram. *Prenat Diagn.* 2011;31:1461-51.

Marder E, Rehm KJ. Development of central pattern generating circuits. *Curr Opin Neurobiol.* 2005;15:86-93.

Masuzaki H, Masuzaki M. Color Doppler imaging of fetal yawning. *Ultrasound Obstet Gynecol* l996;8:355-356.

Palit G, Jacquemyn Y, Kerremans M. An objective measurement to diagnose micrognathia on prenatal ultrasound. *Clin Exp Obstet Gynecol.* 2008;35:121-123.

Petrikovsky BM, Kaplan GP, Holsten N. Fetal yawning activity in normal and high-risk fetuses: a preliminary observation. *Ultrasound Obstet Gynecol* 1999;13:127-130.

Rogers B, Arvedson J.Assessment of infant oral sensorimotor and swallowing function. *Ment Retard Dev Disabil Res Rev.* 2005;11:74-82.

Rose RJ. Prenatal programming of behavior. *Neurosci Biobehav Rev.* 2005;29:321-327.

Rotten D, Levaillant JM, Martinez H., Ducou le Pointe H, Vicaut E. The fetal mandible: a 2D and 3D sonographic approach to the diagnosis of retrognathia and micrognathia. *Ultrasound Obstet Gynecol.* 2002;19:122-130.

Sadler, T.W. Langman's Medical Embriology. Williams & Wilkins, Baltimore. 2009. 414p.

Santagati F, Rijli F. Cranial neural crest and the building of the vertebrate head. *Nature Rev Neurosci* 2003;4:806-8l8.

Sepulveda W, Mangiamarchi M. Fetal yawning. Ultrasound Obstet Gynecol 1995;5:57-59.

van Woerden EE, van Geijn HP, Caron FJ, van der Valk AW, Swartjes JM, Arts NF. Fetal mouth movements during behavioural states 1F and 2F. *Europ J Obstet Gynecol Reprod Biol* 1988;29:97-105.

Walusinski 0, Deputte B. The phylogeny, ethology and nosogeny of yawning. *Rev Neurol* 2004;l60:1011-1021.

Yigiter AB, Kavak ZN. Normal standards of fetal behavior assessed by four-dimensional sonography. *J Matern Fetal Neonatal Med.* 2006;19:707-721.

19

Professional Learning in Sonography

Madeleine Shanahan
School of Medical Sciences, RMIT University
Australia

1. Introduction

The healthcare system is in a state of constant and rapid change as a result of the increase in scientific knowledge and rapid technological advances. To provide the best possible healthcare health practitioners must continue to learn throughout their working life. The notion that professionals must continually update their knowledge is not a new concept (1, 2). For example, Dubin (1 p.486) wrote of professionals:

> *A highly trained person must constantly renew his knowledge. The goal is not merely to keep knowledge already acquired during the period of formal education. Much more than this—for past knowledge may become outdated—the aim is ... self-renewal by keeping abreast of new knowledge that is constantly being added to by research and publication.*

The rate of change of knowledge is increasing and this is reflected in the decreasing 'half-life' of knowledge. The term half-life, borrowed from the field of nuclear physics, represents the process of decay of knowledge such that a half-life of five years indicates that after five years only 50 percent of the body of knowledge acquired at a given point remains relevant to the work task (3). The half-life of knowledge continues to decrease, with, for example, the half-life of medical and scientific knowledge estimated to be between 18 months and three years (4, 5). Akin to medical and scientific knowledge having a short half-life, the knowledge of health professionals is also considered to have a short-half life. Professional obsolescence was the term utilised by Dubin (1) to describe the professionals' reduction in competence to meet the demands of their profession with time. Professional obsolescence, Dubin argues is "almost inevitable ... without continuous updating ... [as] people will carry on their work with increasingly outdated techniques and hypotheses, ignorant of new data, techniques, and principles" (3, p.10). By updating knowledge, professionals grow or appreciate their existing knowledge with new knowledge (3, 6, 7). In essence, to remain competent in their practice, health professionals must advance their knowledge at the same rate as knowledge advances in their field and thus avoid professional obsolescence.

The introduction of CPD requirements within professions formalises the need to update knowledge and counterbalance the effect of professional obsolescence (1, 6). CPD requirements are now common and for many health professionals updating knowledge is now a requirement for practice. The Health Professions Council (HPC) in the United Kingdom regulates 15 health professions and introduced mandatory Continuing Professional Development (CPD) requirements in 2006 (8). The HPC states:

Put simply, CPD is the way health professionals continue to learn and develop throughout their careers so they keep their skills and knowledge up to date and are able to work safely, legally and effectively. (8)

In Australia, CPD linked to registration occurred more recently. For example, the Australian Health Ministerial Council (9) approved the *Continuing professional development registration standard*. This standard took effect from 1 July 2010 for ten health professions and a further four health professionals are to be included from 1 July 2012 (10). Health professions that now have mandated CPD requirements include for example, medicine, medical imaging and nursing and members of these professions perform sonography. With the profound changes in diagnostic ultrasound imaging shown throughout this book, updating knowledge relevant to sonography is an issue of increasing significance for many health professionals. Indeed to provide the best possible sonographic practice, all professionals performing sonography must inform and enhance their individual knowledge with the rapidly changing sonographic discipline knowledge.

2. Professional knowledge

The knowledge base of a profession is composed of the public body of discipline knowledge and the individual knowledge of professionals (11). This distinction between public and individual knowledge is not new. Sir Karl Popper (12) in his writings of the way in which knowledge is created and extended in the scientific community recognised publicly communicated knowledge and the knowledge of the individual. Popper utilised the term objective knowledge to describe publicly shared knowledge artefacts or products and the term subjective knowledge to represent the knowledge of individuals that has not been publicly shared. Other authors (see for example 11, 13-17) have also separated public and individual forms of knowledge. They utilise terms such as explicit, codified or scientific knowledge to describe discipline knowledge that has been communicated, in for example books, journals and conferences. The knowledge of the individual is commonly referred to as tacit knowledge. Higgs and Titchen (17) sub-divide tacit knowledge used by professionals into two categories, professional craft knowledge and personal knowledge. Professional craft knowledge is gained through experience and "embedded in practice" (p.5) and is akin to Schon's (18) 'knowing-in-action' (p.50) and Eraut's (11) process knowledge or 'knowing how' (p.107). Higgs and Titchen (17) contend that through articulation, sharing and critical review, at for example conferences and in journal articles, professional craft knowledge can be transformed from tacit knowledge to public discipline knowledge. According to Higgs and Titchen (17), the second form of tacit knowledge utilised by health professionals, is personal knowledge. This form of knowledge is gained through life experiences, allowing the health professional to "enter the life-world of their patients" (p.6) providing empathic care tailored to the needs of their patient.

Professionals integrate public discipline knowledge and their tacit knowledge in clinical practice (11, 16, 17). As previously noted, public discipline knowledge is communicated through information sources such as books, journals and conferences. With the rapid rate of change of knowledge in diagnostic ultrasound, health professionals must therefore engage in a continuing process of accessing new knowledge disseminated through information sources, internalising it into their tacit knowledge and then utilising it in clinical practice.

3. Learning mediated by information sources

Learning involving the use of information sources is theorised as an activity mediated by tools (19-21). In this mediated learning act, tools such as information sources create a learning environment where higher mental function is achievable than when the learner is left to their own unmediated mental functions (21-23). Learning mediated by tools can be represented by Vygotsky's triangular model. The Vygotskian model of mediated learning has three central elements - subject, tool and object. The *subject* is the learner. *Tools* are utilised by the learner to support the learning process. Tools may be external or internal. External tools are humanly created tools, which support learning such as information sources. Internal tools include processes utilised by individual to support learning such as mnemonic techniques and schemas of events or practice (21, 24). The *object* is the goal or motive (22) of the learning activity. Goals may be set by the individual or by some other such as employer or workplace trainer. In the Vygotskian triad, the learner does not simply react to the external world, a recognised limitation of behaviourist learning theories (24, 25) but is viewed as an active agent purposefully utilising external means or mediating tools to achieve their learning goal (26). The application of the Vygotskian model to health professionals updating their knowledge in diagnostic ultrasound is shown in Figure 1.

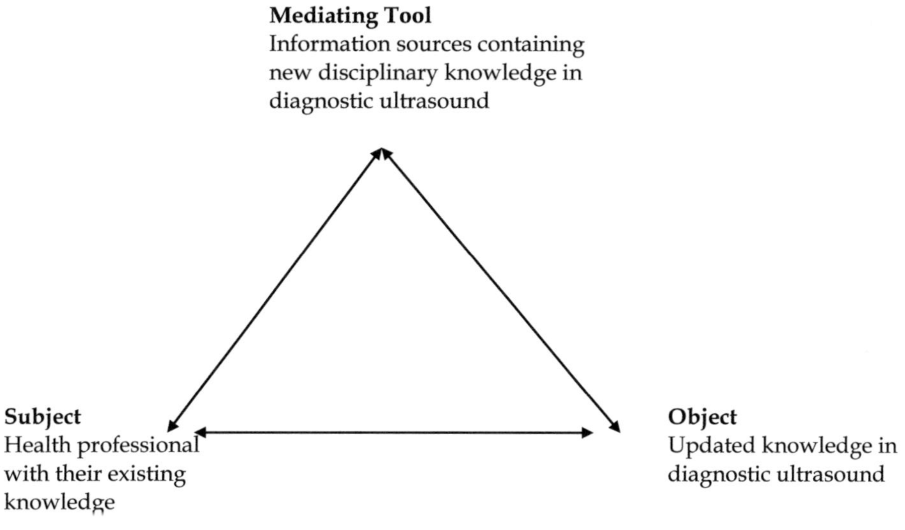

Fig. 1. Adaptation of Vygotskian model of the health professional utilising information sources as a mediating tool to update their knowledge in diagnostic ultrasound

Consider the case where the subject is a health professional involved in sonographic practice. To avoid professional obsolescence this health professional utilises information sources that contain new disciplinary knowledge as mediating tools to update their knowledge in diagnostic ultrasound. As a consequence of this activity the health professional's clinical sonographic practice is based on the latest disciplinary knowledge providing the patient with the best possible healthcare.

Disciplinary knowledge is made public via information sources through a succession of stages (27-30). For example Garvey and Griffith (28) developed a model of knowledge dissemination based on the psychology profession. This study identified a succession of stages through which new research findings are communicated within the profession. Initially research findings are disseminated orally through for example seminars and then to larger audiences at state or national meeting of their professional society. Many psychologists then utilise feedback from seminars and conferences to prepare the manuscript for submission to a journal. Finally, Garvey and Griffith contend that new research findings are cited in other journal articles and appear in books and this stage represents the assimilation of new research into the discipline's public knowledge base. Whilst the Garvey-Griffith model was developed from research based on the psychology profession, the succession of stages is similar across many professional fields (27, 29). The Garvey-Griffith model was developed before the Internet and the World Wide Web transformed the scientific communication process. Describing the Garvey-Griffith model as a model of scientific communication for the print era, Hurd (30) adapted the model for the digital era. Whereas the Garvey-Griffith model had professionals disseminating research findings initially through face-to-face seminars and annual conferences and then through print journals, the Hurd model showed the initial phase of research dissemination occurring primarily through Internet-enabled tools such as listservs, web pages and e-conferences.

The Internet is recognised as an important information source for health professional offering immediate access to the most current health and medical information. Web sites of professional, government, education and commercial organisations are utilised by health professionals to access online journals, health and medical databases, practice guidelines, image banks and case studies as well as information on professional development activities (see for example 31, 32-39). Internet based communication tools of e-mail, listservs and discussion forums are used by health professionals to consult with colleagues nationally and internationally (31, 32, 34, 35, 39).

Whilst the Internet offers access to large quantities of information the lack of quality control over information on the Internet means that its use as a major information source for health professionals has been limited (40). To take advantage of the perceived accessibility of electronic information whilst overcoming the disadvantages of variable quality of information, governments in Australia and internationally have developed Electronic Information Portals to provide health professionals with up-to-date information to inform their clinical practice. Examples of these portals include NHS-net (Internet access for the National Health System) in the UK; National electronic Library for Health (NeLH) in the UK; Hospital Authority Library Information Systems (HALIS) in Hong Kong; Clinical Information Access Program (CIAP), New South Wales, Australia, Clinicians Health Channel, Victoria; Australia and Clinicians Knowledge Network, Queensland, Australia. These portals provide health professionals with access to a range of information sources including health and medical databases, e-journals, e-books and clinical guidelines have also been identified by health professionals as an important information source for updating their professional knowledge (41-46).

The Hurd model and the proliferation of electronic media suggests that to update knowledge in the 21st century health professionals would favour and utilise Internet-based tools over both traditional face-to-face conferences and seminars. However, research examining the use of information sources by health professionals does not support this contention. Keppell and colleagues (45) investigated the use of Clinicians Health Channel, a major online health resource for professionals employed in the public health sector in the Australian state of Victoria. This study (n=233) reported that the four most frequently utilised information sources to refresh knowledge were workshops and seminars (85%), conferences (83%), textbooks (73%) and print journals (72%). When the activity was background research, these health professionals utilise print journals (66%), academic based websites (65%), Internet search engines (61%) and electronic journals (57%). In contrast, when the activity was to assist with clinical diagnosis, the information sources utilised were consultation with colleagues (59%), textbooks (58%), print journals (43%), and academic based websites (36%). Three important aspects of information source use by health professionals at the beginning of the 21st century are demonstrated in this study. First, this study demonstrates that the selection of information sources, or as represented in the Vygotskian model mediating tools, are dependent on purpose of use, or object of activity. Second, seminars and conferences, as identified in the Garvey and Griffth model (28), remain important information sources for updating knowledge. This is evidenced by workshops, seminars and conferences being the top information sources utilised to "refresh knowledge". Third, print journals were, at the time of the study, utilised by a larger number of respondents than electronic journals. Other studies have also demonstrated that health professionals prefer print based information sources such as journals. Davies (47) identified eight studies in which medical practitioners ranked their preference for or identified their use of print and electronic information sources. Each of these studies, published between 2002 and 2005, reported that print-based information sources were preferred or utilised over electronic information sources by medical practitioners. The continued preference for or use of print-based information sources such as journals appears counterintuitive in the digital era where electronic information sources made available through the Internet are considered central to communicating new knowledge (30, 48) and more generally learning (13, 49, 50).

None of the reviewed studies specifically identified health professionals engaged in sonographic practice and so it is not known what information sources they utilise as mediating tools to update their professional knowledge in diagnostic ultrasound. The following section provides research data investigating the use of information sources as mediating tools in professional updating activity by Australian Sonographers.

4. Professional updating activity of Australian Sonographers

The following section discusses research findings from a larger study investigating professional updating activity by Australian Medical Imaging Workers (MIWs). MIWs includes Radiographers, Radiation Therapists, Nuclear Medicine Technologists and Sonographers (51, 52). There were over 10,477 Medical Imaging Workers in Australia in 2006 and of these 2127 were Sonographers. The number of Sonographers increased by 50% between 2001 and 2006 (52) demonstrating one of the most rapid rates of growth of any health profession in Australia. The need to understand how this rapidly growing profession maintains currency of professional knowledge thus is of increasing significance in the 21st century.

4.1 Research study

This study utilised a two-phase sequential exploratory design (53, 54). This two-phase design collected and analysed qualitative data (Phase 1), which was used to inform the quantitative phase (Phase 2) of data collection and analysis (54-56). In the context of this study, interviews were conducted with 28 Medical Imaging Workers, six of whom specialised in Sonography. Interview data was utilised to develop the four-page questionnaire mailed to a random sample of 1142 practitioners holding registration with an Australian Medical Radiation Technologists Board (MRTB). Surveys were returned from 362 MIWs with analysis demonstrating that the sample was representative for area of specialisation and gender (39). Sixty-one survey respondents specialised in Sonography.

The survey data were entered into SPSS 17.0® and descriptive and inferential statistics were used for analysis. Percentages were used to describe survey findings. The collected data allowed for differences between groups to be examined using chi-square analysis using Fisher's exact test. In particular, this paper examines the value Sonographers (N=67) attribute to information sources as tools for updating professional knowledge, frequency of use of these tools within the context of professional knowledge updating activity and identifies factors that afford or constrain access to these information sources,

4.2 Results and discussion

Table 1 displays the demographic characteristics of Sonographers who participated in the survey component of the study. All age ranges were represented in the respondents with 65% of responding Sonographers aged between 30-49 years. This figure is consistent with data from Australian Health and Community Labour Force statistics where the average age for Sonographers was 39 years (52). Over half (56%) of respondents had professional experience of more than 15 years. The majority of Sonographers were female (72.4%), a finding consistent with gender data from Australian Health and Community Labour Force statistics where females account for 77% of Sonographers. The highest qualification for the majority of responding Sonographers practitioners was at the post-graduate level (86%) with 15% (n=9) of respondents undertaking further study. A majority of Sonographers were employed in metropolitan locations (53%) and in the Private Sector (54%).

Almost all Sonographers (97%, n=59)) held membership with one (38%) or more (59%) professional societies. Of the Sonographers holding membership with an Australian professional society, 85% held membership with the Australian Sonographers Association and 46% with Australian Society of Ultrasound in Medicine. Nine percent (n=5) held membership with an overseas professional society. Ninety-three percent (n=57) of responding Sonographers reported they were enrolled in a CPD program.

Mediating tools in professional updating activity

Survey data was examined to determine use of a range of information sources as mediating tools to update professional knowledge. The results are summarised in Table 2.

Conferences

Ninety-seven percent (n=59) of Sonographers identified that they attend national conferences of professional societies, with 51% attending one (36%) or more (15%) conferences each year. Ten percent (n=6) reported attending international conferences to update their professional knowledge with half (n=3) attending at least every second year. Conferences were valued for the intense nature of learning that they enabled "it was 7 in the morning til - we went to lectures until 6 at night and I found that invaluable going to something like that but it is a large, it is a constant sort of impact on you in the fact that it's learning day after day".

Characteristic		No. (%)[a]
Employer	Public	26 (46)
	Private	33 (54)
Work environment [b]	Teaching hospital	28 (48)
	Non-teaching hospital	8 (14)
	Clinic	22 (38)
Geographic location	Metropolitan	32 (53)
	Regional	19 (31)
	Rural and remote	10 (16)
Years of professional experience	< 5 years	6 (10)
	5 - 10 years	12 (20)
	11- 15 years	9 (15)
	>15 years	34 (56)
Level of education	Doctorate	0 (0)
	Master	9 (15)
	Graduate Diploma/ Cert	43 (71)
	Bachelor	3 (5)
	Diploma	5 (8)
	Associate Diploma / Cert	1 (2)
Gender	Female	44 (73)
	Male	16 (27)
Age (years)	20 - 29	6 (10)
	30 - 39	19 (31)
	40 - 49	21 (34)
	50 - 60	12 (20)
	>60	3 (5)

[a] Percentages are based upon number of respondents answering each question.
[b] The responses to this organisation factor exclude Sonographers who indicated they worked in more than one type of these environment and those who selected "other"

Table 1. Demographic characteristics of respondent Sonographers (n=61)

Mediating tool	Percent [a] (No.)
National conference of professional society	97 (59)
Journals	95 (58)
Internet search engines	95 (56)
Web pages	95 (56)
Text and reference books	89 (54)
Health and medical databases	84 (48)
Seminars	68 (41)
Government Electronic Health Information Portal eg CHC, CKN	18 (10)
International conference	10 (6)

[a] Percentages are based upon number of respondents answering each question.

Table 2. Information sources utilised by Sonographers to update professional knowledge

Ninety percent (n=55) of respondents reported that their workplace provided them with leave to attend conferences. The financial cost of attending conferences was shared primarily by the Sonographer who self-funded 45% (Mean) of the cost of attendance and the workplace who provided 45% (Mean) of the cost of conference attendance. Financial support was also received from professional societies, (8% Mean). Difference in support by the workplace, through the provision of leave and financial support to attend conference, was not statistically significant ($p>.05$) across health sector (public, private), geographic location (Metropolitan, regional, rural or remote) or workplace type (teaching hospital, non-teaching hospital, clinic).

Searching for and reading professional literature

The vast majority of Sonographers (98%, n=60) report that they search for and read information on a weekly basis to update professional knowledge. Seventy-four percent (n=45) report reading for one hour or more per week to update their professional knowledge, with 28% (n=17) reading three or more hours per week. Eighty-two percent (n=49) of Sonographers identified that their workplace did not provide dedicated time during work hours to undertake professional reading activities. The greatest variance in the provision of time for professional reading activities by workplaces existed across health sector with 94% (n=30) of Sonographers employed in the private sector not receiving dedicated time for this activity compared to 68% (n=19) of those employed in the public sector, with the difference trending toward statistical significance (Fisher's Exact Test = 6.553, $p=.057$). Sonographers identified that whilst valuable information sources were available in the workplace they lacked time to use them, stating for example, "No time to access the journals at work".

Time is recognised as a major barrier to updating professional knowledge by health professionals (33, 34, 57-59). In recent studies of Australian health professionals the provision of protected time, that is time during work hours when health professionals are not engaged in clinical or teaching duties, have been reported. For example, 58.1% of Australian and New Zealand Radiation Oncologists reported they had access to 'protected time' for non-clinical or teaching activities such as professional reading (60). Over half (52%) of Australian Radiation Therapists reported that they were provided with 'protected time' for professional reading activity (61), a level quite similar to that reported by Radiation Oncologists. In contrast, a minority (20.6%) of Australian Radiographers were provided with 'protected time' to engage in professional reading activity (62). It is apparent from this study that the provision of 'protected time' to Sonographers is low with just 18% reporting that their workplace provides this support. Whilst variation in support across health sector was evident (6-32%), the level of support for 'protected time' for Sonographers was much lower than their colleagues working in Radiation Oncology and Radiation Therapy. Greater provision of 'protected time' for Sonographers should be investigated.

As displayed in Table 2, Sonographers read journals (95%), Internet web pages (95%) and text and reference books (89%) to update their knowledge and they search for professional information using Internet search engines (95%) and health and medical databases (84%).

Journals

Ninety-five percent (n=58) of Sonographers read journals to update their professional knowledge, with 56% reading journals at least several times a month. The majority of

Sonographers report having access to print (97%, n=58) and electronic journals (93%, n=54) in their workplace. Sonographers also identified that there are a number of journals of relevance to diagnostic ultrasound that they could not currently access but needed access. The journal titles and the percent of respondents were: Journal of Diagnostic Medical Ultrasound (43%), American Journal of Obstetrics & Gynaecology (41%), Ultrasound in Obstetrics & Gynaecology (39%), Journal of Vascular Ultrasound (34%), Journal of Ultrasound in Medicine (33%), Journal of Clinical Ultrasound (32%), Ultrasonic Imaging (29%), Seminars in Ultrasound, CT & MRI (28%), and Obstetric & Gynecology Clinics of North America (27%). It is important that professionals engaging in diagnostic ultrasound have access to disciplinary knowledge disseminated through journals. This study identifies that there is a need to review the journals available in the workplace and determine if journals available are meeting the needs of health professionals performing the range of diagnostic ultrasound procedures undertaken in their practice.

Internet web pages and search engines

The majority of Sonographers (95%, n=56) used web sites to update their professional knowledge. National and international professional organisation web sites were valued by Sonographers as they provided access to needed resources "so you can get every article that has been published on the web if you are a member" and "they have guidelines for particular scans that they update so they give you information about minimum requirements for certain types of scans". In addition Sonographers valued online discussion forums "if anyone has a question you have an open forum where you ask how do you deal with things, has anyone seen this before, those sort of daily information, they put it on the website and its open for discussion". Web sites were also valued for providing access to "very good images" demonstrating normal anatomy and pathology. Internet search engines such as Google (95%) and to a lesser extent Google Scholar (40%, n=21) were also utilised to update knowledge. Search engines were used to obtain information on pathologies "we look up various things on the Internet because very often in daily scanning pathology comes through that we are not familiar with and I find I sit down at the computer and look it up". Sonographers also searched for "examples of pictures of what a particular pathology looks like and more information about that pathology" to inform their clinical practice.

The majority of Sonographers (94%, n=57) indicated that there was access to the Internet in the workplace. Half (51%) of the respondents indicated that the Internet was available on all workplace computers. Two-thirds (66%) of Sonographers who reported Internet access on all workplaces computers undertake Internet searches for professional reasons several times a week. However, in workplaces where the Internet was restricted to Offices (17%), only 22% of respondents undertook Internet searches several times a week. As one Sonographer commented "I do have Internet access here but we, this particular practice we just have the one computer, it's the same one that we use for typing our reports and everything so we don't tend to get on that very often". Workplaces can therefore support professional learning through the universal inclusion of the Internet onto all computers.

Books

Eighty-nine percent (n=54) of Sonographers read text and reference books to update their professional knowledge, with 79% using these books at least several times a month. All responding Sonographers reported that they had access to text and reference books in their workplace. Sonographers identified there "are still very good textbooks" but were also cautious about using books stating "by the time the text books are out the information is a couple of years old" and "by the time they are printed the images are fairly old".

Health and medical databases

Eighty-four percent of respondents report utilising health and medical databases to update knowledge. The most commonly utilised databases were Medline (70%, n=40), PubMed (62%, n=36), Informit or Meditext (23%, n=11), Cochrane Library (20%, n=11) and CINAHL (Cumulative Index of Nursing and Allied Health, 16%, n=9). Apart from Medline where only 8% of respondents were unaware of the resource, a large number of Sonographers were unaware of other health and medical databases, EMBASE (88%), CINAHL (77%), Cochrane Library (70%) Informit or Meditext (71%) and PubMed (27%).

Eighteen percent of Sonographers reported that they use government provided electronic health information portals such as Clinicians Knowledge Network (CKN) and Clinicians Health Channel (CHC). Amongst respondents, there was a low level of awareness (33%, n=18) of these government portals. Use of these government health information portals was higher amongst Sonographers employed in the public sector (36%, n=9) compared to the private sector (3%, n=1). This finding is not surprising, as these resources are made available to employees in the public sector only.

Given the low level of awareness of health and medical databases and government electronic information portals, there is an immediate need for professional development activities aimed at expanding the knowledge base of health professionals so they can more fully engage with the electronic health information world that is available.

The majority of Sonographers (69%, n=38) were not able to remotely access electronic information resources available in the workplace such as journals and databases from home. Sonographers identified that professionally relevant information sources could be made more available through the facility of remote access to workplace resources. As the vast majority of Sonographers had Internet access at home (97%), remote access to workplace e-resources would be a useful feature providing these professionals with greater flexibility in terms of when and where they can access needed information sources.

Seminars

Sixty-eight percent of Sonographers attended seminars to update their knowledge. Fifty percent (n=30) attended seminars conducted by a professional society, 22% (n=13) attended seminars organised by their workplace and 15% (n=9) attended seminars organised by Vendors. Seminars were valued as they provided information on "applications for their equipment" and also provided Sonographers with access to leaders in their field "people who do cutting edge stuff and that sort of spreads the word ... in seminars rather than in publishing, here in Australia"

Importance of information sources

A Friedman Test was conducted on survey data (N=61) to determine an ordered ranking for the importance of information sources for professional updating activity. The results are displayed in Table 3.

	Mean Rank
Importance of seminars	2.97
Importance of conference	3.46
Importance of text and reference books	3.56
Importance of Internet	4.08
Importance of print journals	4.38
Importance of electronic journals	4.73
Importance of databases	4.82

Table 3. Ordered ranking of importance of information sources for professional updating activity

The difference in ranking across information sources was statistically significant $\left(\chi^2 = 47.784,\ df = 6,\ p \leq .001\right)$. Seminars, conferences and text and reference books were ranked as the top three information sources for professional updating activity, respectively. This top three ranking is in accord with the study by Keppell and colleagues (45) where health professionals ranked the importance of information sources they used to "refresh knowledge". When we consider the traditional model of scientific communication has new knowledge disseminated initially through seminars and conferences and then through journals and books (27-29), the importance Sonographers attribute to seminars and conferences for updating professional knowledge is not then surprising. Despite the 21st century being described as the electronic age, it is important to recognise that non-electronic information sources continue to be highly valued and used by health professionals to update their professional knowledge.

5. Conclusion

The rapidly changing science and technology underpinning diagnostic ultrasound imaging require professionals to engage in a continued process of updating their knowledge. This process utilises information sources as mediating tools in learning. This study identifies that a range of information sources are utilised to update professional knowledge, with seminars and conferences ranked as most important. A number of recommendations were also identified to support professional updating activity. These include: workplaces examine the journals available to determine if they have adequate coverage of diagnostic ultrasound; universal inclusion of Internet access onto workplace computers; provision of remote access to workplace electronic resources such as journals; greater provision of 'protected time' to support professional learning activities; and professional development activities focused on extending knowledge of electronic resources. As this study was conducted in Australia, the results may not have validity in other settings outside of Australia. The author encourages other researchers to build upon this work so that the body of knowledge on professional learning in Sonography is developed.

6. References

[1] Dubin SS. Obsolescence or lifelong education: A choice for the professional. American Psychologist 1972;27(5):486-498.

[2] Houle CO. Continuing learning in the professions. San Francisco: Jossey-Bass Inc.; 1980.

[3] Dubin SS. Maintaining competence through updating. In: Willis SL, Dubin SS, editors. Maintaining professional competence. San Francisco: Jossey-Bass; 1990. p. 9-43.
[4] Burns R. The adult learner at work: The challenges of lifelong learning in the new millenium. 2nd ed. Warriewood, New South Wales: Business + Publishing; 2002.
[5] Siemens G. Connectivism A learning theory for the digital age. In: International Journal of Instructional Technology and Distance Learning; 2005. p. 3-10.
[6] Candy PC, Crebert G, O'Leary J. Developing lifelong learners through undergraduate education. Canberra: National Board of Employment, Education and Training; 1994. Report No.: 28.
[7] Thistlethwaite J, Spencer J. Professionalism in medicine. Oxon, United Kingdom: Radcliffe Publishing Ltd; 2008.
[8] Health Professions Council. About us. In. London, UK; nd.
[9] Australian Health Workforce Ministerial Council. Communique 22 April, 2010. In; 2010.
[10] Health Practitioner Regulation National Law Act 2009 (and Explanatory Notes). In: Queensland Government; Reprint No. 0A as in force on 3 November 2009.
[11] Eraut M. Developing professional knowledge and competence. London: RoutledgeFalmer; 1994.
[12] Popper KR. Objective knowledge: an evolutionary approach. Oxford: Oxford University Press; 1972.
[13] Jarvis P. Globalisation, lifelong learning and the learning society: Sociological perspectives. London: Routledge; 2007.
[14] Nonaka I, Takeuchi H. The knowledge-creating company: How Japanese companies create the dynamics of innovation. New York: Oxford University Press; 1995.
[15] Polanyi M. The tacit dimension. Gloucester, Mass.: Peter Smith; 1983.
[16] Cheetham G, Chivers G. How professionals learn- the theory. Journal of European Industrial Training 2001;25(5):248-292.
[17] Higgs J, Titchen A. Practice knowledge and expertise in the health professions. Oxford: Butterworth-Heinemann; 2001.
[18] Schon DA. The reflective practitioner: How professionals think in action. London: Ashgate Publishing Ltd; 1991.
[19] Jarvis P. Adult and continuing education: Theory and practice 2nd ed. London: Routledge Falmer; 1995.
[20] Brookfield S. Self-directed learning: A critical review of research In: Brookfield S, editor. Self-directed learning from theory to practice. San Francisco: Jossey-Bass; 1985. p. 6-15.
[21] Vygotsky LS. The instrumental method in psychology. In: Wertsch JV, editor. The concept of activity in Soviet psychology. Armonk, New York: M.E. Sharpe; 1981.
[22] Kaptelinin V, Nardi BA. Acting with technology: Acting theory and interaction design. Cambridge: The MIT Press; 2006.
[23] Brookes BC. The foundations of information science Part 1 Philosophical aspects. Journal of Information Science 1980;2(3/4):125-133.
[24] Merriam SB, Cafarella RS. Learning in adulthood: A comprehensive guide. 2nd ed. San Francisco: Josey-Bass Publishers; 1999.
[25] Jarvis P. Towards a comprehensive theory of human learnng: Lifelong learning and the learning society. London: Routledge; 2006.
[26] Engestrom Y. Expansive learning at work: Toward an activity-theoretical reconceptualisation. London: School of Lifelong Education and International Development, University of London 2001.

[27] Candy PC. Self-direction for lifelong learning. San Francisco: Jossey-Bass Publishers; 1991.

[28] Garvey WD, Griffith BC. Communication and information processing within scientific disciplines: Empirical findings for Psychology. Information Storage and Retrieval 1972;8(3):123-136.

[29] Garvey WD, Lin N, Nelson CE, Tomita K. Research studies in patterns of scientific communication: II. The role of the national meeting in scientific and technical communication. Information Storage and Retrieval 1972;8(4):159-169.

[30] Hurd JM. Scientific communication. Science & Technology Libraries 2004;25(1):5-22.

[31] Bennett NL, Casebeer LL, Kristofco RE, Strasser SM. Physicians' internet information-seeking behaviors. Journal of Continuing Education in the Health Professions 2004;24:31-38.

[32] Herrington A, Herrington J. Effective use of the internet: Keeping professionals working in rural Australia. Barton, ACT: Rural Industries Research and Development Corporation; 2006.

[33] Vorbeck F, Zimmermann C, Vorbeck-Meister I, Kainberger F, Imhof H. Internet use in radiology: results of a nationwide survey. European Journal of Radiology 1999;31(2):141-151.

[34] Masters K. For what purpose and reasons do doctors use the Internet: A systematic review. International Journal of Medical Informatics 2008;77(1):4-16.

[35] Casebeer L, Bennett N, Kristofco R, Carillo A, Centor R. Physician internet medical information seeking and on-line continuing education use patterns. The Journal of Continuing Education in the Health Professions 2002;22:33-42.

[36] Gilmore JA, Scott SD, N. H. Nurses and Internet health information. Journal of Advanced Nursing 2008;61:19-28.

[37] Nail-Chiwetalu BJ, Ratner NB. Information literacy for speech-language pathologists: a key to evidence-based practice. Language, Speech, & Hearing Services in Schools 2006;37(3):157-167.

[38] Veness M, Rikard-Bell G, Ward J. Views of Australian and New Zealand radiation oncologists and registrars about evidence-based medicine and their access to Internet based resources. Australasian Radiology 2003;47:409-415.

[39] Shanahan M, Herrington A, Herrington J. The Internet and the medical radiation science practitioner. Radiography 2009;15(3):233-241.

[40] Estabrooks CA, O'Leary KA, Ricker KL, Humphrey CK. The internet and access to evidence: how are nurses positioned? Journal of Advanced Nursing 2003;42(1):73-81.

[41] Gosling AS, Westbrook JI. Clinicians' awareness and use of online resources: A survey of 5,511 clinicians' use of the Clinical Information Access Program (CIAP). Sydney, NSW: Centre for Health Informatics; 2002.

[42] Hall G. Supporting health professionals in evidence-based practice: a case study of the Clinicians Knowledge Network. In: VALA 2008: 14th biennial conference and exhibition Melbourne Convention Centre Australia; 2008.

[43] Liaw S, Pleteshner C, Deveny E, Guillemin M, Mulcahy D, Arnold M. Peer, paper or online clinical guidelines? The question is the answer. In: Waldruck K, Cesnick B, editors. Twelfth National Health Informatics Conference; 2004; Brunswick East, Vic: Health Informatics Society of Australia; 2004. p. 137-143.

[44] Wilson P, Droogan J, Glanville J, Watt I, Hardman G. Access to the evidence base from general practice: a survey of general practice staff in Northern and Yorkshire Region. Quality in Health Care 2001;10(2):83-89.

[45] Keppell M, Arnold M, Guillemin M, Deveny E, Liaw T, Pearce C, et al. A collaborative inter-disciplinary approach to the evaluation of the Clinicians Health Channel. In: Kennedy G, Keppell M, McNaught C, Petrovic T, editors. Meeting at the Crossroads. Conference proceedings of the 18th Annual Conference of the Australasian Society for Computers in Learning in Tertiary Education; 2001; Melbourne: 9-12 Dec: ASCILITE; 2001.
[46] Turner A, Fraser V, Muir Gray JA, Toth B. A first class knowledge service: developing the National electronic Library for Health. Health Information and Libraries Journal 2002;19:133-145.
[47] Davies K. The information-seeking behaviour of doctors: a review of the evidence. Health Information & Libraries Journal 2007;24(2):78-94.
[48] Bjork BC. A lifecycle model of the scientific communication process. Learned Publishing 2005;18:165-176.
[49] Commission of the European Communities. eEurope An Information Society For All. Lisbon, 23 and 24 March 2000; 2000.
[50] Bonk CJ. The world is open: How web technology is revolutionizing education. San Francisco, CA: Jossey-Bass; 2009.
[51] Australian Institute of Health and Welfare. Health and community services labour force 2001. Canberra: Australian Institute of Health and Welfare (AIHW), National Health Labour Force Series no. 27; 2003.
[52] Australian Institute of Health and Welfare. Health and community services labour force 2006. Canberra: Australian Institute of Health and Welfare (AIHW), National Health Labour Force Series no. 42; 2009.
[53] Creswell JW. Research design: Qualitative, quantitative, and mixed methods approaches. 3rd ed. Thousands Oak, California: SAGE Publications, Inc.; 2009.
[54] Creswell JW, Plano Clark VL, Gutmann ML, Hanson WE. Advanced mixed methods research designs. In: Tashakkori A, Teddlie C, editors. Handbook of mixed methods in social & behavioral research. Thousand Oaks, California: Sage Publications, Inc; 2003. p. 209-240.
[55] Greene JC, Caracelli VJ, editors. Advances in Mixed-Method Evaluation: The Challenges and Benefits of Integrating Diverse Paradigms: New Directions for Evaluation, No. 74; 1997.
[56] Tashakkori A, Teddlie C. Integrating qualitative and quantitative approaches to research. In: Bickman L, Rog DJ, editors. The SAGE handbook of applied social research methods. 2nd ed. Thousand Oaks, California: SAGE Publications, Inc; 2009. p. 283-317.
[57] Newman M, Papadopoulos I, Sigsworth J. Barriers to evidence-based practice. Clinical Effectiveness in Nursing 1998;2(1):11-18.
[58] Gosling AS, Westbrook JI. Allied health professionals' use of online evidence: a survey of 790 staff working in the Australian public hospital system. International Journal of Medical Informatics 2004;73(4):391-401.
[59] Hommelstad J, Ruland CM. Norwegian Nurses' Perceived Barriers and Facilitators to Research Use. AORN 2004;79(3):621-634.
[60] Veness MJ. Evidence based medicine and radiation oncology in Australia and New Zealand in 2000: A survey of consultants and registrars [MPH Treatise]: University of Sydney; 2001.
[61] Shanahan M. Radiation Therapists and the Internet: A perspective from Australia. Journal of Radiotherapy in Practice 2009;8:137-146.
[62] Shanahan M. Radiographers and the Internet: An Australian perspective. Radiologic Technology 2010;81(3):223-232.